Epilepsy Board Review

Epilepsy Board Review

Pradeep N. Modur, MD, MS
Director, Seton Comprehensive Epilepsy Program
Seton Brain and Spine Institute
Associate Professor, Department of Neurology
Dell Medical School at the University of Texas at Austin
Austin, Texas

Puneet K. Gupta, MD, MSE
Epileptologist and Neurohospitalist
Neurology Consultants of Dallas, P.A.
Dallas, Texas

Deepa Sirsi, MD
Assistant Professor
Department of Pediatrics
Department of Neurology and Neurotherapeutics
UT Southwestern Medical Center
Dallas, Texas

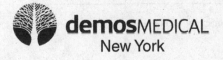
demosMEDICAL
New York

Visit our website at www.demosmedical.com

ISBN: 978-1-6207-0077-8
e-book ISBN: 978-1-6170-5256-9

Acquisitions Editor: Beth Barry
Compositor: diacriTech

Medicine is an ever-changing science. Research and clinical experience are continually expanding our knowledge, in particular our understanding of proper treatment and drug therapy. The authors, editors, and publisher have made every effort to ensure that all information in this book is in accordance with the state of knowledge at the time of production of the book. Nevertheless, the authors, editors, and publisher are not responsible for errors or omissions or for any consequences from application of the information in this book and make no warranty, expressed or implied, with respect to the contents of the publication. Every reader should examine carefully the package inserts accompanying each drug and should carefully check whether the dosage schedules mentioned therein or the contraindications stated by the manufacturer differ from the statements made in this book. Such examination is particularly important with drugs that are either rarely used or have been newly released on the market.

Library of Congress Cataloging-in-Publication Data
Names: Modur, Pradeep N. (Pradeep Narasimhamurthy) author. | Gupta, Puneet K.,
    author. | Sirsi, Deepa, author.
Title: Epilepsy board review / Pradeep N. Modur, MD, MS[JS1], Seton Brain &
    Spine Institute, Austin, Texas Puneet K. Gupta, MD, MSE, Neurology
    Consultants of Dallas, Dallas, Texas, Deepa Sirsi, MD, Plano, Texas.
Description: New York : Demos Medical, [2016] | Includes bibliographical
    references and index.
Identifiers: LCCN 2016015009 | ISBN 9781620700778 | ISBN 9781617052569 (ebook)
Subjects: LCSH: Epilepsy—Examinations, questions, etc.
Classification: LCC RC372.M63 2016 | DDC 616.85/30076—dc23 LC record available at
https://lccn.loc.gov/2016015009

Printed in the United States of America by McNaughton & Gunn.
16 17 18 19 20 / 5 4 3 2 1

To our spouses—Lisa, Paula, and Sudhir—for their continued love, support, and encouragement during our frequent hiatuses from family activities

Contents

Preface

Congratulations! If you are reading *Epilepsy Board Review*, it is quite likely that you have completed your training in epilepsy and you are about to test your mastery. With the recent institution of the epilepsy board examination, we felt the need to provide a self-assessment tool that would help solidify your knowledge and allow you to take the examination with confidence. In this book, we set out to simulate the actual computer-based board examination by writing the material in a question-and-answer format. But we understand that candidates preparing for the examination generally plan their reading in an orderly fashion. Therefore, instead of presenting the material in a completely random manner as done in the examination, we have structured the book into four parts for effective review: (1) Phenomenology of Seizures and Epileptic Disorders, (2) Basic Electroencephalography, (3) Diagnosis of Seizures and Epilepsy, and (4) Treatment of Seizures and Epilepsy. We feel that this division into broad topic areas is logical, and gives you the opportunity to study the material from various sources and then test your knowledge using this book.

At first glance, the epilepsy examination blueprint may appear daunting, but we assure you that we have made every attempt to cover the breadth of material represented in the examination. Epilepsy is an evolving field, in need of constant updates. Although it would be unrealistic to attempt to cover the depth of epilepsy in a volume of this kind, we have tried to provide you with an exposure to the complexities and the latest advances in the field. We have incorporated straightforward questions that can be answered from rote memory as well as those that require meaningful assimilation of data to arrive at the correct answer. Questions are supplemented with illustrations that mirror those found on the board examination. For each question, we provide a discussion of the rationale behind the correct answer and the incorrect answers. We also include references supporting the rationale or suggesting further reading.

PREFACE

Epilepsy Board Review encompasses the basic knowledge you will need to achieve subspecialty certification and models our understanding of adult and pediatric epileptology. It combines the must-know factual information in the field of epilepsy with our own experience, derived from years of interaction with our teachers, students, trainees, and patients. We hope that the 360-plus questions and answers we present will help you reinforce the known concepts, expose the gaps in your knowledge, and provide the confidence to shine in any testing environment.

Pradeep N. Modur, MD, MS
Puneet K. Gupta, MD, MSE
Deepa Sirsi, MD

Acknowledgments

We are grateful to our patients for providing the material from which to learn and to teach. We thank our mentors, colleagues, residents, fellows, students, and technologists for providing us the inspiration. Our special thanks go to Beth Barry at Demos Medical Publishing for having faith in us throughout this journey. Last but not least, we are indebted to our spouses—Lisa, Paula, and Sudhir—and our children—Sara, Maya, Ross, Nayan, Sonali, Shakti, and Devika—for their love and understanding.

Pradeep N. Modur, MD, MS
Puneet K. Gupta, MD, MSE
Deepa Sirsi, MD

Epilepsy Board Review

1

Phenomenology of Seizures and Epileptic Disorders

QUESTIONS

1. According to the Task Force of the International League Against Epilepsy (ILAE) Commission on Therapeutic Strategies, drug resistant epilepsy is defined by treatment failure of how many tolerated and appropriately chosen antiseizure therapies?

   A. One
   B. Two
   C. Three
   D. Four

2. According to the 2014 International League Against Epilepsy (ILAE) definition of epilepsy, which of the following patients is NOT considered to have epilepsy?

   A. A 21-year-old female with two unprovoked generalized tonic–clonic seizures at ages 20 and 21 years
   B. A 70-year-old female with an unprovoked focal seizure 2 months after left hemispheric ischemic infarct
   C. A 16-year-old female with a single unprovoked focal seizure progressing to generalized tonic–clonic seizure and found to have right frontal cortical dysplasia
   D. A 66-year-old male with two generalized tonic–clonic seizures at ages 14 and 66 years

3. A 29-year-old male with epilepsy has been seizure free for 3 years and wants to come off antiepileptic drug (AED) treatment. In counseling this patient regarding relapse following discontinuation of AEDs, all of the following statements are correct EXCEPT:

   A. Adolescent-onset epilepsy has a lower relapse rate compared with childhood-onset epilepsy
   B. Adult-onset epilepsy has a higher relapse rate compared with childhood-onset epilepsy
   C. A single type of focal seizure predicts successful AED withdrawal in adults
   D. Seizure freedom for 2 years predicts successful AED withdrawal in both children and adults

4. Which of the following animal models is best suited for studying epilepsy caused by heterotopia?

   A. Systemic administration of pilocarpine
   B. Systemic administration of kainic acid
   C. Local injection of tetanus toxin
   D. Intraperitoneal injection of methylazoxymethanol

5. Which of the following is true regarding mortality related to sudden unexpected death in epilepsy (SUDEP)?

   A. SUDEP excludes deaths without evidence for a seizure
   B. Rate of SUDEP is twofold higher in patients with epilepsy compared with the general population
   C. Risk of SUDEP can be 100-fold higher in epilepsy surgery patients compared with unselected incident epilepsy patients
   D. SUDEP is an uncommon cause of premature death in patients followed at epilepsy referral centers

6. Regarding epilepsy pharmacogenomics, all of the following statements are correct EXCEPT:

   A. Phenytoin can worsen symptoms in patients with CSTB gene mutation
   B. The ketogenic diet can be successful in treating seizures due to Glut1 transporter deficiency
   C. Valproic acid increases the risk of Stevens–Johnson syndrome (SJS) in patients with HLA-B*1502 allele
   D. Lamotrigine can worsen seizures in patients with SCN1A mutation

7. All of the following statements regarding epidemiology of epilepsy are true EXCEPT:

   A. An estimated 40 million people have epilepsy worldwide
   B. Worldwide mortality from epilepsy is 1%
   C. Incidence of epilepsy is 30 to 80 per 100,000 people per year in developed countries
   D. Prevalence of active epilepsy is 4 to 10 persons per 1,000 population in developed countries

8. According to the 2014 International League Against Epilepsy (ILAE) definition of epilepsy, in which of the following patients is epilepsy considered to have resolved?

    A. A 20-year-old male with a diagnosis of benign rolandic epilepsy who had multiple seizures from age 6 to 13 years, has remained seizure-free since then, and has been off antiseizure medications since age 14
    B. A 52-year-old male with a diagnosis of juvenile absence epilepsy who is currently well controlled on high-dose valproate monotherapy and has remained seizure free for the past 10 years
    C. A 44-year-old female with history of right temporal cavernoma and intractable focal seizures who has remained seizure free for 20 years after lesionectomy and continues on low-dose levetiracetam monotherapy
    D. A 70-year-old female with four generalized tonic–clonic seizures at ages 12, 14, 51, and 64 years, all in association with sleep deprivation, currently on no antiseizure medication

9. Seizure precipitants can be described by all of the following statements EXCEPT:

    A. Stress is the most common seizure precipitant reported by patients
    B. Menstrual effects are likely reported as a precipitant by temporal lobe epilepsy patients
    C. Sleep deprivation is a common precipitant for temporal lobe seizures
    D. Sleep is a common precipitant of extratemporal seizures

10. Which of the following is NOT a risk factor for sudden unexpected death in epilepsy (SUDEP)?

    A. Adult-onset epilepsy
    B. Higher frequency of generalized tonic–clonic seizures (GTCS)
    C. Treatment with two or more antiepileptic drugs
    D. Male gender

11. Which of the following statements best describes the impact of medically intractable epilepsy?

    A. About 10% of patients with epilepsy in the United States are considered to be medically intractable
    B. Disability burden of refractory epilepsy is negligible compared to that of lung cancer
    C. It is estimated that there are >100,000 refractory epilepsy patients in the United States who are potential surgery candidates
    D. About half of refractory mesial temporal lobe epilepsy (MTLE) patients become free of disabling seizures after surgery

12. Which of the following statements is true regarding the epidemiology of epilepsy?

    A. Incidence of acute symptomatic seizures is <50 per 100,000 persons per year
    B. Incidence of single unprovoked seizures is approximately <5 per 100,000 persons per year
    C. Recurrence risk at 2 years after the first seizure is >25% in patients with no risk factors
    D. Recurrence risk at 2 years after the first seizure is similar in idiopathic and remote symptomatic etiologies

13. A 19-year-old boy has absence seizures characterized by staring, sudden impairment of consciousness with complete unresponsiveness, and pause in ongoing activity lasting 20 seconds. The EEG shows 3 Hz spike-wave discharge. About 6 seconds after the onset of the EEG discharge, he has mild myoclonic twitching of eyelids, which persists for a few seconds. His seizure is best classified as:

A. Typical absence seizure
B. Atypical absence seizure
C. Myoclonic absence seizure
D. Eyelid myoclonia with absence seizure

14. Interictal epileptiform discharges are LEAST likely to occur in:

A. N1 sleep
B. N2 sleep
C. N3 sleep
D. REM sleep

15. Which of the following is true regarding the remission of epilepsy?

A. Pooled remission rate for children is 90%
B. Pooled remission rate for adults is 80%
C. Remission is independent of the patient's IQ
D. Length of seizure-free interval on antiepileptic drugs (AEDs) is a predictor of remission

16. Which of the following statements regarding genetic epilepsies is true?

A. The majority of patients with generalized epilepsy with febrile seizures plus (GEFS+) have an identifiable genetic mutation
B. The majority of mutations in Dravet syndrome tend to be inherited
C. Autosomal dominant lateral temporal lobe epilepsy (ADLTLE) is associated with LGI1 mutation in half of the patients
D. Juvenile myoclonic epilepsy (JME) is predominantly inherited in a monogenic manner

17. Which of the following statements best describes the effect of sleep on the manifestation of epilepsy?

A. The longest trains of spike-and-wave discharges are most likely to occur in stage N2 sleep
B. Arousal from sleep is likely to provoke a clinical seizure in juvenile myoclonic epilepsy (JME)
C. Focal clinical seizures are most likely to arise out of slow wave sleep
D. Focal interictal epileptiform discharges are most likely to be seen in light sleep

18. Which of the following statements is true regarding photosensitive seizures?

    A. Both men and women are equally affected by photosensitive seizures
    B. Occipital-predominant photoparoxysmal response (PPR) is more likely to be associ-
       ated with clinical seizures than generalized PPR
    C. More than 90% of patients with photosensitive epilepsy have photic-induced seizures
       only, without spontaneous seizures
    D. Generalized seizures are more common than occipital seizures in patients with
       photosensitivity

19. According to the revised International League Against Epilepsy (ILAE) classification
    published in 2010:

    A. A seizure is defined as being due to abnormal excessive or synchronous neuronal
       activity
    B. Epileptic seizures are differentiated from the nonepileptic seizures
    C. The term "secondarily generalized seizure" is retained
    D. Neonatal seizures are classified as a separate group

20. Regarding West syndrome (WS), all of the following are correct EXCEPT:

    A. Spontaneous remission can occur
    B. Negative MRI predicts favorable outcome
    C. Adrenocorticotrophic hormone (ACTH) has demonstrated efficacy
    D. Gliosis is the most common pathological finding in surgical specimens

21. Which of the following statements is true regarding the description of a seizure in the
    revised International League Against Epilepsy (ILAE) classification published in 2010?

    A. Partial seizures are referred to as localization-related seizures
    B. Generalized seizures are referred to as convulsive seizures
    C. Infantile spasms are referred to as spasms
    D. Dyscognitive seizure corresponds to complex partial seizure

22. Early myoclonic encephalopathy (EME) is characterized by:

    A. Seizure onset between 6 and 12 months after birth
    B. Burst-suppression EEG pattern
    C. Negative family history
    D. Favorable response to valproate

23. The syndrome of benign idiopathic (nonfamilial) neonatal convulsions is characterized
    by all of the following EXCEPT:

    A. Neurologically normal neonate
    B. Focal clonic seizures
    C. Seizure onset after the first week of life
    D. Bursts of theta activity and sharp waves interictally

24. In the International Classification of Diseases, 10th revision (ICD-10) coding system:

   A. There are separate codes for juvenile myoclonic epilepsy (JME) and childhood absence epilepsy (CAE)
   B. Idiopathic and symptomatic focal epilepsies have the same code
   C. Status epilepticus (SE) can be readily identified
   D. Grand mal and complex partial status epilepticus have the same code

25. All of the following statements regarding idiopathic generalized epilepsy (IGE) are true EXCEPT:

   A. It constitutes 15% to 20% of all epilepsies
   B. It constitutes the most frequent group of epilepsies with an adolescent onset
   C. Inheritance is complex and does not follow a well-defined Mendelian pattern
   D. Paternal inheritance has been observed for juvenile myoclonic epilepsy (JME)

26. A 1-year-old boy presented with episodes of sudden extension of upper extremities, quick head drop, and upward rolling of eyes. Initially, the episodes occurred once a day and subsequently increased in frequency to occur in short clusters over 3 seconds. Cognitive development and behavior remained normal. Interictal EEG was normal. During seizures, the EEG showed irregular, generalized polyspike-and-wave discharges. His mother had febrile seizures as a child. Brain MRI was normal. His seizures were controlled after initiation of valproate. Which of the following is the most appropriate diagnosis?

   A. Severe myoclonic epilepsy of infancy
   B. Benign infantile seizures
   C. Benign myoclonic epilepsy of infancy
   D. Epilepsy with myoclonic–atonic seizures

27. Autosomal dominant nocturnal frontal lobe epilepsy (ADNFLE) is characterized by:

   A. Seizure onset in infancy
   B. Seizure remission in the fourth decade of life
   C. Mutations in genes encoding for chloride channel
   D. Normal interictal EEG

28. Progressive myoclonus epilepsy.(PME) syndrome consists of seizures and progressive neurologic dysfunction caused by several distinct disorders. Which of the following features is most compatible with its associated disorder?

   A. Absent electroretinogram in late infantile neuronal ceroid lipofuscinosis (NCL)
   B. Frontal lobe seizures in Lafora body disease (LBD)
   C. Neuropathy in Unverricht–Lundborg disease (ULD)
   D. Lymphocyte vacuolation in myclonic epilepsy with ragged red fibers (MERRF)

29. The syndrome of migrating partial seizures of infancy is characterized by:

   A. Rare partial seizures
   B. Lack of identifiable etiology
   C. Positive family history
   D. Favorable response to conventional antiepileptic drugs (AEDs)

30. Which of the following gene mutations is correctly matched with the associated epilepsy syndrome?

    A. Benign familial neonatal convulsions and KCNQ2 mutation
    B. Glucose transporter type 1 deficiency syndrome and SCN1A mutation
    C. Autosomal dominant lateral temporal lobe epilepsy and CACN1A mutation
    D. Absence epilepsy with episodic ataxia and SCN2A mutation

31. PCDH19-related infantile epileptic encephalopathy is characterized by:

    A. Genetic defect on chromosome X
    B. Restriction of the disorder to males
    C. Normal cognition
    D. Absence seizure as the main seizure type

32. In Lennox–Gastaut syndrome (LGS):

    A. Daily seizures become uncommon over the long term
    B. Nonconvulsive status epilepticus (NCSE) is a risk factor for cognitive impairment
    C. The ketogenic diet is effective in a minority of patients
    D. Vagus nerve stimulation (VNS) is more effective than corpus callosotomy for atonic seizures

33. Nocturnal paroxysmal dystonia is considered to be a:

    A. Movement disorder
    B. Sleep disorder
    C. Epileptic disorder
    D. Psychiatric disorder

34. Mutations in the SCN1A gene are associated with epilepsy syndromes such as severe myoclonic epilepsy of infancy (Dravet syndrome). Which of the following conditions with comorbid seizures is also associated with a mutation in the SCN1A gene?

    A. Familial hemiplegic migraine
    B. Familial cavernous malformations
    C. Neurofibromatosis type 1
    D. Tuberous sclerosis

35. Dravet syndrome is characterized by which of the following?

    A. Childhood onset with tonic seizures
    B. Severe developmental impairment at seizure onset
    C. Ion channel defects
    D. Favorable response to combination of carbamazepine and lamotrigine

36. Which of the following is characteristic of Landau–Kleffner syndrome (LKS)?

    A. Onset under age 1 year
    B. Verbal auditory agnosia at onset of the illness
    C. Cognitive regression
    D. Continuous generalized epileptiform abnormalities in sleep

37. Features of psychogenic nonepileptic seizures (PNES) include all of the following EXCEPT:

    A. Onset is most common in the second decade
    B. Incontinence is seen in >10% of patients
    C. Stererotypic features are seen in a majority of patients
    D. Vocalization is in the middle of the event rather than at onset

38. Epileptic seizures are often confused with sleep disorders. Which of the following statements correctly identifies the sleep-related, nonepileptic paroxysmal disorder?

    A. Sleep paralysis and sleep related hallucinations occur in almost all patients with narcolepsy
    B. Inability to recall dreams suggests REM sleep behavior disorder
    C. Unawareness of nocturnal behavior can be seen in jactatio capitis nocturna (rhythmic movement disorder)
    D. Involuntary muscle contractions before and during sleep suggest restless legs syndrome

39. Which of the following statements best describes the prognosis of psychogenic nonepileptic seizures (PNES)?

    A. Children with PNES have a better prognosis than adults
    B. Females tend to have persistent PNES compared to males
    C. Presence of epileptic seizures predicts persistence of PNES
    D. Convulsive type of PNES is associated with a more favorable prognosis than the limp type

40. Which of the following psychiatric comorbid conditions is most likely to be associated with pure psychogenic nonepileptic seizures (PNES) versus mixed PNES and epilepsy?

    A. Dissociative disorders
    B. Conversion disorders
    C. Affective disorders
    D. Personality disorders

41. When do the compensatory physiological mechanisms typically begin to fail after the onset of status epilepticus (SE)?

    A. Around 5 minutes
    B. Around 10 minutes
    C. Around 30 to 60 minutes
    D. After 90 minutes

42. The common forms of nonconvulsive status epilepticus (SE) can be characterized by all of the following statements EXCEPT:

    A. Most patients with absence SE present with mild to moderate clouding of consciousness
    B. Absence SE can terminate spontaneously without treatment
    C. The primary form of myoclonic SE presents with bilaterally synchronous jerks and preserved consciousness
    D. The symptomatic form of myoclonic SE presents with asymmetric or asynchronous jerks and preserved consciousness

43. What is considered to be the cut-off duration of a discrete seizure in the operational definition of status epilepticus (SE) in adults?

    A. 5 minutes
    B. 10 minutes
    C. 20 to 30 minutes
    D. 30 to 60 minutes

44. All of the following statements regarding status epilepticus (SE) are true EXCEPT:

    A. There is a two-fold higher mortality for seizures lasting 30 minutes or longer compared with those lasting 10 to 29 minutes
    B. One third of SE cases are a manifestation of the initial seizure of epilepsy
    C. Generalized tonic SE is most often seen in children with Lennox–Gastaut syndrome
    D. About 20% of patients with epilepsy experience an episode of SE within 5 years of the diagnosis

45. Regarding the epidemiology of status epilepticus (SE), all of the following statements are true EXCEPT:

    A. Incidence peaks in the first year of life
    B. Incidence peaks in the seventh decade of life
    C. Incidence of generalized convulsive SE (GCSE) is about 7 per 100,000 population per year
    D. Mortality from the first episode of GCSE in adults is about 50%

46. Which of the following statements best reflects the mortality from status epilepticus (SE)?

    A. Mortality of SE is substantially higher in children than adults
    B. Mortality from myoclonic SE is higher than that of generalized tonic–clonic SE
    C. Mortality risk for SE lasting >1 hour is twice that of SE lasting <1 hour
    D. Low antiepileptic drug (AED) levels as the etiology for SE is associated with high mortality

47. Physiological consequences of convulsive status epilepticus (SE) include all of the following EXCEPT:

    A. Elevation of pulmonary arterial pressure, leading to pulmonary edema
    B. Parasympathetic overdrive, leading to bradycardia
    C. Demargination of neutrophils, leading to leucocytosis
    D. Sympathetic overactivity, leading to hyperthermia

48. Which of the following activities can be considered to pose the least amount of risk for a patient with epilepsy to pursue?

    A. Motorbike riding
    B. Hang gliding
    C. Target shooting
    D. Bullfighting

49. The association between idiopathic childhood epilepsy syndromes and cognitive dysfunction affecting school performance is true for all of the following syndromes EXCEPT:

A. Benign childhood epilepsy with centro-temporal spikes is associated with cognitive dysfunction
B. Idiopathic occipital lobe epilepsy is associated with deficits in memory and attention
C. Idiopathic generalized epilepsy is associated with executive dysfunction and impaired psychomotor speed
D. Juvenile myoclonic epilepsy is associated with memory impairment attributed to subtle temporal lobe dysfunction

50. With regard to assessing driving safety in patients with epilepsy, which of the following considerations needs to be entertained?

A. The majority of epilepsy patients tend to be truthful about the presence of epilepsy when asked for driving purposes
B. The majority of epilepsy patients admit to operating a motor vehicle in the recent past
C. Epilepsy patients account for 1% of all automobile accidents
D. A longer period of seizure freedom is likely to be associated with reduced risk of seizure-related automobile accidents

51. A 30-year-old male had a single generalized tonic–clonic seizure 3 months after head trauma for which he did not receive an antiepileptic medication. He had another seizure 8 months later, after which he was started on carbamazepine, which was titrated up to the target dose. He has now remained seizure free for 12 months. According to the International League Against Epilepsy (ILAE) consensus proposal, his treatment outcome can be classified as:

A. Seizure free
B. Treatment failure
C. Undetermined
D. Inadequate

52. A 2-year-old girl with cognitive impairment is seen in the epilepsy clinic. At 9 months of age, she developed clusters of brief seizures associated with apnea that were triggered by fever. Seizures have been refractory to several antiseizure medications. Family history is positive for epilepsy and cognitive impairment in her paternal grandmother. Which of the following gene mutations is likely to be found in this girl?

A. SCN1A mutation on chromosome 2
B. ARX mutation on X chromosome
C. PCDH19 mutation on X chromosome
D. CDKL5 mutation on X chromosome

53. Rett syndrome is characterized by all of the following features EXCEPT:

A. Identifiable mutation in X chromosome in a majority of patients
B. Normal head circumference at birth
C. Short QT interval
D. Breathing irregularities

54. Which of the following occurs in status epilepticus (SE)?

    A. Destruction of gamma-aminobutyric acid (GABA) receptors
    B. Internalization of N-methyl-D-aspartate (NMDA) receptors
    C. Efflux of calcium
    D. Overexpression of neuropeptide Y

55. Which of the following factors is the LEAST likely predictor of poor outcome after refractory status epilepticus (RSE)?

    A. Old age
    B. Etiology
    C. High Acute Physiology and Chronic Health Evaluation-2 (APACHE-2) scale score
    D. Long seizure duration

56. All of the following statements regarding focal cortical dysplasia (FCD) are true EXCEPT:

    A. They can coexist with dysembryoplastic neuroepithelial tumors (DNETs)
    B. They account for the majority of nonlesional focal epilepsies
    C. They can have intrinsic epileptogenicity
    D. They are most commonly found in the temporal lobe

57. A 10-year-old boy presents with medically refractory epilepsy. An extensive diagnostic workup has been negative. Which of the following clinical features should prompt karyotyping for suspected ring chromosome 20 syndrome?

    A. Strong family history of seizures
    B. Dysmorphic facial features
    C. Severe intellectual disability
    D. Nocturnal confusional episodes

58. Autosomal dominant partial epilepsy with auditory features (ADPEAF) is characterized by which of the following features?

    A. Onset during early childhood
    B. Ictal aphasia
    C. Seizures refractory to conventional antiepileptic drugs
    D. Mutation in CHRNA4 gene

59. Which of the following statements is true regarding epilepsy associated with focal cortical dysplasia (FCD)?

    A. FCD is the second most common cause in children undergoing epilepsy surgery
    B. Multilobar type II FCD presents with severe epilepsy at a later age
    C. MRI is negative in 70% of FCD patients
    D. Degree of seizure freedom after epilepsy surgery for FCD is highly variable

60. The long-term sequelae of status epilepticus (SE) can include all of the following EXCEPT:

    A. Nonconvulsive SE can lead to cognitive impairment
    B. Decreased incidence of hemiconvulsion-hemiplegia-hemiparesis syndrome coincides with decreased mortality from SE
    C. Febrile SE is a frequent cause of mesial temporal lobe epilepsy
    D. Acute symptomatic SE leads to development of subsequent seizure disorder in 15% to 30% of cases

61. A 40-year-old male has intractable epilepsy for the past 18 months despite being compliant with carbamazepine and levetiracetam. He reports two focal seizures with impaired consciousness per week and one generalized convulsion, on average, every 3 months. In addition, he has 3 to 4 focal seizures per week on average, associated with brief left-hand twitching, but without loss of consciousness. About 6 months ago, he had three generalized convulsions in 1 month for no obvious reason. Which of the following is true regarding his qualification for disability benefits according to the Social Security Administration?

    A. He qualifies because he has >1 focal seizure with impaired consciousness per week
    B. He qualifies because he has three or more focal seizures with left-hand twitching per week
    C. He qualifies because he had three generalized convulsions in 1 month, 6 months ago
    D. He does not qualify because he has not received treatment for 3 years

62. A 25-year-old male with epilepsy was found deceased one morning. After an investigation, the death was concluded to be sudden unexpected death in epilepsy (SUDEP) by the forensic pathologist. Regarding SUDEP, which of the following is true from a forensic pathologist's perspective?

    A. SUDEP is not considered a "natural death" because the patient had epilepsy
    B. Most victims of SUDEP have a brain lesion to explain the epilepsy
    C. Blood levels of antiseizure medications tend to be therapeutic at the time of death
    D. Specific laws are lacking in the United States for the medical examiners to document SUDEP

63. A new antiepileptic medication approved for adults has been shown to have more than minimal risk. The manufacturer would like to expand the label to include pediatric indication. According to the Pediatric Advisory Committee of the U.S. Food and Drug Administration (FDA), a pediatric clinical trial for this drug:

    A. Can never be conducted
    B. Can be done only if there is the prospect of direct benefit (PDB) to the patient
    C. Can be done due to the importance of the anticipated knowledge even if there is no PDB
    D. Can be done after a 5-year period as long as the risk in adults remains the same over that time

64. A 31-year-old male with history of "intractable spells" has been diagnosed with psychogenic nonepileptic seizures (PNES). Regarding driving restrictions in patients with PNES, all of the following statements are true EXCEPT:

    A. Cultural factors may play a role in placing driving restrictions as there are no clear driving laws for patients with PNES
    B. Studies from different parts of the world suggest that the driving restriction should be similar to that of patients with epilepsy
    C. There is no evidence to suggest a statistically significant increased risk of motor vehicle crashes in patients with PNES
    D. Restriction of driving privileges similar to those with epilepsy could be a motivation to accept the diagnosis and seek appropriate treatment

65. A 16-year-old girl with juvenile myoclonic epilepsy has brief trains of spike-wave discharges lasting 1 to 2 seconds. Her seizures have been controlled with medications for 2 years. She was a competitive swimmer prior to epilepsy onset and would like to learn how to scuba dive. Which of the following would be appropriate in counseling her regarding these activities?

    A. She should not participate in any water activities
    B. She can swim in a pool, but not scuba dive
    C. She can swim in open waters, but not scuba dive
    D. She can swim and scuba with proper precautions

66. Which of the following statements is true regarding operation of vehicles by patients with epilepsy?

    A. Reporting of the epilepsy diagnosis to the motor vehicles department is the responsibility of the driver and not the physician
    B. There is a minimum requirement of 3-month seizure-free period in the United States prior to resuming driving
    C. The U.S. Department of Transportation (DOT) prohibits anyone with a history of epilepsy from ever obtaining a commercial driver's license
    D. The U.S. Federal Aviation Administration (FAA) allows someone with a history of epilepsy to obtain a pilot's license under special circumstances

67. A 21-year-old male with generalized tonic–clonic seizures has been seizure free for a year and wants to play college football. Under what additional circumstance would it be acceptable for him to start playing?

    A. If he underwent weekly processing-speed testing
    B. If he got monthly serum medication levels
    C. Nothing additional is needed
    D. Under no circumstance would it be acceptable for him to play contact sports

68. Which of the following statements is true regarding attention deficit hyperactivity disorder (ADHD) in children with epilepsy?

    A. ADHD may occur before or along with onset of seizures
    B. Prevalence of ADHD in patients with newly diagnosed epilepsy is the same as in the general population
    C. Prevalence of ADHD in epilepsy is <5%
    D. Stimulant therapy for ADHD is associated with high risk for seizure exacerbation

69. A 22-year-old woman has epilepsy. Her seizures are well controlled with levetiracetam, which she takes three times daily to avoid peak dose side effects. Despite being aware of the social stigma and barriers posed by epilepsy, she has applied for a job at the local home improvement store. Which of the following statements is true regarding the legal and social protections provided by the Americans with Disabilities Act (ADA) for patients with epilepsy attending a job interview?

    A. Employer may ask her whether she has epilepsy before making a job offer
    B. Employer may ask her whether she can climb a ladder to stock shelves before making a job offer
    C. She needs to disclose to the employer that she has epilepsy at the time of interview
    D. She is obligated to request special accommodation at the time of interview to be able to take the afternoon dose of medication

70. Regarding the specific patterns of congenital malformations associated with the maternal exposure of antiepileptic drug (AEDs), all of the following statements are correct EXCEPT:

    A. Valproate is associated with hypospadias
    B. Carbamazepine is associated with neural tube defects
    C. Topiramate is associated with cardiac defects
    D. Lamotrigine is associated with cleft lip

71. Which of the following statements is true regarding the cognitive effects in school-age children after in utero exposure to antiepileptic drugs (AEDs)?

    A. Children exposed to valproate are likely to have a significantly lower IQ regardless of the dose
    B. Children exposed to valproate are likely to require a significantly higher level of educational intervention regardless of the dose
    C. Children exposed to lamotrigine are likely to have impaired verbal abilities
    D. Children exposed to carbamazepine are likely to have significantly lower IQ

PHENOMENOLOGY OF SEIZURES AND EPILEPTIC DISORDERS

ANSWERS

1. **B.** Failing two tolerated and appropriately chosen antiseizure therapies defines drug resistant epilepsy according to the Task Force of the ILAE Commission on Therapeutic Strategies. The treatment trials must be adequate in terms of medication dosage and duration.

   Kwan P, Arzimanoglou A, Berg AT, et al. Definition of drug resistant epilepsy: consensus proposal by the ad hoc Task Force of the ILAE Commission on Therapeutic Strategies. *Epilepsia.* 2010;51:1069–1077.

2. **C.** According to ILAE's 2014 "practical clinical definition of epilepsy," epilepsy is a disease of the brain defined by any of the following conditions: (1) at least two unprovoked (or reflex) seizures occurring >24 hours apart; (2) one unprovoked (or reflex) seizure and a probability of further seizures similar to the general recurrence risk (at least 60%) after two unprovoked seizures, occurring over the next 10 years; and (3) diagnosis of an epilepsy syndrome. The last two criteria have expanded the old definition. Based on these criteria, Patients A, B, and D are considered to have epilepsy, whereas Patient C is not. Patients A and D satisfy the criterion 1. Patient B has a risk of >70% of having a recurrent unprovoked seizure, and satisfies criterion 2. The risk of recurrent unprovoked seizures for Patient C remains unknown, although one could argue that it is reasonable to treat a patient with cortical dysplasia; further epidemiologic studies might define the risk more accurately.

   Fisher RS, Acevedo C, Arzimanoglou A, et al. ILAE Official report: a practical clinical definition of epilepsy. *Epilepsia.* 2014;55:475–482.

   Hesdorffer DC, Benn EK, Cascino GD, et al. Is a first acute symptomatic seizure epilepsy? Mortality and risk for recurrent seizure. *Epilepsia.* 2009;50:1102–1108.

3. **A.** Adolescent-onset epilepsy has a higher relapse rate versus childhood-onset epilepsy (relative risk [RR] 1.79). Similarly, adult-onset epilepsy has a higher relapse rate versus childhood-onset epilepsy (RR 1.34). Remote symptomatic epilepsy has a higher relapse rate compared with idiopathic epilepsy (RR 1.55). An abnormal EEG has a higher relapse rate than a normal EEG (RR 1.45). Seizure freedom for 2 to 5 years on AEDs, single type

of focal or generalized seizure, normal neurologic examination, and normal IQ are predictors of successful withdrawal of AED in both children and adults.

American Academy of Neurology, Quality Standards Subcommittee. Practice parameter: a guideline for discontinuing antiepileptic drugs in seizure-free patients—summary statement. *Neurology*. 1996;47:600–602.

Berg AT, Shinnar S. Relapse following discontinuation of antiepileptic drugs: a meta-analysis. *Neurology*. 1994;44:601–608.

4. **D.** Systemic administration of pilocarpine (a muscarinic cholinergic agent) and kainic acid (a glutamate agonist) induce prolonged seizures similar to human temporal lobe epilepsy; thus, both of these models are suitable for studying status epilepticus and temporal lobe epilepsy. Injection of tetanus toxin into the rat hippocampus results in limbic seizures and, therefore, this model is suitable for the study of temporal lobe epilepsy. On the other hand, methylazoxymethanol (MAM) is an alkylating agent that kills neuroblasts in the mitotic phase, resulting in a deranged cortical mantle and structural abnormalities of the radial glia that lead to subcortical heterotopias. It has been shown that intraperitoneal and transplacental administration of MAM to pregnant rats induces structural abnormalities in the offspring that include microcephaly, hippocampal heterotopias, altered neocortical lamination, and large heterotopic aggregates surrounding the ventricular floor; thus, the MAM model is useful for studying epilepsy caused by heterotopia.

Avanzini GG, Treiman DM, Engel J, Jr. Animal models of acquired epilepsies and status epilepticus. In: Engel J, Jr, Pedley TA, eds. *Epilepsy: A Comprehensive Textbook.* Vol 2. 2nd ed. Philadelphia, PA: Lippincott Williams & Wilkins; 2008:415–444.

5. **C.** SUDEP is defined as the sudden, unexpected, witnessed or unwitnessed, nontraumatic, and non-drowning death in patients with epilepsy, with or without evidence of a seizure, after excluding status epilepticus, structural cause or toxicological cause for death. The rate of SUDEP is >20 times higher in patients with epilepsy compared with the general population. Risk of SUDEP can vary by almost 100-fold, depending on the type of epilepsy population studied. The SUDEP rate (per 1,000 person-years) is as follows: 0.09 to 0.35 in unselected cohorts of incident epilepsy patients; 0.9 to 2.3 in general epilepsy populations; 1.1 to 5.9 in the chronic refractory epilepsy population; and 6.3 to 9.3 in epilepsy surgery candidates or in patients who continue to have seizures after surgery. SUDEP is the leading cause of premature death in patients with chronic refractory epilepsy who attend an epilepsy referral center, accounting for 10% to 50% of all deaths.

Shorvon S, Tomson T. Sudden unexpected death in epilepsy. *Lancet.* 2011;378:2028–2038.

6. **C.** CSTB gene mutation is associated with Unverricht-Lundborg disease, a progressive myoclonic epilepsy syndrome. Patients with this mutation tend to have preserved cognition and can mimic juvenile myoclonic epilepsy. Phenytoin can worsen symptoms in this condition. Glucose transporter type 1 (Glut1) transports glucose across the blood-brain barrier. Mutations in SLC2A1, which encodes Glut1, cause reduction of glucose uptake. Glut1 transporter deficiency leads to epilepsy syndromes that are resistant to standard antiepileptic drugs. However, the Glut1 syndromes respond well to the ketogenic diet because the ketones provide an energy source for the brain, bypassing the defective glucose metabolism. Presence of HLAB*1502 predicts the occurrence of SJS with high sensitivity and specificity in people of Asian descent treated with carbamazepine. Such

skin reactions have also been described for phenytoin, lamotrigine, and oxcarbazepine but not for valproic acid. About 80% of patients with Dravet syndrome have SCN1A mutations. In such patients, sodium channel blockers such as carbamazepine, oxcarbazepine, and lamotrigine can exacerbate seizures, whereas valproate, topiramate, levetiracetam, zonisamide, and stiripentol can be beneficial. It has been shown that in the presence of SCN1A mutations, there is substantially reduced sodium current density in inhibitory interneurons; further reduction of this inhibitory component by sodium channel blockers can result in worsening of seizures.

Cavalleri GL, McCormack M, Alhusaini S, et al. Pharmacogenomics and epilepsy: the road ahead. *Pharmacogenomics*. 2011;12:1429–1447.

Lehesjoki A, Kälviäinen R. Unverricht-Lundborg disease. In: Pagon RA, Adam MP, Ardinger HH, et al., eds. GeneReviews® [Internet]. Updated November 26, 2014. http://www.ncbi.nlm.nih.gov/books/NBK1142/. Accessed December 12, 2015.

Weber YG, Nies AT, Schwab M, et al. Genetic biomarkers in epilepsy. *Neurotherapeutics*. 2014;11:324–333.

7. **B.** According to the World Health Organization, an estimated 40 million people have epilepsy worldwide, the mortality from epilepsy is about 0.2%, and epilepsy accounts for 0.5% of disability-adjusted life years worldwide. In developed countries, the incidence of epilepsy is 30 to 80 persons per 100,000 per year and the prevalence of active epilepsy is 4 to 10 persons per 1,000 population.

World Health Organization. *The Global Burden of Disease: 2004 Update*. Geneva, Switzerland: World Health Organization; 2008.

8. **A.** According to the recent "practical clinical definition of epilepsy" issued by the ILAE, epilepsy is considered to be resolved for individuals who had an age-dependent epilepsy syndrome but are now past the applicable age or those who have remained seizure-free for the last 10 years, with no antiseizure medications for the last 5 years. Based on this, the epilepsy in the patient described in A can be considered to have resolved as he has passed the age (i.e., puberty) relevant for his age-dependent epilepsy syndrome (i.e., benign rolandic epilepsy). Patients in B and C are on medication despite meeting the seizure freedom criterion, and therefore, cannot be labeled as resolved. The Patient in D could have been considered resolved had the seizure at age 64 not occurred.

Fisher RS, Acevedo C, Arzimanoglou A, et al. ILAE official report: a practical clinical definition of epilepsy. *Epilepsia*. 2014;55:475–482.

9. **C.** Stress, sleep deprivation, sleep, illness, and fatigue, in that order, are the most frequently reported seizure precipitants. Menstrual effects are reported as major precipitants by 28% of women with temporal lobe epilepsy. Patients with idiopathic generalized epilepsy seem to be more sensitive to seizures during awakening and sleep deprivation, whereas patients with extratemporal epilepsy reported more frequent seizures during sleep. There are no differences in frequency or type of seizure precipitants with regard to gender, seizure duration, seizure frequency, and the number of antiepileptic drugs taken.

Ferlisi M, Shorvon S. Seizure precipitants (triggering factors) in patients with epilepsy. *Epilepsy Beh*. 2014;33:101–105.

Frucht MM, Quigg M, Schwaner C, et al. Distribution of seizure precipitants among epilepsy syndromes. *Epilepsia*. 2000; 41:1534–1539.

10. A. The risk factors for SUDEP include: male gender (1.4 times higher in males than females); early age of onset of epilepsy (1.7 times higher when epilepsy onset is <16 years of age versus 16–60 years); duration of epilepsy (two times higher with epilepsy duration >15 years); history of GTCS versus no GTCS (odds ratio is 2.94 for 1–2 GTCS per year, 8.28 for 3–12 GTCS per year, 9.06 for 13–50 GTCS per year, and 14.51 for >50 GTCS per year); and antiepileptic drug polytherapy (three times higher compared with monotherapy).

Shorvon S, Tomson T. Sudden unexpected death in epilepsy. *Lancet.* 2011;378:2028–2038.

11. C. In the United States, 30% to 40% of patients are considered to have medically intractable epilepsy. According to the World Health Organization, epilepsy-related disability accounts for about 1% of the global burden of disease, comparable to the burden due to breast and lung cancer. The number of epilepsy surgeries performed in the United States was estimated to be 1,500 in 1990, but there are an estimated 100,000 to 200,000 potential surgical candidates in this country. About two thirds of patients can be expected to be free of disabling seizures after temporal resection for refractory MTLE.

Engel J, Jr, Wiebe S, French J, et al. Practice parameter: temporal lobe and localized neocortical resections for epilepsy: report of the Quality Standards Subcommittee of the American Academy of Neurology, in association with the American Epilepsy Society and the American Association of Neurological Surgeons. *Neurology.* 2003;60:538–547.

12. A. The incidence of acute symptomatic seizures is 29 to 39 per 100,000 population per year. The incidence of single unprovoked seizures is 23 to 61 per 100,000 population per year. When several factors are taken into account, recurrence risk at 2 years is <15% in patients with no risk factors, but can reach 100% in patients with two or more risk factors. At 2 years, the recurrence risk is much smaller in idiopathic (32%) versus remote symptomatic (57%) etiologies.

Linehan C, Berg AT. Epidemiologic aspects of epilepsy. In: Wyllie E, ed. *Wyllie's Treatment of Epilepsy: Principles and Practice.* 5th ed. Philadelphia, PA: Lippincott Williams & Wilkins; 2011:2–10.

13. A. The clinical absences along with the 3 Hz spike-wave discharge are characteristic of typical absence seizures. It is important to note that mild eyelid and perioral myoclonia can be seen in typical absence seizures. Atypical absence seizures have slow spike-wave discharges of 2.5 Hz or less. Myoclonic absence seizure is a distinct seizure type included in the 2010 revised seizure classification. It is characterized by clinical absences and severe, repetitive myoclonic jerks of shoulders, arms, and legs with a concomitant tonic contraction. The tonic contraction can cause elevation of arms. Eyelid myoclonia with absence seizure is another distinct seizure type included in the 2010 revised seizure classification. It is characterized by prominent jerking of the eyelids, often associated with upward deviation of eyeballs and retropulsion of the head, followed by mild impairment of consciousness. Myoclonia are triggered by eye closure in a brightly-lit room but disappear in total darkness. Myoclonia can also be photosensitive. The triad of eyelid myoclonia with or without absences, eye closure-induced seizures, and photosensitivity constitutes Jeavons syndrome.

Berg AT, Berkovic SF, Brodie MJ, et al. Revised terminology and concepts for organization of seizures and epilepsies: report of the ILAE Commission on Classification and Terminology, 2005–2009. *Epilepsia.* 2010;51:676–685.

Panayiotopoulos CP. *A Clinical Guide to Epileptic Syndromes and Their Treatment.* Oxford, UK: Bladon Medical Publishing; 2002:114–160.

14. **D.** It has been shown that REM sleep is the least likely and that N3 (slow wave sleep) is the most likely to show interictal epileptiform discharges. The increased synchronization during slow wave sleep and the relative desynchronization during REM sleep are felt to be the underlying mechanisms.

Dworetzky BA, Bromfield EB, Winslow NE. Activation of the EEG. In: Blum AS, Rutkove SB, eds. *The Clinical Neurophysiology Primer*. Totowa, NJ: Humana Press; 2007:73–82.

15. **D.** The pooled remission rates for children and adults are about 69% and 61%, respectively. A normal IQ is associated with a favorable remission as well. Longer seizure-free interval on AEDs is associated with better prognosis of remission. Seizure freedom for 2 to 5 years on AEDs, single type of focal or generalized seizure, normal neurologic examination, and normal IQ are predictors of successful withdrawal of AEDs in both children and adults.

American Academy of Neurology, Quality Standards Subcommittee. Practice parameter: a guideline for discontinuing antiepileptic drugs in seizure-free patients—summary statement. *Neurology*. 1996;47:600–602.

16. **C.** Only about 5% to 10% of patients with GEFS+ have missense mutation of voltage-gated sodium channel SCN1A on chromosome 2q24. Mutations in other sodium channels (SCN1B and SCN2A) and GABA-A receptors (GABRG2 and GABRD) have also been identified in GEFS+. Dravet syndrome (aka severe myoclonic epilepsy of infancy) is also associated with SCN1A gene mutations, with 33% to 100% of patients showing detectable mutations. The majority (95%) of the mutations in Dravet syndrome occur de novo, leading to the introduction of a premature stop codon, which causes truncation and loss of protein function. ADLTLE is associated with LGI1 mutation on chromosome 10q24 in 50% of cases. LGI1 is involved in protein–protein interaction, signal transduction, regulation of cell adhesion, growth, and migration. It also interacts with voltage-gated potassium channels (VGKC) and inhibits fast inactivation of potassium currents. LGI1 also binds to the postsynaptic proteins, possibly enhancing a-amino-3-hydroxy-5-methyl-4-isoxazole-propionic acid (AMPA) receptor-mediated synaptic transmission. About 40% to 50% of patients with JME have a positive family history of epilepsy. Although monogenic mode of inheritance has been reported in JME, in the majority of cases, the mode of inheritance is unknown and is likely polygenic. Mutations in EFHC1 gene on chromosome 6p12.2 and GABRA1 gene on chromosome 5q34 have been reported in JME.

Gallentine WB, Mikati MA. Genetic generalized epilepsies. *J Clin Neurophysiol*. 2012;29:408–419.

Pandolfo M. Pediatric epilepsy genetics. *Curr Opin Neurol*. 2013;26:137–145.

Steinlein OK. Genetics of epilepsy syndromes. In: Engel J, Jr, Pedley TA, eds. *Epilepsy: A Comprehensive Textbook*. 2nd ed. Philadelphia, PA: Lippincott Williams & Wilkins; 2008:195–210.

17. **B.** The longest trains of generalized spike-and-wave complexes, lasting >5 sec, are likely to occur in stage N1 sleep; stage N2 sleep is the next most prominent period. Induced or spontaneous arousals from sleep can provoke clinical seizures in JME. Focal clinical seizures are most likely to occur in light sleep, whereas focal interictal epileptiform discharges are most likely to be seen in slow wave sleep.

Shouse MN, Bazil CW, Malow BA. Sleep. In: Engel J, Jr, Pedley TA, eds. *Epilepsy: A Comprehensive Textbook*. Vol 2. 2nd ed. Philadelphia, PA: Lippincott Williams & Wilkins; 2008:1975–1990.

18. **D.** Photosensitive seizures and epilepsies affect 5% of patients with seizures; two-thirds are women; the peak age at onset is 12 to 13 years. Photosensitivity is genetically determined. PPR can be classified as: (1) generalized spike-waves or polyspike-waves, which are highly correlated with clinical photosensitivity (90%), particularly if they outlast the stimulus train; and (2) posterior spike-waves or polyspike-waves with occipital predominance, which are associated with much lower risk of seizures (50%). Of patients with PPR on EEG, 42% have seizures induced by light stimuli only (i.e., pure photosensitive epilepsy), 40% have spontaneous and photosensitive seizures, and 18% have spontaneous seizures only. Patients with photosensitive epilepsy most commonly have generalized seizures (myoclonic jerks, absences, and generalized tonic–clonic seizures in that order of prevalence) than occipital seizures; extra-occipital focal seizures are exceptional. Video games, television, computer visual display units, discotheques, and natural flickering light are common triggers. Fatigue, sleep deprivation, and prolonged video game playing are facilitating factors. The mechanisms by which video games may induce seizures are photosensitivity, pattern sensitivity, emotional and cognitive excitation, and proprioceptive stimulation.

Panayiotopoulos CP. *A Clinical Guide to Epileptic Syndromes and Their Treatment.* Oxford, UK: Bladon Medical Publishing; 2002:214–239.

19. **A.** There are some significant changes to the definition and classification of seizures in the revised ILAE classification of 2010 as opposed to the older classification of 1981. The revised classification defines an epileptic seizure as "a transient occurrence of signs and/or symptoms due to abnormal excessive or synchronous neuronal activity in the brain." It does not differentiate epileptic seizures from nonepileptic events. The term "secondarily generalized seizure" is no longer included in the revised classification; it is replaced by the expression "evolving to a bilateral, convulsive seizure (involving tonic, clonic, or tonic and clonic components)." Neonatal seizures are no longer classified separately; instead, they are classified within the proposed scheme.

Berg AT, Berkovic SF, Brodie MJ, et al. Revised terminology and concepts for organization of seizures and epilepsies: report of the ILAE Commission on Classification and Terminology, 2005–2009. *Epilepsia.* 2010;51:676–685.

20. **D.** WS starts at 4 to 6 months of age. It is more common in boys than girls. The main seizure type is the epileptic (infantile) spasm, characterized by sudden, brief, flexor/extensor tonic contraction of axial and limb muscles. The spasms occur in clusters throughout the day. Etiology is idiopathic or symptomatic. There are several reports of spontaneous remission within 1 to 12 months of onset of infantile spasms (IS) and WS. Factors reported to be predictive of favorable outcome include the cryptogenic category with normal neuroimaging and normal development before the onset of spasms. About 50% of patients continue to experience seizures on long-term follow-up with higher rates for symptomatic compared with cryptogenic patients (50% vs. 23%). ACTH, prednisone, vigabatrin, valproate, pyridoxine, nitrazepam, topiramate, zonisamide, immunoglobulin, and thyrotropin-releasing hormone have demonstrated efficacy in the treatment of IS. In a comparative trial of vigabatrin and placebo, 10% responded to placebo. There has been greater emphasis on surgical treatment, including focal cortical resection and

hemispherectomy, in patients with focal abnormalities on EEG, MRI, or PET. The most common pathological finding in surgical resections is cortical dysplasia, not gliosis.

Moosa A, Loddenkemper T, Wyllie E. Epilepsy surgery for congenital or early lesions. In: Cataltepe O, Jallo G, eds. *Pediatric Epilepsy Surgery: Preoperative Assessment and Surgical Treatment*. New York, NY: Thieme Medical Publishers; 2010:14–23.

Panayiotopoulos CP. *A Clinical Guide to Epileptic Syndromes and Their Treatment*. Oxford, UK: Bladon Medical Publishing; 2002:50–69.

21. **D.** There are some significant changes to the terminology used to describe seizures in the revised ILAE classification of 2010 as opposed to the older classification of 1981. In the revised classification, the partial seizures (or localization-related seizures) are referred to as focal seizures. However, the generalized seizures are still referred to by the same name. The term "convulsive" is used to describe a seizure with tonic, clonic, or tonic–clonic components. Infantile spasms are referred to as "epileptic spasms" because they can occur past infancy. The subdivision of partial seizures into simple partial and complex partial is eliminated. Instead, the new classification requires a descriptor to denote the degree of impairment of consciousness. Within the new scheme, a dyscognitive seizure corresponds to a complex partial seizure.

Berg AT, Berkovic SF, Brodie MJ, et al. Revised terminology and concepts for organization of seizures and epilepsies: report of the ILAE Commission on Classification and Terminology, 2005–2009. *Epilepsia*. 2010;51:676–685.

22. **B.** EME is a rare epileptic syndrome that starts within a few days of birth. Boys and girls are equally affected. It is characterized by myoclonus, partial seizures, and transient tonic spasms. Erratic or fragmentary myoclonus is the essential symptom and the initial seizure type; it affects face or limbs, and may be restricted to smaller regions. There is rapid cognitive decline. More than half the patients die within months of onset, whereas the rest develop severe neurological deficits. EEG shows burst suppression pattern interictally, which can be replaced by transient hypsarrhythmia but the burst suppression pattern returns. Neuroimaging is normal at onset, but progressive atrophy can be noted. There is a high incidence of familial cases. Etiology is cryptogenic although metabolic errors such as nonketotic hyperglycinemia, molybdedum cofactor deficiency, and Menkes disease have been found. Seizures persist with partial seizures and asymmetric tonic seizures being the main seizure types although tonic spasms can be seen as well. There is no effective treatment. The seizures do not respond to ACTH, clonazepam, nitrazepam, phenobarbital, or valproate. EME should be differentiated from Ohtahara syndrome (OS). OS is characterized by prominent tonic seizures (rare clonic seizures or hemiconvulsions), hypsarrhythmia or burst suppression, structural malformations, and negative family history.

Panayiotopoulos CP. *A Clinical Guide to Epileptic Syndromes and Their Treatment*. Oxford, UK: Bladon Medical Publishing; 2002:36–49.

23. **C.** The syndrome of benign idiopathic (non familial) neonatal convulsions is referred to as "fifth day fits" because of the timing of onset, with 90% of seizures occurring between the fourth and sixth day of life. It is more common in boys (62%) versus girls. Neonates with this syndrome are born full-term with an uncomplicated pregnancy and delivery. It is a self-limited disorder. The seizures are usually focal clonic, with or without associated apnea.

The seizures are typically brief, but recur at frequent intervals, with the entire episode lasting between 2 hours and 3 days, with a median of 20 hours. There is no subsequent recurrence of seizures. There is no family history of neonatal seizures and no etiology for the seizures can be identified. The ictal EEG is characterized by rhythmic spikes. Interictal EEG can be normal or show a "theta pointu alternant" pattern, in which the background is discontinuous, with bursts of rhythmic 4 to 7 Hz theta activity intermixed with sharp waves, alternating between hemispheres. This syndrome is a diagnosis of exclusion.

Panayiotopoulos CP. *A Clinical Guide to Epileptic Syndromes and Their Treatment.* Oxford, UK: Bladon Medical Publishing; 2002:36–49.

24. **C.** The ICD-10 system differs in many ways from the ICD-9 system for coding seizures and epilepsy. In ICD-9 system, CAE is coded 345.0 (generalized nonconvulsive epilepsy) and JME is coded 345.1 (generalized convulsive epilepsy), whereas in ICD-10, both are coded G40.3 (generalized idiopathic epilepsy and epileptic syndromes). In ICD-10, idiopathic and symptomatic focal epilepsies have separate codes: G40.0 codes idiopathic focal epilepsy; G40.1 codes symptomatic focal epilepsy with simple partial seizures; and G40.2 codes symptomatic focal epilepsy with complex partial seizures. In ICD-10, SE can be readily identified by the sixth character, with 1 indicating presence and 9 indicating absence of SE (e.g., G40.201 codes for focal epilepsy, not intractable, with SE and G40.209 codes for focal epilepsy, not intractable, without SE).

American Academy of Neurology. ICD-9 to ICD-10 conversion of epilepsy. https://www.aan.com/uploadedFiles/Website_Library_Assets/Documents/3.Practice_Management/1.Reimbursement/1.Billing_and_Coding/2.ICD-10-CM/AAN%20Epilepsy%20Crosswalk(1).pdf. Accessed December 12, 2015.

Jette N, Beghi E, Hesdorffer D, et al. ICD coding for epilepsy: Past, present, and future—a report by the International League Against Epilepsy Task Force on ICD codes in epilepsy. *Epilepsia.* 2015;56:348–355.

25. **D.** IGE accounts for 15% to 20% of all epilepsies, and constitutes the most frequent group of epilepsies with an adolescent onset. Seizures in IGEs have an onset from childhood to early adulthood. Seizures respond favorably to treatment, with 80% to 90% of patients achieving full seizure control and 50% of patients outgrowing their seizures. There is morning predisposition to convulsive seizures as a general feature. Absence, myoclonic, and generalized tonic–clonic seizures are the main seizure types. Photosensitivity is frequent and can be restricted to an EEG finding (i.e., photoparoxysmal response) or a clinical phenomenon (i.e., photoconvulsive seizure). Inheritance is complex, with many phenotypes, but rare gene defects. Phenotypic expression may vary among family members and can evolve into one another. For JME, maternal, not paternal, inheritance has been observed.

Pal DK, Durner M, Klotz I, et al. Complex inheritance and parent of origin effect in juvenile myoclonic epilepsy. *Brain Dev.* 2006;28:92–98.

Thomas P, Genton P, Gelisse P, et al. Juvenile myoclonic epilepsy. In: Roger J, Bureau M, Dravet C, et al., eds. Epileptic Syndromes in Infancy, Childhood and Adolescence. 4th ed. Montrouge, France: John Libbey Eurotext; 2005:367–388.

26. **C.** The features are consistent with benign myoclonic epilepsy of infancy, which is characterized by onset in a normal infant aged 4 months to 3 years and isolated or brief clusters of bilateral myoclonic jerks associated with generalized polyspike-and-wave discharges.

Interictal EEG shows normal background with rare generalized polyspikes in sleep. Neurological outcome is normal and seizures are easily controlled with valproate, with some patients needing addition of clonazepam or clobazam. It remits in early childhood, but 10% to 20% of children may develop rare generalized tonic–clonic seizures later. Severe myoclonic epilepsy of infancy (Dravet syndrome) has onset in infancy with repeated episodes of febrile status epilepticus. Myoclonic seizures, atypical absences, complex partial seizures, and generalized seizures occur with increasing frequency in the second year of life and are refractory to medications. EEG is normal at onset, but subsequently shows progressive deterioration of background, frequent interictal spikes, and photosensitivity. Stiripentol and the combination of valproate and clobazam have demonstrated efficacy. Prognosis is poor with cognitive decline, refractory seizures, and high mortality. Benign infantile seizures occur in infancy and consist of clusters of focal seizures. Development is normal and the condition resolves by 1 to 3 years of age. Ictal EEG shows focal discharges. Epilepsy with myoclonic–astatic or myoclonic–atonic seizures (Doose syndrome) has onset between ages 1 and 5 years in a normal child with normal MRI. There is strong genetic context with high incidence of idiopathic epilepsy in the family. Myoclonic-atonic seizures manifest as drop attacks, consisting of symmetric myoclonic jerks immediately followed by atonia. Absence seizures can also occur. There is variable response to medication with high efficacy to the combination of valproate and lamotrigine. Prognosis for epilepsy and cognition is variable, ranging from excellent to poor.

Chiron C, Dulac O. The pharmacologic treatment of Dravet syndrome. *Epilepsia.* 2011;52(suppl 2):72-75.

Panayiotopoulos CP. *A Clinical Guide to Epileptic Syndromes and Their Treatment.* Oxford, UK: Bladon Medical Publishing; 2002:50–69.

Panayiotopoulos CP. *A Clinical Guide to Epileptic Syndromes and Their Treatment.* Oxford, UK: Bladon Medical Publishing; 2002:114–160.

27. **D.** ADNFLE is characterized by seizures that begin in childhood, with a mean age at onset of 11 years. Seizures usually persist throughout adult life. Seizures occur in clusters in sleep. Frequently, they are simple partial seizures characterized by vocalization followed by thrashing, hyperkinetic activity, and tonic stiffening with or without clonic activity. Interictal EEG is normal. Ictal EEG is frequently obscured by artifact or may show bifrontal spikes. The seizures may be misdiagnosed as parasomnia, psychiatric disorder or movement disorder. Seizures respond favorably to carbamazepine or oxcarbazepine. It is caused by mutations in CHRNA4 and CNHRNB2, which encode for the nicotinic neuronal acetylcholine receptor subunits on chromosome 20q and 15q.

Panayiotopoulos CP. *A Clinical Guide to Epileptic Syndromes and Their Treatment.* Oxford, UK: Bladon Medical Publishing; 2002:161–168.

28. **A.** PME syndrome can be caused by several distinct disorders including ULD, LBD, MERRF, sialidoses, and NCL. Very prominent myoclonus suggests ULD, MERRF or sialidoses. Absent electroretinogram can be seen in late infantile and juvenile NCL, whereas photosensitivity occurs in late infantile and adult NCL. Partial seizures of occipital origin are often noted in LBD. Vertex epileptiform spikes and neuropathy may occur in sialidoses. Dysmorphic features are usual in sialidoses and may occur in MERRF. The presence of deafness, optic atrophy, lipomas, and myopathy can be seen in MERRF. Lymphocyte vacuolation is seen in sialidosis and sometimes in NCL. Elevated blood and cerebrospinal

fluid lactate levels can be seen in MERRF. Dentatorubropallidian atrophy (DRPLA), a rare autosomal dominant trinucleotide repeat expansion disease, can also present with PME, ataxia, choreoathetosis, dementia, and psychiatric symptoms. A larger number of repeats is associated with younger age at onset and with PME phenotype.

Genton P, Malafosse A, Moulard B, et al. Progressive myoclonus epilepsies. In: Roger J, Bureau M, Dravet C, et al., eds. *Epileptic Syndromes in Infancy, Childhood and Adolescence.* 4th ed. Montrouge, France: John Libbey Eurotext; 2005:441–465.

Girard JM, Turnbull J, Ramachandran N, et al. Progressive myoclonus epilepsy. *Handb Clin Neurol.* 2013;113:1731–1736.

Ikeuchi T, Koide R, Onodera O, et al. Dentatorubral-pallidoluysian atrophy (DRPLA). Molecular basis for wide clinical features of DRPLA. *Clin Neurosci.* 1995;3:23–27.

29. **B.** The syndrome of migrating partial seizures of infancy is characterized by onset between 1 day and 7 months of life with frequent or nearly continuous multifocal partial seizures, intractability to conventional AEDs, and progressive cognitive decline. Potassium bromide has been tried with some success. There is no identifiable etiology or family history. Interictal EEG shows diffuse background slowing with multifocal epileptiform abnormalities. Ictal EEG shows shifting areas of ictal onset, involving both hemispheres and multiple lobes, and overlapping of consecutive seizures. The prognosis is poor.

Coppola G. Malignant migrating partial seizures in infancy: an epilepsy syndrome of unknown etiology. *Epilepsia.* 2009;50(suppl 5):49–51.

Panayiotopoulos CP. *A Clinical Guide to Epileptic Syndromes and Their Treatment.* Oxford, UK: Bladon Medical Publishing; 2002:50–69.

30. **A.** Benign familial neonatal convulsions is associated with KCNQ2 mutation. This syndrome is characterized by early-onset, focal clonic or focal tonic seizures in a neonate with a family history of neonatal seizures and with no other neurological findings. There is autosomal dominant pattern of inheritance with incomplete penetrance. There are two known chromosomal loci: one on chromosome 20q13 (KCNQ2 gene) and the other on chromosome 8q (KCNQ3 gene). Seizure onset is in the first week of life but can recur up to 2 to 3 months of age, when they remit spontaneously. Interictal EEG is normal. There is higher incidence of later seizures in 11% to 16% of patients. Glucose transporter type 1 deficiency syndrome is associated with SLC2A1 gene mutation. Autosomal dominant lateral temporal epilepsy is associated with LGI1 gene mutation. Absence epilepsy with episodic ataxia is associated with CACN1A mutation. Autosomal dominant nocturnal frontal lobe epilepsy is associated with mutations in neuronal acetylcholine receptor subunits (CHRNA4, CHRNA2, and CHRNB2). Glucose transporter type 1 deficiency syndrome is most commonly associated with seizures, which usually begin within the first few months of life. Additional symptoms that can occur include movement disorders, developmental delay, and varying degrees of cognitive, speech, and language impairment. It is caused by mutations in the SLC2A1 gene and is inherited as an autosomal dominant trait. This syndrome does not respond to antiseizure medications but has been successfully treated with the ketogenic diet. Autosomal dominant lateral temporal epilepsy (ADLTE) is characterized by focal seizures with auditory features or aphasia. Mutations in the LGI1 gene have been reported in up to 50% of ADLTE pedigrees.

Pandolfo M. Pediatric epilepsy genetics. *Curr Opin Neurol.* 2013;26:137–145.

Pascual JM, Wang D, Lecumberri B, et al. GLUT1 deficiency and other glucose transporter diseases. *Eur J Endocrinol.* 2004;150:627–633.

Wang D, Pascual JM, De Vivo D. Glucose transporter type 1 deficiency syndrome. Jul 30, 2002 [Updated Jan 22, 2015]. In: Pagon RA, Adam MP, Ardinger HH, et al., eds. *GeneReviews [Internet].* Seattle, WA: University of Washington; 1993–2015. http://www.ncbi.nlm.nih.gov/books/NBK1430. Accessed December 14, 2015.

31. **A.** PCDH19-related infantile epileptic encephalopathy is an X-linked disorder. PCDH19 encodes protocadherin 19 on chromosome Xq22.3, a protein that is highly expressed during brain development and is believed to play a significant role in neuronal migration or establishment of synaptic connections. PCDH19 mutations are linked to epilepsy and mental retardation only in heterozygous females, whereas hemizygous males are asymptomatic. Typical features include generalized or focal seizures, high sensitivity to fever, and brief seizures occurring in clusters, repeating over several days. PCDH19 has been reported to be the second most relevant gene in epilepsy after SCN1A.

Depienne C, LeGuern E. PCDH19-related infantile epileptic encephalopathy: an unusual X-linked inheritance disorder. *Hum Mutat.* 2012;33:627–634.

32. **B.** In LGS, seizures persist on a daily basis in two thirds of patients, 10 years after diagnosis. Risk factors for severe cognitive impairment in patients with LGS include NCSE, previous diagnosis of West syndrome, symptomatic etiology, and early age of onset of epilepsy. Of these, NCSE appears to be the most important risk factor. The ketogenic diet and VNS are effective with 50% of children experiencing >50% reduction in seizures. Some patients can have >90% seizure reduction with the ketogenic diet. Corpus callosotomy and VNS have similar rates of seizure reduction, but corpus callosotomy is felt to be more effective for atonic seizures.

Bourgeois BFD, Douglass LM, Sankar R. Lennox-Gastaut syndrome: a consensus approach to differential diagnosis. *Epilepsia.* 2014;55(suppl 4):4–9.

Douglass LM, Salpekar J. Surgical options for patients with Lennox–Gastaut syndrome. *Epilepsia.* 2014;55(suppl 4):21–28.

Kossoff EHW, Shields DW. Nonpharmacologic care for patients with Lennox–Gastaut syndrome: ketogenic diets and vagus nerve stimulation. *Epilepsia.* 2014;55(suppl 4):29–33.

33. **C.** Nocturnal paroxysmal dystonia is considered an epileptic disorder. It is characterized by recurrent episodes of complex behavior, including repetitive stereotyped dystonic, ballistic, or choreoathetoid movements involving one or more extremities and neck during non-REM sleep. They last from seconds to minutes. Although the scalp EEG is often negative, the spells are felt to be nocturnal frontal lobe epileptic seizures. The other disorders listed are considered nonepileptic paroxysmal disorders, which make up 20% to 25% of patients seen in epilepsy clinics and monitoring units. It is important to recognize these nonepileptic disorders in order to avoid unnecessary treatments and delay appropriate treatments. Nonepileptic paroxysmal events differ significantly by age group: neonates have apnea, benign neonatal sleep myoclonus, and hyperekplexia; infants have breath-holding spells, benign myoclonus of infancy, shuddering attacks, Sandifer syndrome, benign torticollis in infancy, spasmus nutans, and head banging; children have vasovagal syncope, migraine, benign paroxysmal vertigo, tic disorders, and parasomnias; adolescents and adults have narcolepsy, periodic limb movement in sleep, paroxysmal

dyskinesia, hemifacial spasm, stiff person syndrome, and psychogenic nonepileptic seizures; and the elderly have cardiogenic syncope, transient global amnesia, and REM sleep behavior disorder.

Andermann F. Overview: disorders that can be confused with epilepsy. In: Engel J, Jr, Pedley TA, eds. *Epilepsy: A Comprehensive Textbook*. 2nd ed. Philadelphia, PA: Lippincott Williams & Wilkins; 2008:2696–2697.

34. **A.** Familial hemiplegic migraine has been associated with gene mutations in CACNA1A (FHM1), ATP1A2 (FHM2), and SCN1A (FHM3). Familial cavernous malformations are associated with mutations in KRIT1 (CCM1), CCM2 (CCM2), or PDCD10 (CCM3). Specifically, KRIT1 is a protein that is involved in multiple signaling pathways including cell death and angiogenesis. Neurofibromatosis type 1 is caused by a gene mutation on chromosome 17 that is responsible for cell division. Tuberous sclerosis has been associated with mutations in TSC-1 (chromosome 9) and TSC-2 (chromosome 16), which encode for hamartin and tuberin, respectively, both of which act as tumor suppressor genes.

Friedman JM. Neurofibromatosis 1. October 2, 1998 [Updated Sep 4, 2014]. In: Pagon RA, Adam MP, Ardinger HH, et al., eds. *GeneReviews [Internet]*. Seattle, WA: University of Washington; 1993–2015. http://www.ncbi.nlm.nih.gov/books/NBK1109. Accessed December 12, 2015.

Morrison L, Akers A. Cerebral cavernous malformation, familial. February 24, 2003 [Updated May 31, 2011]. In: Pagon RA, Adam MP, Ardinger HH, et al., eds. *GeneReviews [Internet]*. Seattle, WA: University of Washington; 1993–2015. http://www.ncbi.nlm.nih.gov/books/NBK1293. Accessed December 12, 2015.

Northrup H, Koenig MK, Pearson DA, et al. Tuberous sclerosis complex. July 13, 1999 [Updated Sep 3, 2015]. In: Pagon RA, Adam MP, Ardinger HH, et al., eds. GeneReviews [Internet]. Seattle, WA: University of Washington; 1993–2015. http://www.ncbi.nlm.nih.gov/books/NBK1220. Accessed December 12, 2015.

Vanmolkot KR, Babini E, de Vries B, et al. The novel p.L1649Q mutation in the SCN1A epilepsy gene is associated with familial hemiplegic migraine: genetic and functional studies. *Hum Mutat*. 2007;28:522.

35. **C.** Dravet syndrome (severe myoclonic epilepsy of infancy) in most patients is due to de novo mutations that lead to loss of function of the SCN1A channel. The clinical onset is in a normal infant aged 3 months to 2 years with repeated, prolonged, unilateral, clonic seizures during febrile illnesses. This is followed by myoclonic, atypical absence, and focal seizures around age 2 years. EEG is normal at onset; subsequently, progressive deterioration of background, generalized and multifocal spikes, and photosensitivity are seen. Seizures are frequent and resistant to antiseizure medications. Progressive cognitive decline is common. Stiripentol, in combination with valproate and clobazam, has demonstrated efficacy in controlling convulsive seizures. Other effective treatments include topiramate, felbamate, and ketogenic diet. Lamotrigine, carbamazepine, and vigabatrin can worsen myoclonus.

Dravet C, Bureau M, Oguni H, et al. Severe myoclonic epilepsy of infancy (Dravet syndrome). In: Roger J, Bureau M, Dravet C, et al., eds. *Epileptic Syndromes in Infancy, Childhood and Adolescence*. 4th ed. Montrouge, France: John Libbey Eurotext; 2005:89–114.

36. **B.** LKS usually occurs in children ages 3 to 10 years and may first manifest as apparent word deafness or verbal auditory agnosia. Seizures and behavioral disturbances occur in two thirds of children. The majority of cases are idiopathic, but any process affecting the auditory cortex can cause symptomatic LKS. Classic features include word

deafness, language regression, and seizures in a previously normal child. In contrast to LKS, the syndrome of epilepsy with continuous spike waves during slow wave sleep (CSWS) is characterized by regression in cognition and behavior in addition to language. Electrographic status epilepticus of sleep (ESES) can be seen with more focal epileptiform feature in LKS, whereas ESES with generalized epileptiform pattern is seen in CSWS. Activation of epileptiform abnormalities occurs in NREM sleep.

McVicar KA, Shinnar S. Landau–Kleffner syndrome, electrical status epilepticus in slow wave sleep, and language regression in children. *Ment Retard Dev Disabil Res Rev.* 2004;10:144–149.

Tassinari CA, Rubboli G, Volpi L, et al. Electrical status epilepticus during slow sleep (ESES and CSWS) including acquired epileptic aphasia (Landau–Kleffner syndrome). In: Roger J, Bureau M, Dravet C, et al., eds. *Epileptic Syndromes in Infancy, Childhood and Adolescence.* 4th ed. Montrouge, France: John Libbey Eurotext; 2005:295–314.

37. **A.** PNES typically occur in the third or fourth decades of life although onset in children and the elderly has been noted. PNES are more common in women; in most studies, 60% to 75% of patients with PNES are women. Incontinence has been reported to occur in 10% to 44% of patients with PNES; most of which consist of urinary incontinence, but fecal incontinence has also been described. Presence of non stereotypic semiology strongly suggests PNES, but the presence of stereotypic semiology does not rule it out. In fact, it has been shown that 60% to 90% of patients with PNES have stereotypic features although the duration of the events may vary. Vocalization (e.g., screaming, sobbing) occurs during PNES; it is more likely to be seen in the middle of the event in contrast to epileptic seizures, where the vocalization occurs at onset.

Kanner AM, Lafrance WC, Jr, Betts T. Chapter 282: psychogenic non-epileptic seizures. In: Engel J, Jr, Pedley TA, eds. *Epilepsy: A Comprehensive Textbook.* 2nd ed. Philadelphia, PA: Lippincott Williams & Wilkins; 2008: 2795–2810.

38. **C.** Jactatio capitis nocturna (rhythmic movement disorder) is a disorder mainly of infancy and childhood in which patients have involuntary, repetitive movements of large muscles groups immediately before and during sleep, often involving the head and neck. These patients are unaware of their behavior. The majority of these occur out of non-REM sleep, although its occurrence in REM sleep has been reported. Sleep paralysis and hypnagogic (or hypnopompic) hallucinations are seen in about 25% and 30% of patients with narcolepsy, respectively. On the other hand, more common clinical features include automatic behaviors (50%), cataplexy (70%), and excessive daytime sleepiness (90%). Sleep paralysis and sleep related hallucinations can also be seen in other conditions that can cause sleep deprivation. Patients with REM sleep behavior disorder can recall their dreams, and therefore, many of their behaviors witnessed during sleep can be explained. Restless legs syndrome is characterized by an urge to move before sleep, and therefore involves voluntary muscle contractions. In contrast, periodic limb movements of sleep involve involuntary movements that occur in non-REM sleep.

Frenette E, Guilleminault C. Nonepileptic paroxysmal sleep disorders. *Handb Clin Neurol.* 2013; 112:857–860.

Mahowald MW, Schenck CH. Sleep disorders. In: Engel J, Jr, Pedley TA, eds. *Epilepsy: A Comprehensive Textbook.* 2nd ed. Philadelphia, PA: Lippincott Williams & Wilkins; 2008:2757–2764.

39. **A.** Children tend to have a better prognosis than adults, which could be due to early intervention (time of spell onset to diagnosis is shorter) and differences in psychopathology. Predictors of persistent PNES include history of comorbid psychiatric disorders (e.g., mood disorder, personality disorder, dissociative disorder), history of abuse, and longer duration of symptoms before diagnosis. Nonpredictors of persistent PNES include gender, presence of epileptic seizures, and extent of psychotherapy. Once the diagnosis of PNES is made, continued persistence of PNES suggests underlying dissociative disorder, whereas transient improvement with later recurrence suggests underlying conversion or somatoform disorders; complete remission is typically seen in patients with mild or no underlying psychopathology. The limp or catatonic type of PNES is associated with a better prognosis than the convulsive or thrashing type.

Benbadis SR. Psychogenic nonepileptic attacks. In: Wyllie E, ed. *Wyllie's Treatment of Epilepsy: Principles and Practice*. 5th ed. Philadelphia, PA: Lippincott Williams & Wilkins; 2011:486–494.

Kanner AM, Lafrance WC, Jr, Betts T. Psychogenic non-epileptic seizures. In: Engel J, Jr, Pedley TA, eds. *Epilepsy: A Comprehensive Textbook*. 2nd ed. Philadelphia, PA: Lippincott Williams & Wilkins; 2008: 2795–2810.

40. **A.** Dissociative disorders and posttraumatic stress disorders were found to be significantly associated with pure PNES, whereas conversion, affective, and personality disorders were equally associated with both pure PNES and mixed PNES and epilepsy. In addition, patients with pure PNES are more likely to have the following features: female gender, older age, longer history of PNES, prior psychiatric hospitalization, and prior psychiatric medication treatment.

D'Alessio L, Giagante B, Oddo S, et al. Psychiatric disorders in patients with psychogenic non-epileptic seizures, with and without comorbid epilepsy. *Seizure*. 2006;15:333–339.

41. **C.** Seizures, in general, place metabolic demands on the body. When seizures progress into SE, the metabolic demands on the body are increased, leading to more reliance on the compensatory mechanisms. Although in some patients these mechanisms can start to fail during early SE, the majority of failure tends to occur when the SE is established or refractory (i.e., 30–60 minutes). Once malignant SE (>60 minutes) sets in, there is minimal compensation and organ failure starts.

Foreman B, Hirsch LJ. Epilepsy emergencies: diagnosis and management. *Neurol Clin.* 2012;30:11–41.

42. **D.** Absence SE has been classified into four grades based on the continuum of alteration of consciousness: (1) "slight clouding of consciousness" (19% of cases) is associated with simple slowing of thought and expression, sometimes so subtle that only the patient may be able to recognize it; (2) "marked clouding of consciousness" (64%) is associated with a more obvious confusional state affecting alertness, attention, memory, judgment, and language, leading to severe disorientation with delayed responses; (3) "profound clouding of consciousness" (7%) is associated with motionless behavior, inability to move, and inability to feed; and (4) "lethargic stupor" (8%) is associated with a catatonic stupor, motionless staring, upward eye deviation, and incontinence. The duration of each episode is variable, typically lasting 6 to 72 hours. Spontaneous cessation of absence SE can occur, resulting in sudden clinical improvement. In other cases, the patients fall asleep and awaken normal or it progresses to a generalized tonic–clonic convulsion. Myoclonic SE is divided into two forms: pure (primary; seen in patients with known generalized epilepsies) and symptomatic (secondary; seen in

patients with degenerative encephalopathies). The primary form presents with generalized bilaterally synchronous jerks with preservation of consciousness despite long-lasting seizures. The secondary form presents with asymmetric or asynchronous jerks and variable impairment of consciousness.

Ohtahara S, Ohtsuka Y. Myoclonic status epilepticus. In: Engel J, Jr, Pedley TA, eds. *Epilepsy: A Comprehensive Textbook.* 2nd ed. Philadelphia, PA: Lippincott Williams & Wilkins; 2008:725–729.

Thomas P, Snead OC, III. Absence status epileptics. In: Engel J, Jr, Pedley TA, eds. *Epilepsy: A Comprehensive Textbook.* 2nd ed. Philadelphia, PA: Lippincott Williams & Wilkins; 2008:693–703.

43. A. In the operational definition of SE in children over 5 years and adults, it is proposed that seizures lasting 5 minutes or more should be considered SE. This shorter time duration is used for a number of reasons. Studies have shown that almost all discrete seizures last less than 120 seconds. In addition, prolonged seizures are likely to become more difficult to treat, and in animal models, histopathological damage has been shown to occur after 15 to 30 minutes of continuous seizure activity. The term "status epilepticus" is applicable when there are two or more discrete seizures with incomplete cognitive recovery between them. If recovery occurs between the events, then the events could be classified as acute repetitive seizures (i.e., cluster or serial seizures), which lie on the spectrum of discrete seizures and SE. Acute repetitive seizures have the potential to progress into SE.

Hirsch LJ, Gaspard N. Status epilepticus. *Continuum (Minneap Minn).* 2013;19:767–794.

Treiman DM. Generalized convulsive status epilepticus. In: Engel J, Jr, Pedley TA, eds. *Epilepsy: A Comprehensive Textbook.* 2nd ed. Philadelphia, PA: Lippincott Williams & Wilkins; 2008:665–676.

44. A. There is a 10-fold or greater mortality for seizures lasting ≥30 minutes compared with those lasting 10 to 29 minutes. Among all cases of SE, about one third are a manifestation of the initial seizure of epilepsy, one third occur in patients with established epilepsy, and one third occur as a result of an acute isolated brain insult. SE occurs in 0.5% to 6.6% of patients with an established diagnosis of epilepsy. About 20% of patients with epilepsy experience an episode of SE within 5 years of the diagnosis. Generalized tonic SE is most often seen in children with Lennox-Gastaut syndrome, and can be precipitated by administration of benzodiazepines.

Leszczyszyn D, Pellock J. Status epilepticus and acute seizures. In: Pellock J, Bourgeos B, Dodson E, eds. *Pediatric Epilepsy: Diagnosis and Therapy.* 3rd ed. New York, NY: Demos; 2008:461–476.

45. D. The annual incidence of SE ranges from 7 to 41 cases per 100,000 population per year. Most population-based studies define SE based on a 30-minute duration. The wide range of incidence rates is most likely due to differences in case ascertainment, the populations being studied, and inconsistencies regarding inclusion of convulsive and nonconvulsive SE. When only generalized convulsive SE (GCSE) is included, the incidence rate is about 7 per 100,000 population per year. Incidence of SE has a bimodal distribution, peaking before 1 year of age and after 60 years of age. The mortality rate for adults who present with a first episode of GCSE is about 20%.

Drislane FW. Convulsive status epilepticus in adults: classification, clinical features, and diagnosis. UpToDate [Updated November 20, 2015]. http://www.uptodate.com/contents/convulsive-status-epilepticus-in-adults-classification-clinical-features-and-diagnosis?source=search_result&search=status+epilepticus&selectedTitle=2%7E150. Accessed January 19, 2016.

Drislane FW. Convulsive status epilepticus in adults: treatment and prognosis. UpToDate [Updated December 11, 2015]. http://www.uptodate.com/contents/convulsive-status-epilepticus-in-adults-treatment-and-prognosis?source=search_result&search=status+epilepticus&selectedTitle=1%7E150. Accessed January 19, 2016.

46. **B.** Fever and infection are the most common causes of SE in children, whereas epilepsy and stroke are the most common causes in adults. Three risk factors that independently predict SE mortality are older age, longer duration of SE, and etiology of SE. Mortality risk from SE rises with duration of SE. Mortality risk for SE lasting >1 hour is 10 times higher than SE lasting <1 hour, emphasizing the need for rapid treatment. About 80% of patients respond to initial treatment administered within 30 minutes; in contrast, 60% of patients treated 2 hours after the onset of SE fail to respond to medication. Mortality is 3% in children, 26% in adults younger than age 60, and 39% in adults age 60 and older. Mortality is nearly 50% for adults 80 years and older. Myoclonic SE has the highest mortality (50%–86%) when compared with generalized tonic–clonic SE (30%) or simple partial SE (17%–24%). In terms of etiology, low AED levels are associated with low mortality, whereas acute symptomatic causes are associated with high mortality.

Waterhouse E. Status epilepticus. *Continuum (Minneap Minn)*. 2010;16:199–227.

47. **B.** There are many physiological consequences of SE. There tends to be sympathetic overdrive that leads to tachycardia, and potentially fatal arrhythmias have been reported. In animal studies, pulmonary arterial pressure was found to be elevated, contributing to pulmonary edema. The increase in plasma catecholamines leads to demargination of neutrophils, leading to leukocytosis in patients without evidence of underlying infection. Hyperthermia is a very common accompaniment of major motor SE. The convulsing muscles and the sympathetic overactivity due to the heat result in hyperthermia. Core temperatures up to 107°F have been reported in humans. Continued muscle activity leads to conversion to anaerobic metabolism contributing to lactic acidosis. Metabolic and respiratory acidosis leads to low pH, in the range of 6.28 to 7.5.

Shorvon SD, Pellock JM, DeLorenzo RJ. Acute physiologic changes, morbidity, and mortality of status epilepticus. In: Engel J, Jr, Pedley TA, Eds. *Epilepsy: A Comprehensive Textbook*. 2nd ed. Philadelphia, PA: Lippincott Williams & Wilkins; 2008:737–749.

Simon RP. Physiologic consequences of status epilepticus. *Epilepsia*. 1985;26(suppl 1):S58–S66.

48. **C.** Motorbike riding and hang gliding are rather prolonged activities, and pose a relatively high risk for epilepsy patients during the entire time they are involved in such activities. Bullfighting is inherently dangerous even if it lasts for a relatively brief period. On the other hand, target shooting poses some risk to the patient (the shooter) or others around the patient for the very short time when the shooter is squeezing the trigger. Among the choices presented, target shooting is the least risky activity for a patient with epilepsy.

Drazkowski JF, Sirven JI. Driving and social issues in epilepsy. In: Wyllie E, ed. *Wyllie's Treatment of Epilepsy: Principles and Practice*. 5th ed. Philadelphia, PA: Lippincott Williams & Wilkins; 2011:1051–1056.

49. **D.** Impairments in language, memory, and learning of auditory material and academic skills have been noted during the active phase in benign childhood epilepsy with

centro-temporal spikes. Idiopathic occipital lobe epilepsy has been associated with lower scores on intellectual functioning, memory, and attention. Idiopathic generalized epilepsy is associated with mildly decreased measures of intelligence, executive function, and psychomotor speed. Juvenile myoclonic epilepsy has been associated with subtle structural abnormalities in the mesial frontal lobes, with evidence of frontal lobe dysfunction demonstrated by PET scan with corresponding impairments in abstract reasoning and planning noted on neuropsychologic testing.

Hwang S, Ettinger A, So E. Epilepsy comorbidities. *Continuum* (Minneap Minn). 2010;16:86–104.

50. **D.** The actual number of patients with epilepsy who drive is unknown. Only 14% of individuals were found to be truthful about the presence of epilepsy on their driving license application. A prospective survey of 367 patients indicated that about 30% of respondents reported having operated a motor vehicle in the previous 12 months. Reports suggest that epilepsy patients account for approximately 0.02% to 0.04% of all reported car accidents. It is presumed that longer periods of seizure freedom translate into reduced risk of seizure-related automobile accidents. A self-reported survey suggested that the risk of motor vehicle crashes reduced by 85% and 93% if the patient did not have a seizure at 6 months and 12 months, respectively.

Drazkowski JF, Sirven JI. Driving and social issues in epilepsy. In: Wyllie E, ed. *Wyllie's Treatment of Epilepsy: Principles and Practice*. 5th ed. Philadelphia, PA: Lippincott Williams & Wilkins; 2011:1051–1056.

51. **C.** In 2010, the ILAE provided a definition for drug resistant epilepsy. Based on that, the pretreatment interseizure interval was 8 months in this patient. Although the patient has remained seizure free for 12 months, the duration is less than three times the pretreatment interseizure interval. Therefore, the treatment outcome is "undetermined" and drug responsiveness of epilepsy is "undefined." If this patient remains seizure free for 24 months (i.e., three times the pretreatment interseizure interval), then the treatment outcome would be "seizure free" and drug responsiveness of epilepsy would be "drug responsive." Note that the term "inadequate" is not used in the description of treatment outcome.

Kwan P, Arzimanoglou A, Berg AT, et al. Definition of drug resistant epilepsy: consensus proposal by the ad hoc Task Force of the ILAE Commission on Therapeutic Strategies. *Epilepsia*. 2010;51(6):1069–1077.

52. **C.** Seizures triggered by fever raise the possibility of epilepsy due to mutations in the sodium channel such as PCDH19 and SCN1A. PCDH19 mutations are responsible for a disorder also known as epilepsy limited to females with mental retardation (EFMR). Girls with EFMR typically present in infancy with clusters of 10 or more brief focal or generalized seizures over a few days and epilepsy is often refractory to medications. Development is normal at onset with regression at seizure onset. Autistic features are seen in severely affected girls. The mode of inheritance is X linked, from normal transmitting carrier fathers or affected mothers. De novo mutations can also be present. PCDH19 syndrome has similarities with Dravet syndrome, which is caused by SCN1A mutations. However, Dravet syndrome typically presents in infancy with hemiclonic or generalized status epilepticus triggered by fever. More often the SCN1A mutations are de novo in Dravet syndrome, but a family history of epilepsy or febrile seizures is reported in 25% to 50% of families. Lack of hemiclonic convulsions suggests PCHD19 mutation in

this child. Mutations in the ARX gene can cause X-linked infantile spasm syndrome, which begins in the first year of life. ARX mutations are also associated with Partington syndrome (intellectual disability and dystonia) and X-linked lissencephaly with abnormal genitalia (lissencephaly, epilepsy, and abnormal genitalia). Mutations in the CDKL5 gene also cause X-linked infantile spasm syndrome, which is characterized by infantile spasms and intellectual disability. This is more common in females, but it has been identified in a small number of males. Some cases of X-linked infantile spasm syndrome are caused by a deletion involving part of or the entire CDKL5 gene; others result from mutations that alter the function of the CDKL5 protein or prevent the production of any functional protein. Patients with CDKL5 encephalopathy may develop stereotypic hand movements that are seen in Rett syndrome. However, CDKL5 encephalopathy is recognized as a separate clinical entity. The regression seen in Rett syndrome is typically not seen in patients with CDKL5 encephalopathy who have delayed development from birth.

Dravet C, Bureau M, Oguni Y, et al. Severe myoclonic epilepsy of infancy (Dravet syndrome). In: Roger J, Bureau M, Dravet C, et al., eds. *Epileptic Syndromes in Infancy, Childhood and Adolescence.* 4th ed. Montrouge, France: John Libbey Eurotext; 2005:89–114.

Duszyc K, Terczynska I, Hoffman-Zacharska D. Epilepsy and mental retardation restricted to females: X-linked epileptic infantile encephalopathy of unusual inheritance. *J Appl Genet.* 2015;56:49–56.

Genetics Home Reference. ARX. http://ghr.nlm.nih.gov/gene/ARX. Accessed January 22, 2016.

Genetics Home Reference. CDLK5. http://ghr.nlm.nih.gov/gene/CDKL5. Accessed January 22, 2016.

53. **C.** Rett syndrome is a progressive neurodevelopmental disorder and one of the most common causes of mental retardation in females. Classical Rett syndrome is caused by an X-linked dominant mutation at Xq28 involving the methyl-CpG binding protein 2 (MECP2) gene with lethality in hemizygous males. This mutation is identified in 90% to 95% of affected children. Skewing of X inactivation can modulate the severity of the disorder. Children with classical Rett syndrome have normal development and head circumference until 6 months of age, after which there is arrest of development. Progressive loss of speech and purposeful hand use occur, along with microcephaly, autism, ataxia, and stereotypic hand movements. Seizures and breathing irregularities then follow. The condition stabilizes for a while, but late motor deterioration occurs. Prolonged QT interval and cardiac arrhythmias can be present. Severe, early onset of seizures is felt to be associated with CDKL5 rather than MECP2 mutation. Breathing irregularities such as breath holding and hyperventilation, episodes of motor activity such as trembling and jerking, and cardiac arrhythmias from prolonged QT interval are often confused with seizures.

Weaving LS, Ellaway CJ, Gecz J, et al. Rett syndrome: clinical review and genetic update. *J Med Genet.* 2005;42:1–7.

54. **A.** In SE, there is receptor trafficking resulting in self-sustaining seizures. There is internalization of clathrin-coated GABA-A receptors into endosomes, which are destroyed in the lysosomes or recycled in the Golgi apparatus. In addition, there is mobilization of NMDA receptors to the synaptic membrane resulting in additional receptors. There is influx of Na^+ and Ca^{2+} due to activation of NMDA and a-amino-3-hydroxy-5-methyl-4-isoxazolepropionic acid (AMPA) receptors, leading to altered mitochondrial function, and eventually, apoptosis or necrosis. There are anecdotal reports of decreased hippocampal

neurons in patients dying from SE, increase in neuron specific enolase (NSE) after SE, and atrophy on MRI. Depletion of inhibitory peptides (e.g., dynorphin, galanin, somatostatin, neuropeptide Y) and increased expression of proconvulsant peptides (e.g., substance P, neurokinin B) also occur.

Chen JW, Wasterlain CG. Status epilepticus: pathophysiology and management in adults. *Lancet Neurol.* 2006;5:246–256.

55. **D.** Factors associated with poor outcome after RSE include underlying etiology, older age (>50 years), long seizure duration, and high APACHE-2 scale scores. However, after correcting for underlying etiology, coma, and type of status epilepticus seizure, the duration has been shown not to be associated with outcome. The APACHE score system is designed to measure the severity of disease in patients admitted to the intensive care unit. This score ranges from 0 to 71 points and the APACHE score is the sum of acute physiologic scale, age, and chronic health points. Ongoing studies might clarify this further.

Brophy GM, Bell R, Claassen J, et al. Guidelines for the evaluation and management of status epilepticus. *Neurocrit Care.* 2012;17:3–23.

56. **D.** Malformations of cortical development range from the minor FCDs to more extensive malformations such as pachygyria, polymicrogyria, schizencephaly, and lissencephaly. Histologically, FCD is categorized as: mild malformation of cortical development (mMCD), FCD type 1a (isolated architectural abnormalities), type 1b (with additional immature or giant neurons), type 2a (with additional dysmorphic neurons), and type 2b (with additional balloon cells). In type 1a, the MRI is negative or shows focal gray–white blurring; in type 2b, the MRI shows increased signal intensity extending from the cortex to the ventricular surface. The cytomegalic neurons exhibit epileptogenic potential due to dendritic and axonal overgrowth. Repetitive calcium spikes suggest hyperexcitability. FCDs account for the majority of nonlesional surgical cases. The major pathologies found in extratemporal resection include FCD (38%), tumors (28%), chronic infarct (18%), and vascular malformations (3%). The most frequent locations for FCD are frontal (68%), temporal (28%), and multilobar (4%). FCD can coexist with DNETs, which becomes an important consideration when planning surgical resection.

Mirzaa G, Kuzniecky R, Guerrini R. Malformations of cortical development and epilepsy. In: Wyllie E, ed. *Wyllie's Treatment of Epilepsy: Principles and Practice.* 5th ed. Philadelphia, PA: Lippincott Williams & Wilkins; 2011:339–351.

57. **D.** A ring chromosome is a chromosomal anomaly in which the tip of the short arm of a chromosome merges with the tip of the long arm, and chromosomal material is lost in the subtelomeric region of one or both chromosomal arms. Ring chromosomes are unstable; during mitosis, the ring may be lost or duplicated, resulting in mosaic karyotypes. Most cases of ring chromosome 20 syndrome are sporadic, only a few are inherited. This syndrome is associated with epilepsy, mild intellectual deficit, and behavioral problems. In rare cases, brain, kidney, or heart malformations may be present. There is no recognizable dysmorphism, but strabismus and microcephaly have been reported. Seizure onset is from late infancy to early adulthood, usually around 4 to 8 years of age. This syndrome is characterized by focal seizures, nocturnal frontal lobe seizures, and prolonged episodes of nonconvulsive status epilepticus. Semiology consists of motionless stare, complex automatisms, wandering, hypomotor or hypermotor behavior, and prolonged nocturnal

confusional events. The seizures tend to be refractory to treatment. The mosaicism ratio is believed to be associated with age at seizure onset, IQ, dysmorphism, and malformation, but not with the response to antiepileptic drug treatment.

Radhakrishnan A, Menon RN, Hariharan S, et al. The evolving electroclinical syndrome of "epilepsy with ring chromosome 20". *Seizure.* 2012;21:92–97.

58. **B.** Onset of ADPEAF is typically during adolescence or early adulthood although it can start from age 4 to 50 years. The most common auditory symptoms include simple unformed sounds such as humming, buzzing, or ringing. Ictal receptive aphasia, consisting of inability to understand language in the absence of general confusion, is also prominent. Secondary generalized seizures are common. Seizures may be precipitated by sounds such as a ringing telephone. The clinical course is usually benign with seizures responding well to treatment with antiepileptic drugs at low doses. Interictal EEG may show abnormalities in two thirds of patients. Imaging is usually normal. It is inherited as an autosomal dominant disorder with incomplete penetrance. It is associated with a mutation in LGI1 gene, not CHRNA4; the latter mutation is associated with autosomal dominant nocturnal frontal lobe epilepsy.

Ottman R. Autosomal dominant partial epilepsy with auditory features. 2007 Apr 20 [Updated 2015 Aug 27]. In: Pagon RA, Adam MP, Ardinger HH, et al., eds. *GeneReviews [Internet].* Seattle, WA: University of Washington; 1993–2015. http://www.ncbi.nlm.nih.gov/books/NBK1537/. Accessed December 27, 2015.

59. **D.** FCD is the most common cause in children and the third most common cause in adults undergoing epilepsy surgery. The International League Against Epilepsy (ILAE) classification grades isolated FCD into mild type I (cortical dyslamination), severe type II (dyslamination plus dysmorphic neurons and balloon cells), and dysplasia associated with other epileptogenic lesions (type III). Multilobar type II lesions present at an earlier age and with more severe epilepsy compared with focal type I abnormalities, often in the temporal lobe. Patients with severe type II dysplasia have a higher frequency of seizures per day including status epilepticus, and more extratemporal lesions than those with mild type I dysplasia. Interictal and ictal scalp EEG localizes FCD with 50% to 66% accuracy. MRI findings include abnormally thick cortical gray matter, loss of the gray–white differentiation, and white matter FLAIR hyperintensity. MRI is negative in approximately 30% of cases, most often linked with mild type I cases. Fluorodeoxyglucose(FDG)-PET scan can be 80% to 90% accurate, but is not 100% sensitive. About 60% of patients with cortical dysplasia achieve seizure freedom after epilepsy surgery, with a much higher rate of seizure freedom with complete (80%) compared with incomplete (20%) resection.

Hauptman JS, Mathern GW. Surgical treatment of epilepsy associated with cortical dysplasia: 2012 update. *Epilepsia.* 2012;53(suppl 4):98–104.

60. **C.** Although complex febrile seizures is a risk factor for development of mesial temporal sclerosis and epilepsy, the majority of patients with febrile SE do not have unprovoked seizures, as shown in population and prospective studies. There are reports suggesting lasting cognitive impairment after both convulsive and nonconvulsive (complex partial and absence) SE. It is generally accepted that much of the morbidity and mortality is associated with the precipitating acute neurologic insult. Hemiconvulsion-hemiplegia-hemiparesis syndrome was common in children with convulsive SE lasting >1 hour.

Recent studies have noted a near absence in the past two decades for unclear reasons. However, it seems to coincide with the decrease in the mortality from SE. About 15% to 30% of patients with acute symptomatic SE develop a subsequent seizure disorder (even years later) depending on the severity of the underlying insult.

Shinnar S, Babb TL, Moshé SL, et al. Long-term sequelae of status epilepticus. In: Engel J, Jr, Pedley TA, eds. *Epilepsy: A Comprehensive Textbook.* 2nd ed. Philadelphia, PA: Lippincott Williams & Wilkins; 2008:751-759.

61. **A.** In the United States, the Social Security Administration lists the requirements to qualify for disability. There are two listings for epilepsy: Listing 11.02 for convulsive epilepsy (primarily refers to grand mal seizures or psychomotor seizures) and Listing 11.03 for nonconvulsive epilepsy (refers to petit mal, psychomotor, or focal seizures). In order to qualify for disability benefits for convulsive epilepsy, an adult should have a seizure frequency of >1 seizure per month despite taking prescribed treatment for at least 3 months; there needs to be documentation of daytime episodes (loss of consciousness and convulsive seizures) or nocturnal episodes manifesting significant residual interference with daytime activity. Adults with nonconvulsive epilepsy should have a seizure frequency of >1 seizure per week despite taking prescribed treatment for at least 3 months; there needs to be documentation of alteration of awareness or loss of consciousness and transient postictal manifestations of unconventional behavior or significant interference with daytime activity.

Disability Evaluation Under Social Security: 11.00 Neurological—Adult. https://www.ssa.gov/disability/professionals/bluebook/11.00-Neurological-Adult.htm#11_02. Accessed January 22, 2016.

62. **B.** Sudden death refers to natural unexpected death occurring within 1 hour of new symptoms. Although cardiac causes are the leading cause of sudden death, the exact incidence from other causes is not well established. SUDEP is the main cause of death in individuals with epilepsy, but the term is underused in death certification. It represents approximately 1% to 1.5% of all "natural" deaths certified by the medical examiner or coroner. Following the increasing awareness of SUDEP, in 2013, two U.S. states (New Jersey and Illinois) have signed SUDEP measures into law, which require the medical examiners to inquire about history of epilepsy as part of the autopsy. SUDEP is most commonly encountered by the forensic pathologist rather than the clinician. Due to the strict requirements for the diagnosis of SUDEP, there cannot be an obvious anatomic cause for the death at autopsy. However, 60% to 70% of cases have been found to have a lesion in the brain (e.g., old trauma) to explain the epilepsy. Most victims have little or no blood levels of anticonvulsant medications at the time of death.

de la Grandmaison GL. Is there progress in the autopsy diagnosis of sudden unexpected death in adults? *Forensic Sci Int.* 2006;156:138–144.

Leestma JE, Hughes JR, Teas SS, et al. Sudden epilepsy deaths and the forensic pathologist. *Am J Forensic Med Pathol.* 1985;6:215–218.

Smithson WH, Colwell B, Hanna J. Sudden unexpected death in epilepsy: addressing the challenges. *Curr Neurol Neurosci Rep.* 2014;14:502.

63. **B.** Trials involving children that pose more than low risk must offer PDB; trials cannot be justified by the importance of the anticipated knowledge. However, a study can be done if there is no PDB as long as the allowable risk exposure for an intervention or

procedure is restricted to low risk. This is contrary to the trials involving adult subjects, where the risks of research participation can be justified either by the PDB to the patient or by the importance of the anticipated knowledge.

Roth-Cline M, Gerson J, Bright P, et al. Ethical considerations in conducting pediatric research. *Handb Exp Pharmacol*. 2011;205:219–244.

64. **B.** Although clear driving laws do not exist for patients with PNES, the motor vehicles department in the United Kingdom provides some guidance. Cultural factors may play a role in placing driving restrictions as noted by surveys in the United States and Germany. Surveys of providers suggest that the proportion of providers enforcing driving restrictions in patients with PNES is variable although most feel that the length of restriction should be less than that of patients with epilepsy. Sampling driving records of patients with PNES revealed no statistically significant increase in motor vehicle crashes. Some providers believe that restricting driving privileges similar to patients with epilepsy could be a motivation to accept the diagnosis and seek appropriate treatment. Interestingly, similar provider surveys conducted in different countries showed differences in what providers recommend in terms of driving restrictions, which may reflect national or cultural differences.

Benbadis SR, Blustein JN, Sunstad L. Should patients with psychogenic nonepileptic seizures be allowed to drive? *Epilepsia*. 2000;41:895–897.

Morrison I, Razvi SS. Driving regulations and psychogenic nonepileptic seizures: perspectives from the United Kingdom. *Seizure*. 2011;20:177–180.

Specht U, Thorbecke R. Should patients with psychogenic nonepileptic seizures be allowed to drive? Recommendations of German experts. *Epilepsy Behav*. 2009;16:547–550.

65. **D.** Although water poses special dangers for people with seizures, there is usually a way to make this a safer activity. Those with intractable epilepsy could still be in a shallow pool or body of water with a life jacket and with a buddy who knows basic lifesaving techniques. The lifeguards should know that they must keep their eyes on the pool while the child is swimming. People with controlled seizures can be encouraged to swim with reasonable safety tips. Competitive swimming practices and matches are usually well supervised, so they can be encouraged. Swimming in open waters (e.g., lake, bay, or ocean) is much more dangerous than swimming in a pool, and in general, swimming should be allowed only in clear water where they are in sight with a lifejacket. Snorkeling in relatively calm water with a buddy should be safe. Patients with well-controlled seizures can snorkel and scuba dive as long as they are accompanied by someone with lifesaving skills.

Wheless JW, Sirven JI. Playing sports and other activities. http://www.epilepsy.com/learn/seizures-youth/about-kids/playing-sports-and-other-activities. Accessed January 22, 2016.

66. **D.** Responsibility for mandatory reporting varies by state. A person with epilepsy may be civilly or criminally liable for a motor vehicle accident caused by seizures. Liability may occur when a person drives against medical advice, without a valid license, without notifying the state department of motor vehicles of the medical condition, or with the knowledge that he or she is prohibited from driving. Some states (California, Delaware, Nevada, New Jersey, Oregon, and Pennsylvania) have "mandatory reporting laws." These laws require doctors and other health care providers to report persons with active

epilepsy and other disorders that may make driving hazardous. These laws generally mandate the doctor to notify the Department of Motor Vehicles of the person's name, age, and address. There are special exceptions to the driving rules (depending on location) pertaining to nocturnal seizures, presence of simple partial sensory seizures, or seizure occurrence in the setting of medication adjustment rather than noncompliance. The required seizure-free period prior to resumption of driving varies by state. Most states require a 3 to 6 months seizure-free period, but it can be as long as 1 year. The U.S. DOT allows people with a history of epilepsy who have been seizure-free off medication for 10 years to obtain a commercial driver's license (CDL). People with epilepsy cannot get a CDL if they have ongoing seizures or are seizure-free while taking medication. Although the FAA often prohibits patients with epilepsy from obtaining a pilot's license even if controlled by medication or in remission, there are a few exceptions to this rule: those with rolandic seizures may be eligible for certification if they are seizure-free for 4 years and have normal EEG; and a license may be issued to those with a history of single febrile seizure prior to age 5 years if they are seizure-free off all medications for at least 3 years.

Drazkowski J. An overview of epilepsy and driving. *Epilepsia.* 2007;48(suppl 9):10–12.

Guide for Aviation Medical Examiners. *Decision Considerations—Aerospace Medical Dispositions. Item 46. Neurologic—Neurologic Conditions.* http://www.faa.gov/about/office_org/headquarters_offices/avs/offices/aam/ame/guide/app_process/exam_tech/item46/amd/nc/. Accessed January 22, 2016.

Wheless, JW, Shafer PO, Sirven JI. *Driving and Transportation.* http://www.epilepsy.com/get-help/staying-safe/driving-and-transportation. Accessed January 22, 2016.

67. **C.** Contact sports (e.g., football, basketball, soccer, rugby, and ice hockey) are generally safe for people with epilepsy. Although the main concern with these sports is the chance of injury, the risk is not necessarily more than others, even if an absence or complex partial seizure were to occur during a game. Tackle football, rugby, and ice hockey have a higher incidence of injuries, and thus should probably be limited to those with well-controlled seizures.

Wheless JW, Sirven JI. *Playing Sports and Other Activities.* http://www.epilepsy.com/learn/seizures-youth/about-kids/playing-sports-and-other-activities. Accessed January 22, 2016.

68. **A.** ADHD may develop before or along with onset of seizures. ADHD is about 2.5-fold more common among children with newly diagnosed seizures than controls. The prevalence of ADHD in epilepsy is 10% to 40%, which is higher than the general population. Contributing factors include underlying cause for epilepsy, effects of antiepileptic drugs, and effects of interictal EEG abnormalities. Stimulant therapy is generally safe and effective in the treatment of ADHD in children with epilepsy, but anecdotal reports of seizure exacerbation exist.

Hwang S, Ettinger A, So E. Epilepsy comorbidities. *Continuum* (Minneap Minn). 2010;16:86–104.

69. **B.** An employer may not ask a job applicant whether she has epilepsy or about her treatment related to epilepsy before making a job offer. However, an employer may ask questions pertaining to the qualifications for, or performance of, the job such as whether she has a driver's license; whether she can climb a ladder to stock shelves, and so on. The ADA does not require applicants to voluntarily disclose that they have epilepsy or another disability unless they will need a reasonable accommodation for the application

process. Some individuals may choose to disclose their condition because they want their coworkers or supervisors to know what to do if they have a seizure. Often the decision to disclose depends on the type of seizure a person has, the need for assistance during or after a seizure, the frequency of seizures, and the type of work for which the person is applying. Sometimes the decision to disclose depends on whether an individual will need a reasonable accommodation to perform the job (e.g., breaks to take medication). A person with epilepsy, however, may request an accommodation after becoming an employee even if she did not do so when applying for the job or after receiving the job offer.

Questions & Answers about Epilepsy in the Workplace and the Americans with Disabilities Act (ADA). http://www.eeoc.gov/laws/types/epilepsy.cfm. Accessed January 22, 2016.

70. **C.** Cardiac malformations, hypospadias, and cleft palate and cleft lips are associated with maternal exposure to carbamazepine, phenytoin, phenobarbital, lamotrigine, and valproate. Studies have shown an increase in the risk of neural tube defects associated with maternal use of valproate, and possibly carbamazepine. Infants exposed to lamotrigine in early pregnancy have been noted to have 10-fold increased rate of cleft palate or cleft lip. Infants exposed to topiramate have been noted to have a 10-fold increased risk of cleft lip than unexposed infants.

Tomson T, Battino D. Teratogenic effects of antiepileptic medications. *Lancet Neurol.* 2012;11:803–813.

71. **B.** The effects of in utero exposure to AEDs were studied in school-age children at age 6. In children who were exposed in utero to high-dose valproate (>800 mg daily), it has been shown that the mean IQ is about 10 points lower and the need for educational intervention is eightfold higher compared with control children. Exposure to valproate doses of <800 mg daily was not associated with lower IQ, but was associated with impaired verbal abilities and a 6-fold increase in educational intervention. Exposure to carbamazepine or lamotrigine in utero is not associated with a significant effect on IQ, but carbamazepine is associated with impaired verbal abilities. These data are consistent with the data from younger cohorts, and suggest that school-age children exposed to higher doses of valproate in utero experience significantly poorer cognitive development than control children or children exposed to lamotrigine and carbamazepine.

Baker GA, Bromley RL, Briggs M, et al. IQ at 6 years after in utero exposure to antiepileptic drugs: a controlled cohort study. *Neurology.* 2015;84:382–390.

Basic Electroencephalography

1. A 32-year-old female with new-onset seizures undergoes a routine EEG as shown in the following (filter: 1–70 Hz). Point 1 and Point 2, respectively, correspond to:

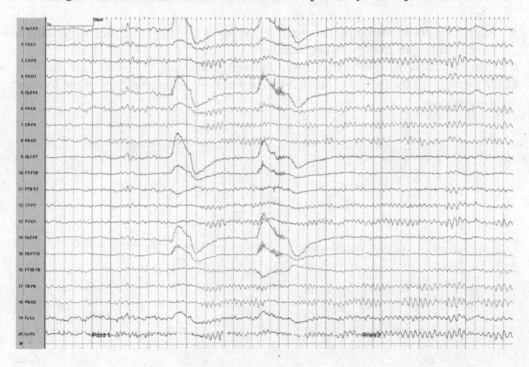

    A. Eyes open and eyes closed
    B. Stage N2 sleep and arousal
    C. Eyes closed resting and eyes open reading
    D. Stage N1 sleep and stage N2 sleep

2. In the EEG in Question 1, the amplitude of the activity seen at Point 2:

    A. Is higher on the left side in the majority of normal individuals
    B. Can show side-to-side asymmetry of up to 20% in normal individuals
    C. Diminishes with age
    D. Can increase while doing simple arithmetic

3. T-type calcium channels can be characterized by all of the following EXCEPT:

    A. They remain open for short periods of time
    B. They contribute to the rhythmic firing patterns in the thalamus
    C. They are the target for ethosuximide
    D. When open, they allow for calcium to exit the cell

4. Which of the following produces a surface-negative field potential on the scalp?

    A. Superficial excitatory postsynaptic potential (EPSP)
    B. Superficial inhibitory postsynaptic potential (IPSP)
    C. Deep excitatory postsynaptic potential (EPSP)
    D. None of the above

5. Which of the following is true regarding the current flow across an activated neuronal membrane?
    A. Local extracellular potential produced by an excitatory postsynaptic potential (EPSP) is positive
    B. Inhibitory postsynaptic potential (IPSP) occurs when negative ions flow intracellularly, resulting in an outward current flow
    C. Current sink occurs at the site of neuronal activation
    D. Orientation of the dipole generated by current flow is independent of the location of the synapse

6. An 11-year-old girl with seizures consisting of brief eye fluttering is admitted for video-EEG monitoring. Her EEG is shown in the following (filter: 1–70 Hz). Which of the following statements is true regarding the predominant waveforms seen in this segment?

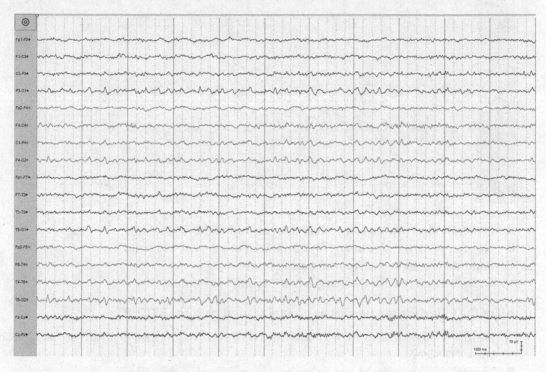

A. They are seen during light sleep

B. They are normal during wakefulness in young children

C. They appear when during scanning or reading

D. They are associated with an increased risk of epilepsy

7. Detection of spontaneous EEG activity by scalp electrodes requires meeting all of the following conditions EXCEPT:

A. Synchronous activation of the regularly arranged pyramidal neurons

B. Summation of transverse components of the extracellular current flow

C. Summation of longitudinal components of the extracellular current flow

D. Laminar current flow along the main axes of the neurons

8. The frequency of the posterior dominant rhythm (PDR) is:

A. 3 Hz by age 3 months

B. 4 Hz by age 12 months

C. 6 Hz by 3 years

D. 10 Hz by 8 years

9. The EEG segment shown in the following (filter: 1–70 Hz; sensitivity: 15 mcV/mm; solid vertical lines are 1-second apart) is most consistent with:

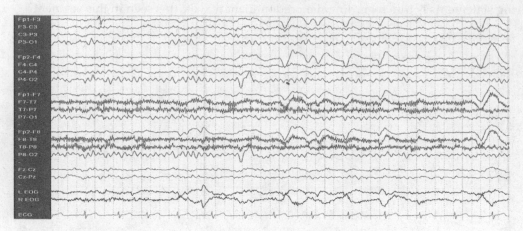

A. Posterior slow waves of youth in a 1-year-old child
B. Normal posterior dominant rhythm (PDR) in a 4-year-old child
C. Lambda waves in a 15-year-old adolescent
D. Occipital spike-wave discharges in a 2-month-old infant

10. All of the following can be seen as normal arousal patterns EXCEPT:

A. Diffuse 4- to 6-Hz activity with intermixed slower frequencies in adults arousing from stage N1 sleep
B. Frontal rhythmic sharp and spiky activity in a 3-year-old child
C. Short duration, diffuse theta activity in older children
D. Rapid transition to waking rhythm in adolescents

11. In the bipolar derivation of G1 to G2, if G1 is positive and G2 is negative, the net voltage and waveform deflection, respectively, will be:

A. Negative and upward
B. Positive and downward
C. Negative and downward
D. Positive and upward

12. In the 10–20 International System of electrode placement for recording EEG, the:

A. Distance between two adjacent electrodes is either 10 or 20 cm
B. Distance between two adjacent electrodes is either 10% or 20% of the total measured length
C. Distance is measured between superior orbital margin and base of the occiput
D. Letter "C" corresponds to the "central region" between the two hemispheres

13. Age-related EEG slowing in the elderly is characterized by all of the following EXCEPT:

A. It is usually in the range of 1.5- to 3-Hz activity
B. It has greater predominance over the left temporal region
C. It occurs in trains of 1 to 3 slow waves
D. It can occur during wakefulness and light sleep

14. Lambdoid waves are:

A. Periodic, surface-negative waveforms in the occipital region
B. Seen during deeper stages of sleep
C. Most common in young children
D. Can be seen in blind, otherwise healthy, individuals

15. Intermittent photic stimulation (IPS) can induce different responses. All of the following statements are correct regarding those responses EXCEPT:

A. Photosensitive response refers to EEG changes without clinical correlate
B. Photoconvulsive response refers to spike-wave discharges correlated to clinical manifestations
C. Photomyoclonic response refers to muscle twitching timed to the stimulus
D. Photoelectric response refers to changes induced by chemical reaction

16. Which of the following statements most accurately describes the photic driving response?

A. It has a one-to-one frequency relationship with the flash
B. It is typically seen with 5- to 30-Hz flash frequency range
C. It is attenuated in individuals with prominent lambda waves
D. It is always time locked with the onset and offset of the flash stimulus

17. A 10-year-old boy was undergoing hyperventilation (HV) with good effort during EEG recording as shown in the following (filter: 1–70 Hz; sensitivity: 15 mcV/mm; solid vertical lines are 1 second apart). The technologist was concerned and called the epilepsy fellow for guidance. The patient was able to recall the code words provided. Which of the following actions will be most helpful in this situation?

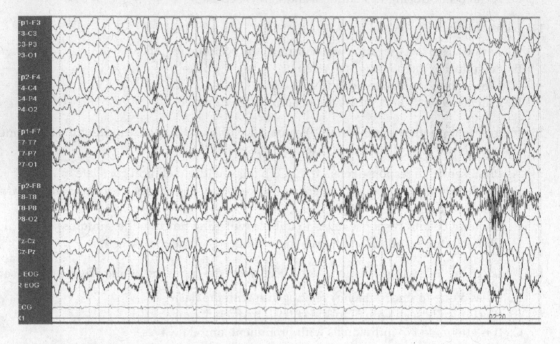

A. Administering lorazepam immediately

B. Waking the patient up

C. Inquiring about the time of the child's last meal

D. Prescribing an antiseizure medication

18. Which of the following characteristic occipital responses can be seen with photic stimulation using slow (<5 Hz) flash rates?

A. Low amplitude, focal spikes in a 22-year-old normal male

B. Low amplitude, focal spikes in a 2-year-old child with congenital blindness

C. High amplitude, focal epileptiform spikes in a 3-year-old child with intellectual disability and myoclonus

D. High-amplitude driving response in a 54-year-old male in alcohol withdrawal

19. Which of the following statements is true regarding pharmacological activation of seizures?

   A. Antiepileptic drugs (AEDs) have no effect on the frequency of interictal epileptiform discharges (IEDs)

   B. Increased seizure frequency after abrupt AED discontinuation is due to rebound phenomenon rather than AED subtherapeutic level

   C. AED withdrawal may unmask a seizure focus that is different from where the habitual seizures originate

   D. AED withdrawal is free from complications as long as it is performed in the epilepsy monitoring unit (EMU)

20. The value of sleep or sleep deprivation as an activation procedure can be characterized by all of the following statements EXCEPT:

   A. When the initial routine EEG is normal, a repeat sleep-deprived EEG captures interictal epileptiform discharges (IEDs) 30% to 70% of the time

   B. Nearly all patients with IEDs during a daytime nap recording have their first IED within 30 minutes of sleep onset

   C. IEDs seen during REM sleep are more localizing than those seen in NREM sleep

   D. Following sleep deprivation, IEDs continue to appear exclusively in sleep

21. The following EEG segment is recorded during intermittent photic stimulation (IPS) at 6 Hz flash rate. The activity at Fp1 and Fp2 was also seen at 3 Hz flash rate but disappeared at flash rates of 9 Hz and higher. What does this activity represent?

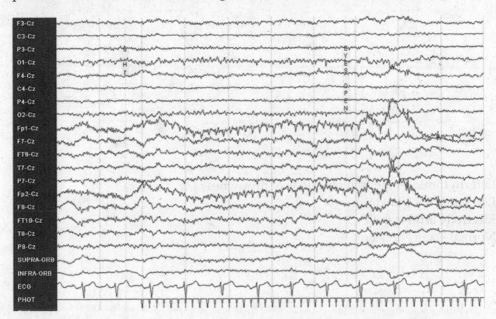

   A. A low-voltage response to the light stimulation of the retina

   B. A train of spike-wave discharges arising from a frontal lobe seizure focus

   C. Muscle twitching due to heightened brainstem reflexes

   D. A photochemical reaction between the electrode and the light

22. Shut eye waves are:

    A. Seen in the frontal region
    B. Associated with scanning complex picture
    C. Seen in children under 10 years of age
    D. Surface-positive waveforms

23. Which of the following patterns is seen in the following EEG from a 17-year-old girl with suspected left temporal lobe epilepsy?

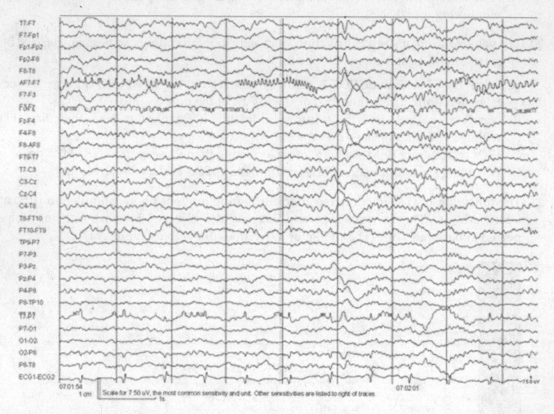

    A. Left rhythmic temporal theta bursts of drowsiness
    B. Left temporal ictal discharge
    C. Electrode artifact in F7
    D. Normal stage N2 sleep

24. A 23-year-old female undergoes a routine EEG after she had a generalized tonic–clonic seizure witnessed by her coworkers. Which of the following statements best describes the activity seen in the following EEG segment (filter: 1–70 Hz)?

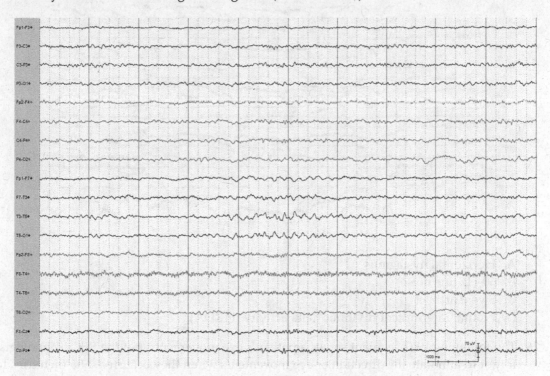

A. It can have shifting asymmetry from side to side
B. It is most prominent during deep sleep
C. It can evolve into delta-frequency activity
D. It correlates with mesial temporal lobe epilepsy

25. The slow activity seen in the anterior channels in the following EEG (filter: 0.1–70 Hz) most likely represents:

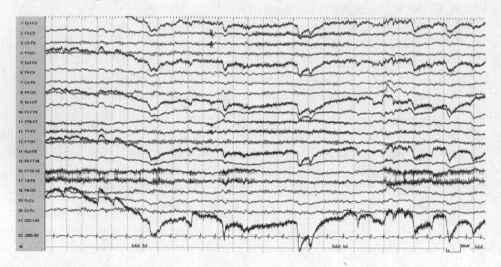

A. Horizontal nystagmus
B. 60-Hz line noise
C. Sweat artifact
D. Frontal intermittent rhythmic delta activity (FIRDA)

26. The following EEG segment shows a patient's eye movements, but the EEG technologist forgot to annotate the direction of eye movements when they occurred. She then tries to figure out which way the patient is looking by using the polarities of the homologous channels. Markers 1 to 4 are placed immediately before the eye movement of interest. Which of the following statements regarding the eye movements is correct?

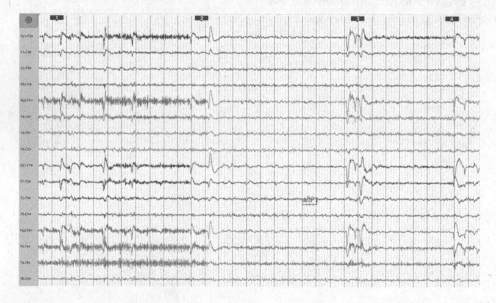

A. Marker 1 corresponds to downward eye movement
B. Marker 2 corresponds to downward eye movement
C. Marker 3 corresponds to right eye movement
D. Marker 4 corresponds to left eye movement

27. 14- and 6-Hz positive bursts:

A. Increase in incidence with age
B. Have posterior temporal distribution
C. Become prominent during deeper stages of sleep
D. Usually last 5 to 8 seconds

28. Which of the following is true regarding lambda waves?

A. They are most often seen in young adults
B. They are triggered by eye closure
C. They persist in dim lighting conditions
D. They can be seen in occipital, parietal, or posterior temporal regions

29. The waveforms seen at time instants 1, 2, and 3 in the following EEG segment (filter: 1–70 Hz) can be characterized by all of the following features EXCEPT:

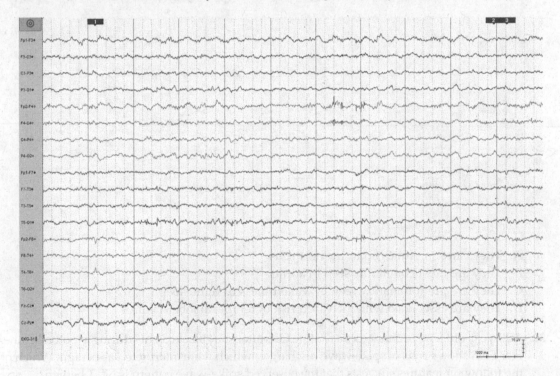

A. They are most prominent during deeper stages of sleep
B. They typically have steep descending limbs
C. They may or may not have an aftergoing slow wave
D. They may have opposite polarities in the two hemispheres

30. Subclinical rhythmic electrographic discharge of adults (SREDA) is characterized by all of the following EXCEPT:

A. Occurrence in young adults
B. Temporo-parietal distribution
C. Sudden buildup of theta activity
D. Initial evolution from delta to theta-frequency activity

31. A 35-year-old woman with long history of epilepsy undergoes an EEG (filter: 1–70 Hz). The waveforms enclosed by the rectangle can be characterized by all of the following statements EXCEPT:

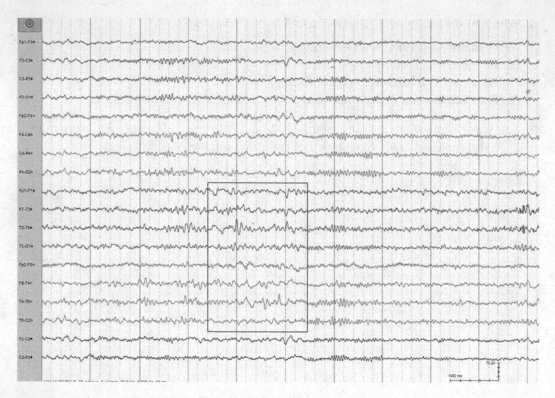

A. They can sometimes occur in short runs
B. They are most commonly seen in adults
C. They are predominantly seen in wakefulness or light sleep
D. They are associated with increased risk of temporal lobe seizures

32. A 22-year-old female undergoes a routine EEG after she "blacked out" during a football game. Her EEG shows runs of spike-wave discharges, which were interpreted as benign. Which of the following features suggests that the observed spike-wave pattern is NOT benign?

A. Discharge frequency of 4 Hz
B. Occurrence in wakefulness and light sleep
C. Spike component is much smaller than the wave component
D. Burst duration of 1 second

33. Waveforms occurring in the temporal region can be considered epileptiform if they have which of the following features?

A. Diphasic morphology with steep ascending and descending limbs
B. Occurrence in light sleep
C. Persistence during slow-wave sleep
D. Accompanied by aftergoing slow waves

34. A 51-year-old male with a history of anaplastic astrocytoma, status postresection 6 months ago, was admitted for spells of left-hand twitching. Which of the following is seen on his routine EEG shown (filter: 1–70 Hz)?

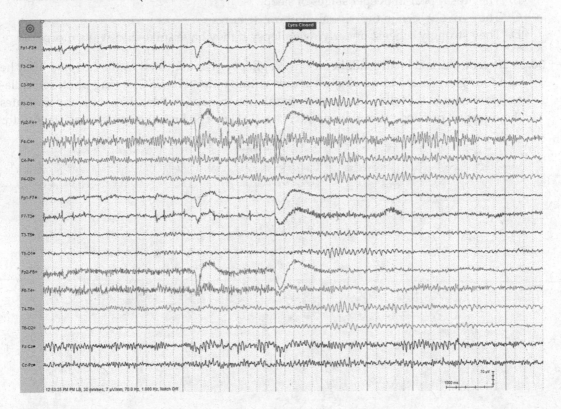

A. Breach rhythm
B. Seizure discharge
C. Wicket rhythm
D. Subclinical rhythmic electrographic discharge of adults (SREDA)

35. Which of the following features is most helpful in differentiating epileptiform discharges from wicket spikes?

A. Persistence in deeper stages of sleep
B. Occurrence in trains
C. Aftergoing slow wave
D. Disruption of background

36. Which of the following patterns can be seen upon arousal?

    A. 10-Hz rhythmic discharge with notched appearance in the frontal region

    B. 12-Hz rhythmic discharge in the occipital region

    C. 6-Hz rhythmic discharge with notched appearance in the occipital region

    D. 6-Hz rhythmic discharge with notched appearance in the temporal region

37. Which of the following statements is true regarding interictal epileptiform discharges (IEDs)?

    A. Spikes are generated by synchronous depolarization of neurons within 6 mm^2 of the cortex

    B. They disappear in deeper stages of sleep

    C. They are not seen in individuals without seizures

    D. They strongly suggest underlying epilepsy if they have spike-and-wave morphology

38. A 20-year-old male with childhood-onset epilepsy was admitted to the hospital after he had four generalized tonic–clonic seizures within a day. His EEG during photic stimulation is shown in the following (photic stimulation frequency: 9 Hz; bar at the top indicates the duration of photic stimulation; filter: 1.6–70 Hz). The finding is most consistent with:

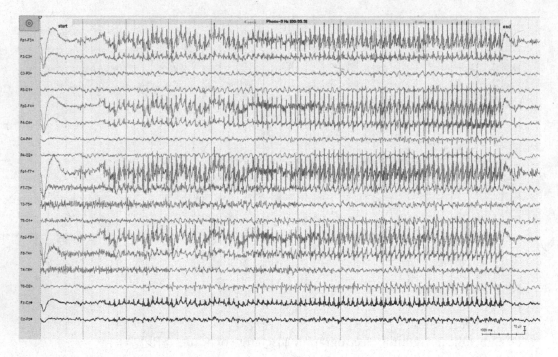

    A. Photomyoclonic response

    B. Photoparoxysmal response

    C. Photoconvulsive response

    D. Photoelectric response

39. Which of the following interictal EEG patterns is associated with a risk for seizures?

A. Small sharp spikes (SSS) with an aftergoing slow wave
B. Frontal phantom spike-wave discharges
C. Occipital phantom spike-wave discharges
D. Rudimentary spike-wave discharges (pseudo-petit mal discharges)

40. The condition characterized by the interictal abnormality shown in the following EEG (filter: 1.6–70 Hz) can be associated with which of the following seizure types?

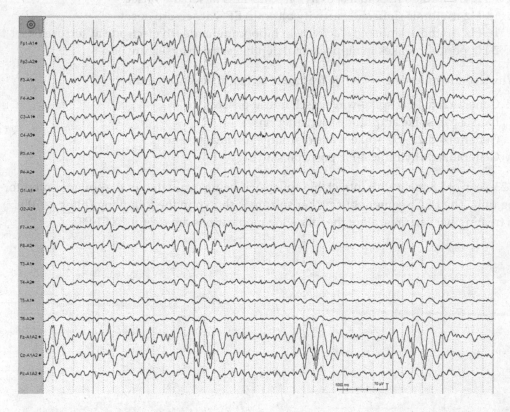

A. Atonic seizures
B. Tonic seizures
C. Myoclonic seizures
D. Myoclonic-atonic seizures

41. Atonic seizures can be characterized by all of the following ictal patterns EXCEPT:

A. Generalized attenuation
B. Generalized slow rhythmic discharge
C. Generalized fast rhythmic discharge
D. Generalized spikes or sharp waves

42. Which of the following ictal patterns is most likely to be seen with a tonic seizure?

A. Generalized 2-Hz spike-wave discharge
B. Generalized, bifrontally predominant 4-Hz rhythmic discharge
C. Generalized 16-Hz rhythmic discharge
D. Generalized 4-Hz polyspike-wave discharge

43. Which of the following ictal patterns is LEAST likely to be seen in temporal lobe seizures?

A. 7-Hz rhythmic sinusoidal activity on scalp EEG at seizure onset
B. 18-Hz rhythmic sinusoidal activity on scalp EEG at seizure onset
C. 16-Hz rhythmic sinusoidal activity in hippocampal depth electrode at seizure onset
D. 2-Hz periodic spikes in hippocampal depth electrode at seizure onset

44. Which of the following is NOT a feature of a typical absence seizure?

A. Generalized 4-Hz spike-wave discharge at onset
B. Increase in spike amplitude soon after onset
C. Generalized 2.5-Hz spike-wave discharge toward the end
D. Generalized rhythmic 4-Hz postictal slowing

45. A 23-year-old female with intractable epilepsy is being evaluated in the epilepsy monitoring unit. The EEG segment during her seizure is shown in the following (filter: 1–70 Hz). In treating her seizures, all of the following medications are useful EXCEPT:

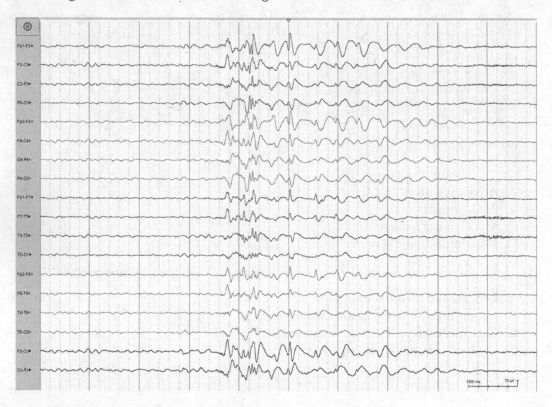

A. Lamotrigine
B. Felbamate
C. Carbamazepine
D. Topiramate

46. A 17-year-old female has the following finding on her EEG during one of her seizures (filter: 1–70 Hz). Her clinical presentation can include all of following EXCEPT:

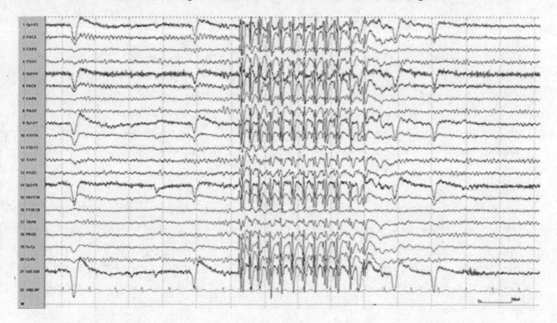

A. Sudden pause while talking
B. Twitching of eyelids
C. Severe intellectual disability
D. Blank stare

47. A 60-year-old male is admitted for evaluation of altered mental status and has the EEG shown in the following figure (filter: 1–70 Hz). The abnormality seen is:

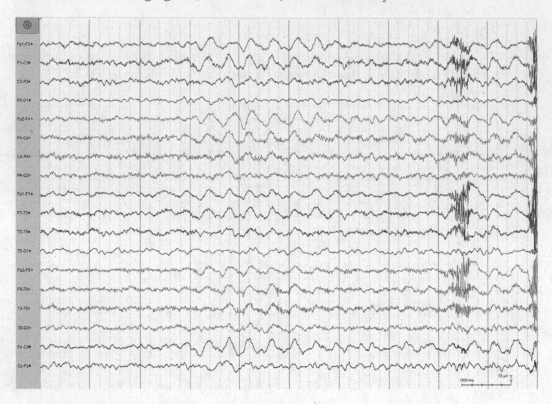

A. Indicative of bifrontal gray matter dysfunction

B. More common in patients with chronic versus acute conditions

C. More commonly seen in patients with metabolic encephalopathy versus structural lesions

D. Identified by out-of-phase deflections in fronto-polar and infraorbital electrodes

48. The following figure shows an EEG obtained from a patient being evaluated for suspected brain death. Prior to the interpretation of the EEG, the physician looks at the recording parameters. Which of the listed parameters would disqualify the study from being interpreted as compatible with electrocerebral inactivity (ECI)?

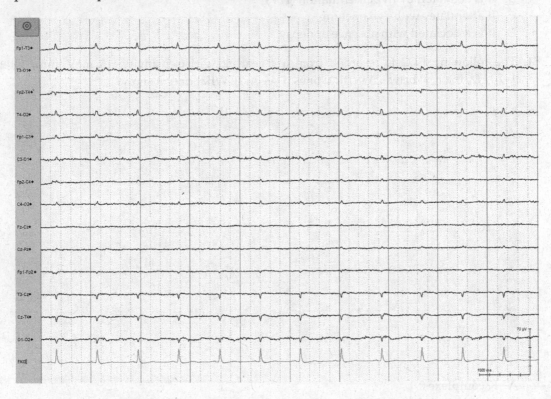

A. Study duration of 30 minutes
B. Recording sensitivity of 2 mcV/mm
C. Impedance between 100 and 10,000 Ω
D. Low frequency filter of 1.6 Hz, high frequency filter of 70 Hz

49. Which of the following statements is true of slow activity on the EEG seen in brain tumors?

A. Focal slowing is seen in cortical tumors but not white matter tumors
B. Focal slow delta-range activity is more likely to be seen with slowly growing tumors
C. Generalized delta activity is not a feature of brain tumors
D. Rhythmic delta activity can be seen with a tumor in the deep frontal white matter

50. Occipital intermittent rhythmic delta activity (OIRDA) is characterized by all of the following features EXCEPT:

  A. It is activated by deeper stages of sleep
  B. It is activated by hyperventilation (HV)
  C. It attenuates with eye opening
  D. It is associated with absence epilepsy

51. The following EEG is recorded from a 4-year-old girl (sensitivity: 15 mcV/mm; filter: 1–70 Hz; interval between vertical lines: 1 second). What does it show?

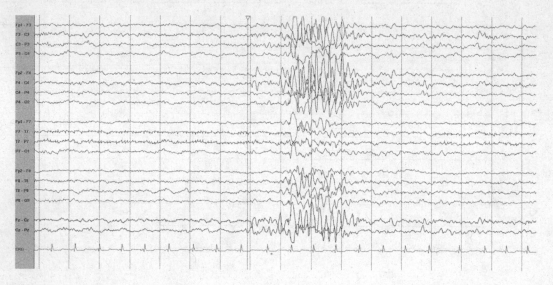

  A. K complexes
  B. Hypnagogic hypersynchrony
  C. Irregular generalized spikes
  D. Generalized paroxysmal fast activity (GPFA)

52. The following EEG segment is recorded from a 7-year-old girl during hyperventilation (HV) (sensitivity: 15 mcV/mm; filter: 1–70 Hz; interval between vertical lines: 1 second). What does it show?

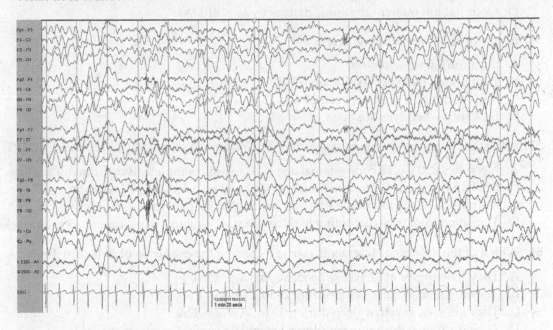

A. Generalized, slow spike-wave discharge
B. Onset of drowsiness
C. Occipital intermittent rhythmic delta activity (OIRDA)
D. Frontal intermittent rhythmic delta activity (FIRDA)

53. The following EEG segment is from a 2-year-old boy in stage 2 sleep (sensitivity: 10 mcV/mm; filter: 1–70 Hz; interval between vertical lines: 1 second). What do the prominent waveforms in the posterior head region represent?

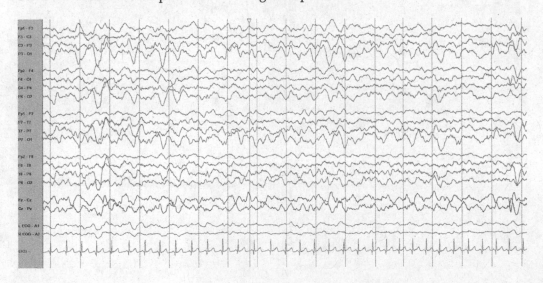

A. Cone waves
B. Positive occipital sharp transients of sleep (POSTS)
C. Shut eye waves
D. Occipital intermittent rhythmic delta activity (OIRDA)

54. Posterior slow waves of youth are:

A. Seen during wakefulness
B. Suppressed by hyperventilation (HV)
C. Most commonly seen between 16 and 25 years of age
D. Best seen when eyes are open

55. All of the following statements regarding maturation of neonatal EEG are true EXCEPT:

A. Neonates <30 weeks conceptional age (CA) exhibit complete asynchrony of activity
B. Median duration of interburst interval (IBI) at 24 weeks CA is 10 seconds
C. Amplitude of activity in the IBIs of trace discontinu pattern is <25 mcV
D. Transition from trace discontinu to trace alternant pattern occurs around 35 to 36 weeks

56. Which of the following statements is true regarding the evolution of delta brushes?

A. They first appear at 22 weeks conceptional age (CA)
B. They are seen in quiet sleep during 29 to 33 weeks CA
C. They are seen in active sleep during 33 to 38 weeks CA
D. They disappear during wakefulness beyond 38 weeks CA

57. A healthy 3-year-old boy is being evaluated for daydreaming spells. The following EEG (sensitivity: 10 mcV/mm; filter: 1–70 Hz; interval between vertical lines: 1 second) was recorded soon after a loud noise occurred in the hallway. There were no obvious behavioral changes in the child. What does the EEG show?

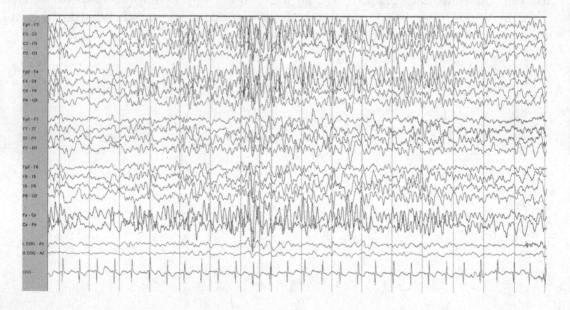

A. Fast alpha variant
B. Arousal from sleep
C. Ciganek rhythm
D. Electrographic seizure

58. An EEG from a 14-month-old child in stage 2 sleep is shown in the figure (sensitivity: 10 mcV/mm; filter: 1–70 Hz; interval between two vertical lines: 1 second). Which of the following statements is true regarding the sleep spindles?

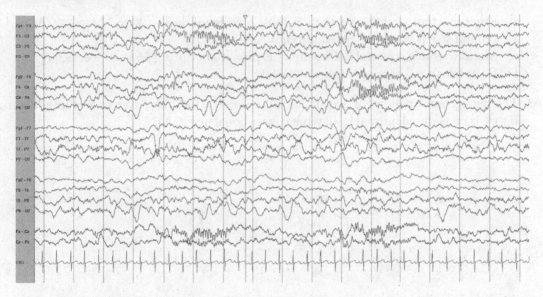

A. Spindle duration is abnormally prolonged
B. Spindle frequency is abnormally high
C. Interhemispheric asynchrony of the spindles is normal
D. Comb-shaped spindle morphology is abnormal

59. Which of the following statements is true regarding the evolution of sleep spindles?

A. They are first seen around age 3 months
B. They exhibit midline (vertex) predominance at 6 months
C. They reach a frequency of 14 Hz by 1 year
D. They have a burst duration of <1 second by 2 years

60. Which of the following statements is true regarding the maturation of the posterior dominant rhythm (PDR)?

A. PDR is first discernible with a frequency of 3 Hz at 6 months of age
B. PDR frequency decreases with age but the mean frequency remains at or above 9 Hz
C. PDR has higher voltage on the left side in both children and adults
D. PDR is better regulated in young adults than children

61. Seizures in the neonates are characterized by which of the following?

    A. Seizures have an erratic EEG evolution, shifting from one area to another

    B. Isolated seizures tend to be prolonged

    C. Status epilepticus presents with brief, recurrent seizures from a single focus

    D. Electroclinical dissociation is seen in <10% of neonatal seizures

62. Which of the following neonatal EEG features is correctly matched with the conceptional age (CA)?

    A. Rhythmic temporal theta activity is most prominent during 30 to 32 weeks CA

    B. Frontal sharp waves disappear around 36 weeks CA

    C. Monorhythmic occipital delta activity is prominent during 36 to 40 weeks CA

    D. Delta brushes disappear around 40 weeks

63. The background pattern of a neonatal EEG (filter: 0.5–70 Hz) shown in the following figure is considered normal until what conceptional age (CA)?

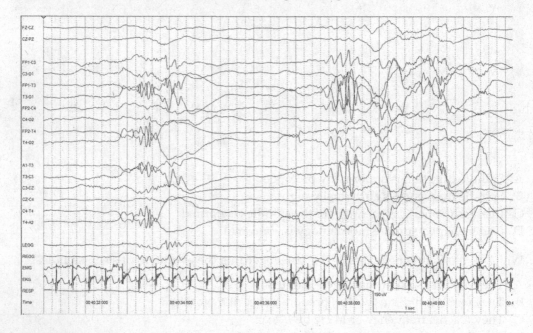

    A. 31 to 32 weeks

    B. 33 to 34 weeks

    C. 35 to 36 weeks

    D. 37 to 38 weeks

64. Which of the following statements is true regarding epilepsy syndromes seen in the neonatal period?

    A. Benign familial neonatal seizures (BFNS) are associated with LRG1 gene mutations

    B. Ohtahara syndrome (OS) is characterized by predominant tonic spasms

    C. Early myoclonic epilepsy (EME) responds favorably to vigabatrin

    D. Migrating partial seizures of infancy (MPSI) is associated with a favorable prognosis

65. A 64-year-old female is being evaluated for rapidly progressive dementia with myoclonus over the past several months. Which of the following EEG abnormalities suggests a specific clinical diagnosis in this patient?

  A. 2-Hz triphasic waves
  B. 0.5-Hz unilateral periodic lateralized epileptiform discharges (PLEDs)
  C. 1-Hz bisynchronous, generalized periodic epileptiform discharges (GPEDs)
  D. Frontal intermittent rhythmic delta activity (FIRDA)

66. All of the following periodic EEG patterns can be associated with a specific underlying neurological disorder EXCEPT:

  A. Periodic generalized sharp waves occurring at 1-Hz frequency and accompanied by occasional myoclonic jerks
  B. Periodic generalized sharp waves occurring every 10 to 15 seconds and accompanied by occasional myoclonic jerks
  C. Left parieto-central periodic lateralized epileptiform discharges occurring at 1-Hz frequency
  D. Bitemporal independent periodic lateralized sharp waves occurring at 1- to 1.5-Hz frequency

67. The following EEG is recorded from a behaviorally asleep term neonate (sensitivity: 7 mcV/mm; filter: 0.5–70 Hz; interval between vertical lines: 1 second). Which of the following patterns is it most consistent with?

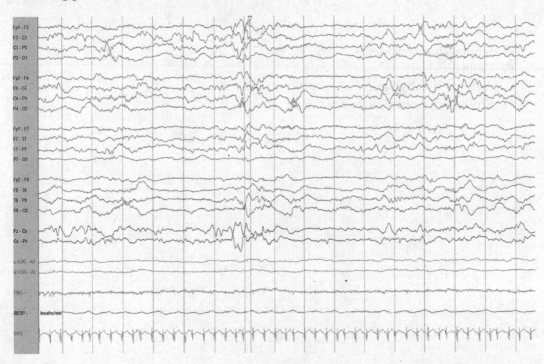

A. Burst suppression
B. Continuous slow-wave sleep
C. Trace alternant
D. Activité moyenne

68. The following neonatal EEG is consistent with which of the following patterns (sensitivity: 7 mcV/mm; filter: 0.5–70 Hz; interval between vertical lines: 1 second)?

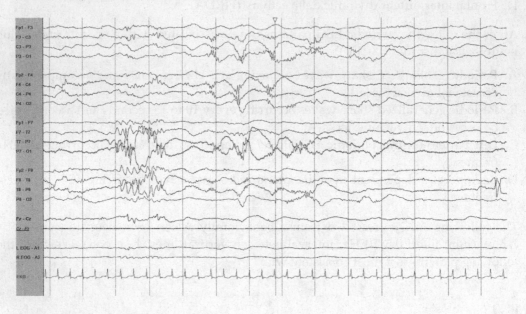

A. Frontal sharp transients
B. Delta brushes
C. Anterior dysrhythmia
D. Rhythmic occipital delta activity

69. A patient with altered mental status presented to the emergency department. Based on the following EEG (filter: 1–70 Hz), what is the most likely clinical correlate?

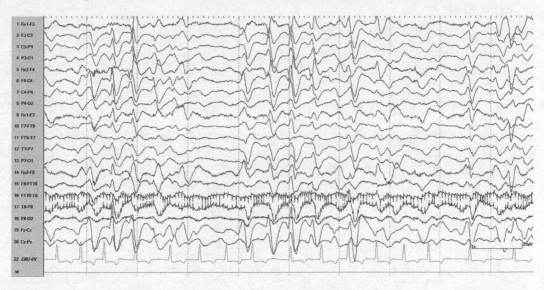

A. A 70-year old with an acute right middle cerebral artery (MCA) ischemic stroke

B. A 14-year old with herpes simplex virus (HSV) encephalitis

C. A 45-year old with focal status epilepticus due to medication noncompliance

D. A 29-year old with bipolar disorder on lithium after an attempted suicide

70. Normal variants that are often misinterpreted as epileptiform patterns include all of the following EXCEPT:

A. Subclinical rhythmic electrographic discharge of adults (SREDA)

B. 6-Hz spike-and-wave complexes

C. Temporal intermittent rhythmic delta activity (TIRDA)

D. Small sharp spikes (SSS)

71. The following EEG (filter: 1–70 Hz) is shown without the montage labels. Which of the following statements best describes the clinical significance of the rhythmic activity seen in the EEG?

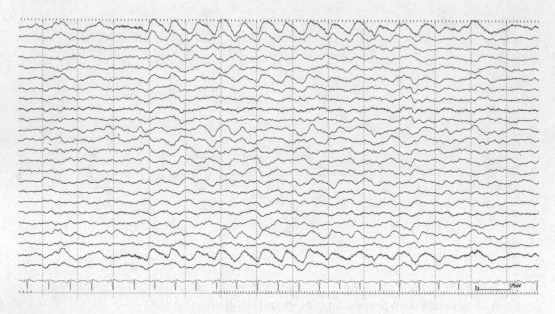

   A. It suggests nonspecific dysfunction if seen in the temporal region in a 70-year-old
   B. It is considered a normal sleep variant if seen in the frontal region in a 35-year-old
   C. It is associated with absence epilepsy if seen in the occipital region in a 6-year-old
   D. It is associated with poor prognosis if seen in a generalized distribution in a 15-year-old

72. Which of the following is NOT an identifiable pattern of progressive EEG changes described in patients with untreated generalized convulsive status epilepticus (GCSE)?

   A. Merging seizures
   B. Periodic epileptiform discharges
   C. Continuous ictal activity
   D. Continuous background suppression

73. A 20-year-old male is admitted to the ICU because of coma of unclear etiology. There was no history of trauma and no structural lesion was seen on imaging. Which of the following findings on his EEG would be associated with a relatively favorable prognosis?

   A. Bursts of high-amplitude, mixed-frequency activity alternating with low-voltage background
   B. Spindle-like discharges with cyclic variability and reactivity
   C. Diffuse, monomorphic, nonreactive alpha activity
   D. Anteriorly predominant, mixed theta and alpha activity, invariant to stimulation

74. A 35-year-old woman was admitted to the ICU after being found unresponsive. She was placed on continuous video-EEG monitoring (cVEEG) for suspected seizures. Her quantitative EEG (qEEG) consists of the following panels from top to bottom: fast Fourier transform (FFT) spectrogram of the left hemisphere; FFT spectrogram of the right hemisphere; amplitude-integrated EEG; and peak envelope. The color bar at the top indicates the power (black = lowest power; white = highest power). The red vertical lines represent 5-minute intervals. Three raw scalp EEG segments are also shown (P1, P2, and P3). Which of the following lists the correct chronological order of the scalp EEG patterns that best correlate with the activity indicated by the three blue vertical lines on the spectrogram?

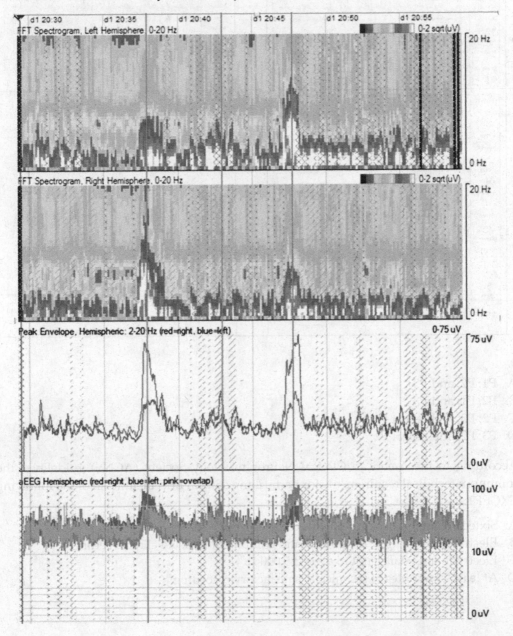

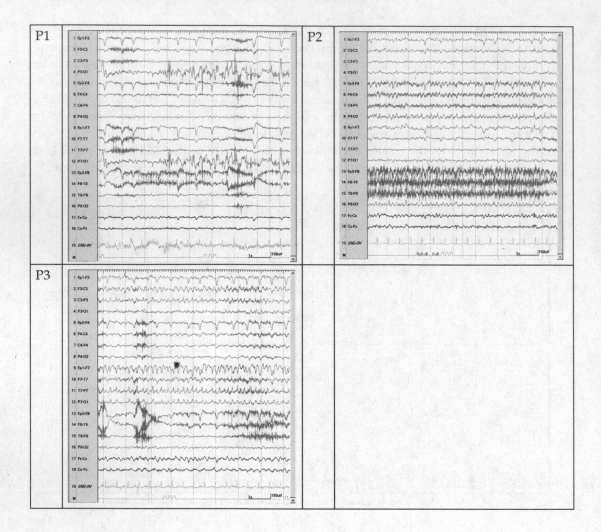

A. P1; P2; and P3
B. P2; P1; and P3
C. P2; P3; and repeat P3
D. P3; P2; and repeat P2

75. According to the American Clinical Neurophysiology Society (ACNS) guidelines, the minimum technical requirements for performing clinical EEG include all of the following EXCEPT:

A. Sixteen channels of simultaneous recording
B. Electrical shielding of the patient and equipment in usual clinical settings
C. Electrode impedance not to exceed 5,000 Ω
D. At least 20 minutes of technically satisfactory recording

76. The ictal EEG patterns are associated with the subtypes of status epilepticus (SE) include all of the following EXCEPT:

    A. Bilaterally synchronous and symmetric 4- to 6-Hz spike-wave discharges in absence SE
    B. Localized high-frequency activity in simple partial SE
    C. Periodic lateralized discharges in complex partial SE
    D. Arrhythmic spike-wave discharges separated by high-amplitude slow activity in myoclonic SE

77. A 54-year-old male, with history of brain tumor resection several years ago, is admitted to the ICU after an episode of chest pain. He undergoes continuous video-EEG monitoring (cVEEG) for altered mental status and suspected seizures. His quantitative EEG (qEEG) consists of the following panels from top to bottom: fast Fourier transform (FFT) spectrogram of the left hemisphere; FFT spectrogram of the right hemisphere; amplitude-integrated EEG; and peak envelope. The color bar at the top indicates the power (black = lowest power; white = highest power). The red vertical lines represent 2-minute intervals. For illustrative purposes, three different time periods are spliced together as indicated by the time at the top. Which of the following scalp EEG patterns best correlates with the activity indicated by the blue vertical line in the 01:28 time block?

(continues on pages 70 and 71)

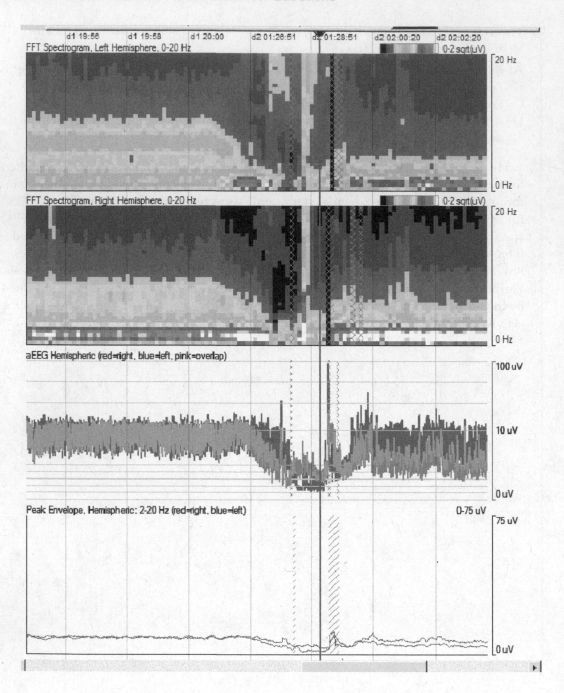

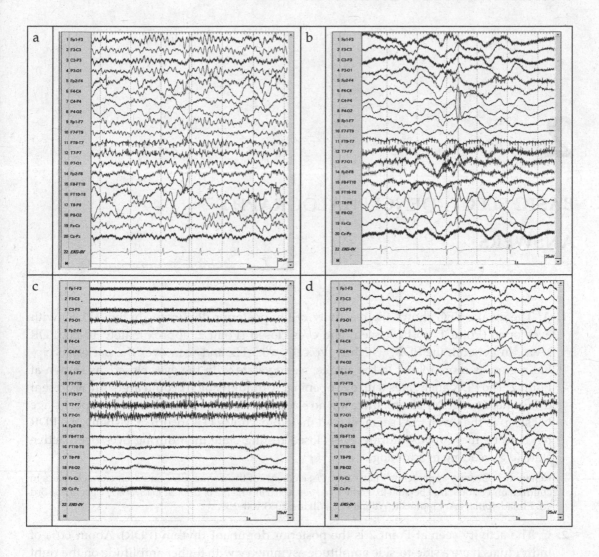

2

BASIC ELECTROENCEPHALOGRAPHY

ANSWERS

1. **A.** The awake EEG shows the reactivity of the posterior dominant rhythm (PDR) with eyes open (Point 1, no PDR seen) and eyes closed (Point 2, approximately 10-Hz PDR seen). In general, the PDR, which is typically >8.5 Hz and seen over the parieto-occipital region, is more robust in the awake, resting state with the eyes closed, as shown at Point 2. The PDR attenuates with eye opening. Although Point 1 could arguably represent drowsiness (stage N1 sleep), there are no sleep spindles or K complexes to support stage N2 sleep in the given EEG segment, and therefore, choice D is incorrect. Usually, the PDR tends to be more robust during eyes closed resting state than during eyes open active state (e.g., reading or scanning).

   Kellaway P. Orderly approach to visual analysis: elements of the normal EEG and their characteristics in children and adults. In: Ebersole JS, Pedley TA, eds. *Current Practice of Clinical Electroencephalography*. 3rd ed. Philadelphia, PA: Lippincott Williams & Wilkins; 2003:100–159.

2. **C.** The activity seen at Point 2 is the posterior dominant rhythm (PDR). About 60% of individuals have a side-to-side amplitude asymmetry with higher amplitude on the right side except in some left-handed people (although there is no consistent correlation with handedness). Up to 50% amplitude asymmetry is considered normal. The amplitude of the PDR tends to decrease with age because of thickening of the skull, which attenuates the amplitude. In most people, the PDR amplitude decreases with eye opening and with mental effort, such as doing simple arithmetic.

   Kellaway P. Orderly approach to visual analysis: elements of the normal EEG and their characteristics in children and adults. In: Ebersole JS, Pedley TA, eds. *Current Practice of Clinical Electroencephalography*. 3rd ed. Philadelphia, PA: Lippincott Williams & Wilkins; 2003:100–159.

3. **D.** T-type calcium channels are important for rhythmic firing patters in the thalamus, resulting in thalamocortical oscillations. When a membrane is depolarized, these channels mediate calcium influx. They tend to open for short, or transient, periods of time and hence the name T-type; this is in contrast to the L-type or long-lasting calcium channels. They play a role in absence epilepsy and are the target of ethosuximide.

Heinemann U, Mody I, Yaari Y. Control of neuronal excitability. In: Engel J, Jr, Pedley TA, eds. *Epilepsy: A Comprehensive Textbook.* 2nd ed. Philadelphia, PA: Lippincott Williams & Wilkins; 2008:223–231.

Stefan H, Snead OC III, Eeg-Olofsson O. Typical and atypical absence seizures, myoclonic absences, and eyelid myoclonia. In: Engel J, Jr, Pedley TA, eds. *Epilepsy: A Comprehensive Textbook.* 2nd ed. Philadelphia, PA: Lippincott Williams & Wilkins; 2008:574–584.

4. **A.** A negative field potential is seen at the scalp surface when there is a superficial EPSP (i.e., at the apical dendrites) or a deep IPSP (i.e., at the cell body or basal dendrites). A positive field potential is seen at the surface when there is a superficial IPSP or a deep EPSP. At the macroscopic level, the field potential generated by synchronous activation of a population of pyramidal neurons functions in a similar manner. The dendrites of the pyramidal cells are perpendicular to the cortical surface. Accordingly, at the cortical apex, the generators are oriented perpendicular to the scalp surface, resulting in radial dipoles. In contrast, within the walls of the sulci, the generators are oriented parallel to the scalp surface, resulting in tangential dipoles (e.g., the centro-temporal spikes of rolandic epilepsy).

Lagerlund TD, Rubin DI, Daube JR. Volume conduction. In: Daube JA, Rubin DI, eds. *Clinical Neurophysiology.* 3rd ed. New York, NY: Oxford University Press; 2009:33–54.

5. **B.** The direction of current flow across an activated neuronal membrane is dependent on whether the synapse is excitatory or inhibitory. An EPSP occurs when positive ions flow intracellularly (i.e., inward current flow), whereas an IPSP occurs when negative ions flow intracellularly (i.e., outward current flow). Because of this, the local extracellular potential produced by an EPSP is negative and the one produced by an IPSP is positive. In addition to the local synaptic transmembrane current flow, there is current flow in the opposite direction further along the dendritic tree, referred to as the passive source or sink. The combination of these current flows results in a dipole, the orientation of which depends on the type of the synapse (i.e., excitatory or inhibitory) and the location of the synapse (i.e., superficial or deep).

Lagerlund TD, Rubin DI, Daube JR. Volume conduction. In: Daube JA, Rubin DI, eds. *Clinical Neurophysiology.* 3rd ed. New York, NY: Oxford University Press; 2009:33–54.

6. **A.** The EEG segment in the figure shows slow background with no posterior dominant alpha rhythm, consistent with drowsiness or light sleep. The predominant waveforms seen in the EEG segment are positive occipital sharp transients of sleep (POSTS), which are surface positive and localized to the bioccipital region. POSTS tend to occur in trains with a frequency of 4 to 5 Hz. They should not be confused with lambda waves, which are also positive and occipital in location, but they occur when the patient is actively reading or scanning during wakefulness. POSTS are a normal variant and are not associated with epilepsy.

Kellaway P. Orderly approach to visual analysis: elements of the normal EEG and their characteristics in children and adults. In: Ebersole JS, Pedley TA, eds. *Current Practice of Clinical Electroencephalography.* 3rd ed. Philadelphia, PA: Lippincott Williams & Wilkins; 2003:100–159.

7. **B.** Spontaneous EEG activity is generated by the pyramidal neurons. A potential generated by a population of neurons is equal to the sum of individually generated neuronal potentials. The dendritic trees allow for multiple synapses, which contribute to

the overall potentials. Recording of these potentials at a distance (e.g., on the scalp surface) requires neuronal generators to be arranged in a regular manner and activated synchronously. Pyramidal neurons are arranged with their main axes parallel to one another and perpendicular to the cortical surface. They are also activated relatively synchronously by synapses initiated by a single axon or small group of axons. This leads to extracellular current flow with two components, longitudinal and transverse. The transverse components cancel each other out, whereas the longitudinal components summate, resulting in laminar current flow along the main axes of the pyramidal neurons.

Lagerlund TD, Rubin DI, Daube JR. Volume conduction. In: Daube JA, Rubin DI, eds. *Clinical Neurophysiology*. 3rd ed. New York, NY: Oxford University Press; 2009:33–54.

8. **A.** The frequency of the PDR evolves from infancy to adolescence. A simplified way of remembering it is: 3 Hz by age 3 months, 6 Hz by age 12 months, 8 Hz by 3 years, 9 Hz by age 9 years, and 10 Hz by age 15 years. The PDR frequency can decline with age, as early as 58 years in some studies, but the overall frequency still remains >8 Hz and typically >9 Hz.

Kellaway P. Orderly approach to visual analysis: elements of the normal EEG and their characteristics in children and adults. In: Ebersole JS, Pedley TA, eds. *Current Practice of Clinical Electroencephalography*. 3rd ed. Philadelphia, PA: Lippincott Williams & Wilkins; 2003:100–159.

9. **B.** The EEG segment shows a PDR with a frequency of approximately 9 Hz, which is normal in a 4-year-old child. Once mature, a normal PDR is typically between 8.5 and 12 Hz and follows a normal distribution, centering around 10 Hz. However, in <2% of individuals, no overt PDR is appreciable, and in <7% of individuals, a low-voltage PDR is seen. In such cases, increasing the interelectrode distances can increase the sensitivity of detecting a PDR. Normal PDR attenuates with eye opening. Change in cerebral blood flow can vary the PDR by up to 2 Hz. Some studies have shown that the PDR may slow down by 1 Hz every decade after the age of 50 years. The PDR is typically most prominent over the posterior head regions. In about one-third of healthy adults, the PDR can have a broader field, and can be seen over the parietal and posterior temporal head regions, but it does not extend to the frontal region. Posterior slow waves of youth, lambda waves, or spike-wave discharges are not seen in this EEG.

Kellaway P. Orderly approach to visual analysis: elements of the normal EEG and their characteristics in children and adults. In: Ebersole JS, Pedley TA, eds. *Current Practice of Clinical Electroencephalography*. 3rd ed. Philadelphia, PA: Lippincott Williams & Wilkins; 2003:100–159.

10. **A.** In adults, the pattern of arousal depends on the stage of sleep preceding the arousal. From stage N1, there is typically only a reversion to the waking alpha rhythm pattern. In children, arousal from sleep can be characterized by prolonged, diffuse, high-voltage 4- to 6-Hz activity with intermixed slower frequencies, called hypnopompic hypersynchrony. In addition, prolonged rhythmic sharp or spiky activity over the midline frontal region can be seen in children aged 2 to 4 years, called frontal arousal rhythm (FAR). Although FAR is rare (occurring in 0.22% of children) and considered to be a normal variant, it is reported to be associated with epileptic seizures in 70% of cases, including the occurrence of eyelid flutter and chewing. By 6 to 12 years, arousal is characterized by short duration,

high-voltage theta activity. A mature pattern of arousal with rapid transition from sleep to waking rhythm is seen in adolescents.

Kellaway P. Orderly approach to visual analysis: elements of the normal EEG and their characteristics in children and adults. In: Ebersole JS, Pedley TA, eds. *Current Practice of Clinical Electroencephalography*. 3rd ed. Philadelphia, PA: Lippincott Williams & Wilkins; 2003:100–159.

11. **B.** In a bipolar montage channel G1 to G2, the resultant voltage equals the difference between G1 and G2. Thus, if G1 is positive and G2 is negative, the net voltage will be positive. Furthermore, there is a universally accepted polarity convention in EEG. According to the convention, if the G1 input is more positive than the G2 input, the pen deflection will be downward and vice versa. It follows that either a positive event at G1 or a negative event at G2 leads to a downward deflection. Similarly, a negative event at G1 or a positive event at G2 leads to an upward deflection. A flat line (i.e., an equipotential) occurs if both G1 and G2 have equal inputs.

Connolly MB, Sharbrough FW, Wong PKH. Electrical fields and recording techniques. In: Ebersole JS, Pedley TA, eds. *Current Practice of Clinical Electroencephalography*. 3rd ed. Philadelphia, PA: Lippincott Williams & Wilkins; 2003:72–99.

12. **B.** The 10–20 International System of EEG electrode placement was developed to ensure standardized reproducibility so that a subject's EEG recordings could be compared over time and subjects could be compared to each other. This system is based on the relationship between the location of an electrode and the underlying area of cerebral cortex. The "10" and "20" refer to the fact that the actual distances between the adjacent electrodes are either 10% or 20% of the total front-to-back or right-to-left distances of the skull. Each site has a letter to identify the lobe and a number to identify the hemisphere location. The letters F, T, C, P, and O stand for frontal, temporal, central, parietal, and occipital lobes, respectively. Note that there is no central lobe but the "C" letter is used for identification purposes only. A "z" (zero) refers to an electrode placed on the midline between the two hemispheres. Even numbers (2, 4, 6, and 8) refer to electrode positions over the right hemisphere, whereas odd numbers (1, 3, 5, and 7) refer to those over the left hemisphere. Two anatomical landmarks are used for the essential positioning of the EEG electrodes: nasion is the point between the forehead and the nose; inion is the lowest point of the skull from the back of the head and is normally indicated by a prominent bump. The figure to show the electrode positions is drawn as if standing at the subject's head of the bed looking down onto the patient (e.g., opposite to typical axial neuroimaging).

Connolly MB, Sharbrough FW, Wong PKH. Electrical fields and recording techniques. In: Ebersole JS, Pedley TA, eds. *Current Practice of Clinical Electroencephalography*. 3rd ed. Philadelphia, PA: Lippincott Williams & Wilkins; 2003:72–99.

13. **A.** Low voltage, intermittent temporal theta is felt to be an age-related pattern in the elderly, and has been estimated to occur with an incidence of approximately 35%. It is usually in the range of 4 to 5 Hz in the temporal region, more prevalent over the left hemisphere. It is felt to represent a subharmonic of the 8- to 10-Hz background rhythm, which is often seen in the elderly. However, this rhythm is distinct from the alpha rhythm in that it persists with eye opening (although attenuated) and even into drowsiness and light sleep (when it may be augmented). Hyperventilation also augments its voltage

and persistence. Temporal theta in the elderly usually occurs as a brief fragment lasting only one to three waves, rarely more than seven. The clinical significance of this pattern remains controversial. Some regard these waveforms as normal variants, but others have suggested that they signify underlying subclinical vascular insufficiency.

Markand ON, Brenner RP. Organic brain syndromes and dementias. In: Ebersole JS, Pedley TA, eds. *Current Practice of Clinical Electroencephalography*. 3rd ed. Philadelphia, PA: Lippincott Williams & Wilkins; 2003:378–404.

14. **B.** Lambdoid waves, also known as positive occipital sharp transients of sleep (POSTS), are surface-positive triangular waves that occur in the bilateral occipital region during light and deeper stages sleep, but not in rapid eye movement (REM) sleep. They are similar if not identical to the lambda waves in morphology and distribution, and therefore, referred to as lambdoid waves. Unlike lambda waves, they are not seen during wakefulness. They are relatively common, being seen in 50% to 80% of healthy adults. They are usually symmetric and occur in runs at a frequency of 4 to 5 Hz. They are most commonly seen in individuals 15 to 35 years old, but they can be seen in children as young as 4 years. It is believed that the POSTS might represent a "playback" of information to the visual cortex to reexamine the visual material collected during the day. They are absent in blind or severely amblyopic individuals.

Kellaway P. Orderly approach to visual analysis: elements of the normal EEG and their characteristics in children and adults. In: Ebersole JS, Pedley TA, eds. *Current Practice of Clinical Electroencephalography*. 3rd ed. Philadelphia, PA: Lippincott Williams & Wilkins; 2003:100–159.

15. **A.** Photic stimulation can be traced back to ancient Greece, where the potter's wheel was used to screen for seizures. The use of IPS for EEG was reported around 1934. The responses that can be seen during IPS include photic driving, photoparoxysmal (photoconvulsive) response, photomyogenic (photomyoclonic) response, and photoelectric response. Photic driving response refers to activity in the posterior head regions time locked to the photic stimulus and occurs at the same, subharmonic, or supraharmonic frequency of the stimulus frequency. Photoparoxysmal response refers to the generalized, bisynchronous, spike-and-wave or polyspike-and-wave discharges that occur during IPS and typically outlast the stimulus by a few seconds. They may be accompanied by impairment of consciousness or brisk jerks involving predominantly the upper extremities and head. Photomyoclonic response refers to the appearance of brief repetitive muscle spikes over the anterior head regions. They often increase in amplitude as stimulation continues and stop promptly when the stimulus is withdrawn. It can be associated with eyelid flutter or discrete muscle twitches involving the face and head. High impedance electrodes can cause photoelectric (photovoltaic) artifact during IPS, where each flash causes a photochemical reaction in the electrode. This is seen as brief spike-like transients in the high impedance electrodes simultaneously with the flash and it disappears when the involved electrode is covered. In contrast, a photosensitive response is not a specifically defined response during IPS.

Dworetzky B, Herman S, Tatum WO. Artifacts of recording. In: Schomer DL, Lopes da Silva FH, eds. *Niedermeyer's Electroencephalography: Basic Principles, Clinical Applications, and Related Fields*. 6th ed. Philadelphia, PA: Lippincott Williams & Wilkins; 2011:239–266.

Fisch BJ, So EL. Activation methods. In: Ebersole JS, Pedley TA, eds. *Current Practice of Clinical Electroencephalography*. 3rd ed. Philadelphia, PA: Lippincott Williams & Wilkins; 2003:246–270.

Klem GH. Artifacts. In: Ebersole JS, Pedley TA, eds. *Current Practice of Clinical Electroencephalography*. 3rd ed. Philadelphia, PA: Lippincott Williams & Wilkins; 2003:271–287.

16. **B.** The photic driving response is usually one-to-one with the flash frequency, but can also be a subharmonic or supraharmonic of the flash frequency. The photic driving tends to occur in response to flash frequencies in the 5 to 30 Hz range, with the driving response typically in the theta range in younger patients. This is likely due to the fact that the most robust response is typically seen when the flash frequency is close to the patient's posterior dominant rhythm (PDR). A prominent photic driving response can be seen in individuals with large lambda waves or positive occipital sharp transients of sleep (POSTS). Slower flash frequencies of <5 Hz result in flash evoked potentials rather than photic driving. The onset of the driving may be delayed by 70 to 150 milliseconds compared with the flash stimulus. The photic driving may briefly outlast the stimulus, especially when the posterior background rhythm is entrained.

Fisch BJ, So EL. Activation methods. In: Ebersole JS, Pedley TA, eds. *Current Practice of Clinical Electroencephalography*. 3rd ed. Philadelphia, PA: Lippincott Williams & Wilkins; 2003:246–270.

17. **C.** The EEG shows diffuse slowing, which is consistent with a normal HV response. HV causes the subject to exhale excessive amounts of CO_2, resulting in drop in $PaCO_2$ and hypocapnia. The hypocapnia can cause mild cerebral vasoconstriction and mild cerebral hypoxia. HV may bring out focal or generalized slowing in patients with structural disease and diffuse encephalopathic disorders. HV-induced diffuse slowing usually disappears after stopping HV, but it may persist for up to 30 seconds in normal adults; further persistence at any age, by itself, is not necessarily abnormal. HV-induced slowing is enhanced by an upright position as opposed to a recumbent position probably because of relative cerebral anoxia. In adults, a low blood glucose level (<80 mg/dL) tends to enhance the slow waves, whereas a high level (>120 mg/dL) tends to suppress them. Therefore, inquiring about the child's last meal will be most helpful in this situation. HV can also bring out interictal epileptiform discharges (IEDs) or trigger more overt seizures. In the given EEG, there was no convincing evolution to support a seizure. In addition, the boy recalled the code words, which also fails to support the diagnosis of seizure. No spikes were noted to support IEDs. Therefore, administration of lorazepam or prescription of an antiseizure medication would not be appropriate. Although hypnogogic hypersynchrony could have a similar appearance, it is not likely as the patient was already awake and performing HV with good effort.

Fisch BJ, So EL. Activation methods. In: Ebersole JS, Pedley TA, eds. *Current Practice of Clinical Electroencephalography*. 3rd ed. Philadelphia, PA: Lippincott Williams & Wilkins; 2003:246–270.

18. **C.** At <5-Hz flash rates, the photic response consists of a diffuse, not focal, light-evoked potential; this is not an induced rhythm and is not considered true photic driving. Needle-like occipital spikes can be seen in most congenitally blind children at baseline, not necessarily in response to photic stimulation. These spikes are not indicative of predisposition to epileptic seizures, and are probably due to functional deafferentation. High-amplitude photic driving at very slow flash rates can be seen in adults with progressive degenerative neurological disorders. High-amplitude epileptiform spikes, time locked to very

slow flash rates, suggest progressive degenerative or acute structural disorders in any age group. Such disorders include mitochondrial encephalomyopathy, lactic acidosis, and stroke-like episodes (MELAS) syndrome and late-infantile neuronal ceroid lipofuscinosis (NCL). NCL is characterized by intellectual decline, myoclonus, intractable seizures, and optic atrophy. Alcohol withdrawal is not associated with photic driving response at low flash rates.

Fisch BJ, So EL. Activation methods. In: Ebersole JS, Pedley TA, eds. *Current Practice of Clinical Electroencephalography*. 3rd ed. Philadelphia, PA: Lippincott Williams & Wilkins; 2003:246–270.

Nordli DR, Jr, Riviello JJ, Jr, Niedermeyer E. Seizures and epilepsy in infants to adolescents. In: Schomer DL, Lopes da Silva FH, eds. *Niedermeyer's Electroencephalography: Basic Principles, Clinical Applications, and Related Fields*. 6th ed. Philadelphia, PA: Lippincott Williams & Wilkins; 2011:479–540.

19. C. AED withdrawal is a valuable activation method for recording seizures. The effect of AEDs on the frequency of IEDs is unclear; however, valproate is widely accepted as suppressing generalized spike-wave discharges, with the discharges reappearing after valproate discontinuation. Abrupt discontinuation of AEDs is widely accepted as a cause for increased seizure frequency, but the mechanism by which this occurs is controversial. The two leading theories are rebound phenomenon (similar to that seen in abstinence in drug addiction) and loss of therapeutic effect (i.e., the increased seizure frequency occurs not as levels fall from their baseline, but as AED levels become subtherapeutic). Drug withdrawal may unmask a seizure focus that is different from where the habitual seizures originate. It is unclear whether the unmasked seizure focus would be a de novo seizure focus. There are well-documented complications related to AED discontinuation, whether done in the EMU setting or outside; they include status epilepticus, fractures (especially vertebral body compression fractures in those with osteoporosis), dislocated joints, and external or internal soft tissue injuries.

Fisch BJ, So EL. Activation methods. In: Ebersole JS, Pedley TA, eds. *Current Practice of Clinical Electroencephalography*. 3rd ed. Philadelphia, PA: Lippincott Williams & Wilkins; 2003:246–270.

20. D. When the initial routine EEG is normal, a repeat sleep-deprived EEG captures IEDs 30% to 70% of the time. Nearly all patients with IEDs during a daytime nap recording have their first IED within 15 to 30 minutes of sleep onset, thus supporting the role of capturing at least 30 minutes of sleep in the study. IEDs seen during REM sleep are more localizing than those seen in non-REM sleep and most closely represent the location of IEDs seen during wakefulness. Following sleep deprivation, IEDs are not exclusively seen during sleep, but may appear during wakefulness, and are felt to be independent of the occurrence of sleep during the recording. Of note, sleep deprivation is not typically needed on routine outpatient EEG studies if IEDs have been seen on previous studies or if the diagnosis of epilepsy has been clinically confirmed. Although the role of sleep deprivation in the activation of seizures (e.g., during inpatient video-EEG monitoring) is debatable, its role in increasing the seizure frequency in the setting of stressful life situations has been reported.

Fisch BJ, So EL. Activation methods. In: Ebersole JS, Pedley TA, eds. *Current Practice of Clinical Electroencephalography*. 3rd ed. Philadelphia, PA: Lippincott Williams & Wilkins; 2003:246–270.

21. A. The activity in Fp1 and Fp2 electrodes is the electroretinogram (ERG), which is a low-voltage (typically <50 mcV using a contact lens type of electrode) response to photic-induced light stimulation of the retina. The ERG consists of two peaks that occur about 12 and 35 ms following the flash. This activity can be confused with a faulty electrode (e.g., pop) or photoelectric response. The photoelectric response is actually an artifact during IPS, where each flash causes a photochemical reaction in the exposed metallic surface of the silver electrode, resulting in brief spike-like transients in the electrode simultaneously with the flash. Photoelectric artifact disappears when the involved electrode is shielded from the light. Another way to determine the source of the artifact is to increase the flash frequency to about 30 Hz, which tends to diminish the ERGs because the retinal response is physiologically unable to respond to faster frequencies. The activity does not have the spike-wave morphology. Muscle twitching in the anterior head regions during IPS can represent photomyoclonic response, which often increases in amplitude as stimulation continues and stops when the stimulus is withdrawn. This is felt to be caused by heightened brainstem reflexes. However, the observed activity does not have the features of muscle artifact.

Klem GH. Artifacts. In: Ebersole JS, Pedley TA, eds. *Current Practice of Clinical Electroencephalography*. 3rd ed. Philadelphia, PA: Lippincott Williams & Wilkins; 2003:271–287.

22. **C.** Shut eye waves (also known as slow lambda waves of youth) are seen in the occipital region in children <10 years of age. They occur in association with eye blinks. They occur singly as surface-negative, high-amplitude (100–200 mcV), broad (200–400 ms), monophasic or diphasic waves.

Cervone RL, Blum AS. Normal variant EEG patterns. In: Blum AS, Rutkove SB, eds. *The Clinical Neurophysiology Primer*. Totowa, NJ: Humana Press; 2007:83–100.

23. **D.** This EEG shows an artifact in the AF7–F7 channel in the setting of normal stage N2 sleep. The artifact affects the electrode AF7, not F7, because the channel F7–F3 does not show the same artifact. Electrode artifacts have a variable presentation. An electrode pop presents with a rapid rise followed by a slower fall. The amplitude of the pop tends to be larger than the surrounding electrodes suggesting that the field is limited to that one electrode. There is typically recurrence within a short time if the electrode is not fixed. At times, the pop may have pseudo-evolution (as seen in this EEG at AF7), which may be confused with a seizure. The pop reflects the inability of the electrode and skin interface to function as a capacitor and store the electrical charge across the electrolyte gel applied under the electrode. When the charge is released, there is a change in impedance resulting in a sudden potential in the channels containing that electrode.

Klem GH. Artifacts. In: Ebersole JS, Pedley TA, eds. *Current Practice of Clinical Electroencephalography*. 3rd ed. Philadelphia, PA: Lippincott Williams & Wilkins; 2003:271–287.

24. **A.** The EEG shows rhythmic temporal theta bursts of drowsiness (RTTBD), also known as psychomotor variant or rhythmic midtemporal theta bursts of drowsiness (RMTD). It is found in <2% of EEG recordings. It consists of notched or arciform, sharply contoured, or flat-topped theta activity with shifting asymmetry from side to side. It is most prominent during drowsiness, but can rarely be seen during wakefulness. It is most prominent in the midtemporal region, but may spread to involve parasagittal or occipito-temporal regions. It can occur in runs, lasting from a few seconds up to a minute. The RTTBD pattern may begin and end with a gradual increase or decrease in amplitude, but does not evolve into other frequencies. This feature differentiates it from a true seizure

discharge which tends to show evolution in frequency. Although historically it was associated with psychomotor seizures, this has not been proven and the pattern is now felt to be of unclear significance.

Edwards JC, Kutluay E. Patterns of unclear significance. In: Schomer DL, Lopes da Silva FH, eds. *Niedermeyer's Electroencephalography: Basic Principles, Clinical Applications, and Related Fields*. 6th ed. Philadelphia, PA: Lippincott Williams & Wilkins; 2011:267–280.

25. **C.** The EEG is compressed to show 30 seconds on the page (note the calibration mark at the bottom). It shows slow undulating waves (<0.5 Hz) in the frontal region with super-imposed normal activity, most consistent with sweat artifact. The large baseline sways are due to the sodium chloride and lactic acid in the sweat. The use of standard low frequency filters (e.g., 0.5 or 1 Hz) minimizes this artifact. Lateral eye movements as seen in horizontal nystagmus appear in the homologous anterior channels (i.e., F7/F8 > Fp1/Fp2) with out-of-phase deflections due to the dipole effect of the eyeball (i.e., the cornea is relatively positive compared with the retina). The activity is too slow for the 60-Hz line noise (or its subharmonics) or FIRDA.

Klem GH. Artifacts. In: Ebersole JS, Pedley TA, eds. *Current Practice of Clinical Electroencephalography*. 3rd ed. Philadelphia, PA: Lippincott Williams & Wilkins; 2003:271–287.

26. **B.** The markers 1 to 4 correspond to upward, downward, left, and right eye move-ments, respectively. Eye movements are appreciated on the scalp EEG due to the dipole effect of the eyeball, with the cornea being relatively positive compared with the retina. This generator produces a direct current (DC) potential of about 50 to 100 mcV during eye movements. Vertical eye movements lead to the same polarity on the homologous anterior channels (i.e., FP1/FP2). When looking up (marker 1), Fp1/Fp2 show positive deflections due to the corneal positivity. When looking down (marker 2), the electrodes show negative deflections due to the retinal negativity. The lateral eye movements lead to opposite polarities on the homologous anterior channels (i.e., F7/F8). When looking left (marker 3), F7 shows positive deflection due to the corneal positivity, whereas F8 shows negative deflection due to the retinal negativity. When looking right (marker 4), F8 shows positive deflection due to the corneal positivity, whereas F7 shows negative deflection due to the retinal negativity. Oblique eye movements are more difficult to detect and can be misinterpreted as focal abnormalities.

Klem GH. Artifacts. In: Ebersole JS, Pedley TA, eds. *Current Practice of Clinical Electroencephalography*. 3rd ed. Philadelphia, PA: Lippincott Williams & Wilkins; 2003:271–287.

27. **B.** 14- and 6-Hz positive bursts (also known as 14- and 6-Hz positive spikes or ctenoids) are named after the frequency of bursts. They appear around age 3 to 4 years, but are more commonly seen in children and adolescents, especially those age 13 to 14 years. The 6-Hz positive bursts predominate in children <1 year and in adults >40 years, whereas the 14-Hz positive bursts predominate or combine with 6-Hz spikes in the other age groups. They are still seen during adulthood, but the incidence decreases with advanced age, with a reported incidence of 58% in normal teenagers and 12% in healthy adults. The bursts are of medium amplitude (20–60 mcV), and occur in short runs (0.5–1 sec long). They are best seen in the posterior temporal regions, unilaterally or bilaterally with shift-ing predominance. They are typically seen during drowsiness or light sleep. They are comb-shaped rather than sinusoidal in appearance. The 14- and 6-Hz positive spikes may

be distinguished from temporal spikes by their characteristic positive polarity (compared with the negative polarity of epileptiform discharges) and their typical frequency.

Edwards JC, Kutluay E. Patterns of unclear significance. In: Schomer DL, Lopes da Silva FH, eds. *Niedermeyer's Electroencephalography: Basic Principles, Clinical Applications, and Related Fields*. 6th ed. Philadelphia, PA: Lippincott Williams & Wilkins; 2011:267–280.

28. **D.** Typically, lambda waves are confined to the occipital leads, but spread to the parietal and posterior temporal areas is common. They can be seen in any age group, but are most common in children and adolescents. They are most evident when an awake subject scans a complex picture in a well-lit room, and are time locked to saccadic eye movements. They tend to disappear with eye closure, removal of the visual stimuli, or dimming the lights. They are usually bisynchronous waveforms with biphasic or triphasic morphology with the most prominent phase being surface positive.

Chang BS, Schomer DL, Niedermeyer E. Normal EEG and sleep: adults and elderly. In: Schomer DL, Lopes da Silva FH, eds. *Niedermeyer's Electroencephalography: Basic Principles, Clinical Applications, and Related Fields*. 6th ed. Philadelphia, PA: Lippincott Williams & Wilkins; 2011:183–214.

29. **A.** The EEG segment shows small sharp spikes (SSS) at the marked time instants. They are also known as benign epileptiform transients of sleep (BETS) or benign sporadic sleep spikes (BSSS). They are considered to be benign nonepileptiform variants. They are not associated with epilepsy, but they have been correlated with psychotic disorders. They are mainly seen in adults in up to 25% of normal EEG records. Their duration is usually <50 ms and the amplitude is <50 mcV. SSS typically occur in drowsiness or light sleep and tend to disappear in deeper stages of sleep. They tend to have a broad field of distribution with anterior or midtemporal predominance, and are best seen in derivations with long interelectrode distances. They are unilateral, bilaterally independent, or bilaterally synchronous in distribution. The morphology tends to be monophasic or diphasic with a steep descending limb (this is unlike epileptiform discharges, which tend to have a steep ascending limb and a gradual descending limb). Although SSS may be associated with an aftergoing slow wave, they do not disrupt the EEG background unlike the epileptiform discharges. On a transverse montage, they may exhibit a transverse oblique dipole with opposite polarities in the two hemispheres, which is not typical for epileptiform discharges.

Edwards JC, Kutluay E. Patterns of unclear significance. In: Schomer DL, Lopes da Silva FH, eds. *Niedermeyer's Electroencephalography: Basic Principles, Clinical Applications, and Related Fields*. 6th ed. Philadelphia, PA: Lippincott Williams & Wilkins; 2011:267–280.

30. **A.** SREDA is best seen in older adults (average age 61 years) in the temporo-parietal region. It usually occurs during relaxed wakefulness or drowsiness, but can also be seen during sleep. It is usually bilateral, but asymmetric. It is characterized by sudden buildup of rhythmic, monomorphic theta or delta activity that evolves. The discharge may begin as a single or series of sharp transients, initially at the delta frequency, then increasing to a well-defined 4- to 7-Hz rhythm. The discharge may end abruptly or dissipate gradually. There is no "postictal" slowing following SREDA. The average duration is 40 to 80 seconds. SREDA is not associated with clinical symptoms, is not considered a seizure discharge, and does not increase the risk of epileptic seizures.

Edwards JC, Kutluay E. Patterns of unclear significance. In: Schomer DL, Lopes da Silva FH, eds. *Niedermeyer's Electroencephalography: Basic Principles, Clinical Applications, and Related Fields*. 6th ed. Philadelphia, PA: Lippincott Williams & Wilkins; 2011:267–280.

31. **D.** The waveforms enclosed by the rectangle are most consistent with wicket spikes. Wicket spikes are seen in 1% to 3% of EEGs, and are most common in adults older than 30 years. They occur in wakefulness, light sleep, and REM sleep. They usually occur singly or in short runs with a frequency of 6 to 11 Hz (wicket rhythm). They typically occur in the temporal regions with shifting predominance. Wicket spikes are sharp, monophasic, or arciform waveforms, resembling the Greek letter "mu." They do not disrupt the background and are not associated with an aftergoing slow wave. They are considered to be a normal variant, not associated with underlying seizures.

Edwards JC, Kutluay E. Patterns of unclear significance. In: Schomer DL, Lopes da Silva FH, eds. *Niedermeyer's Electroencephalography: Basic Principles, Clinical Applications, and Related Fields*. 6th ed. Philadelphia, PA: Lippincott Williams & Wilkins; 2011:267–280.

32. **A.** Sometimes the phantom spike-wave discharges, a benign variant, are confused with epileptiform spike-wave discharges. Phantom spike waves occur in bursts lasting 1 to 2 seconds with a frequency of 5 to 7 Hz (typically 6 Hz). They are usually seen in adolescents and adults with an incidence of 1% to 2.5%. They occur during relaxed wakefulness and drowsiness, but disappear during deeper stages of sleep (unlike epileptiform discharges, which persist or become more prominent in deep sleep). The spike component tends to be of short duration (<30 ms) and low amplitude (<25 mcV) compared with the aftergoing slow wave, which is of much higher amplitude. The evanescent nature of the spikes gives rise to the term "phantom" spike wave. There are two variants of phantom spike waves: wake, high amplitude, anterior location, male gender (WHAM) and female gender, occipital location, low amplitude, drowsiness (FOLD). Current consensus is that this EEG pattern is of unclear clinical significance; however, high spike amplitude, rate <6 Hz, and persistence in deeper stages of sleep are more likely associated with seizures.

Edwards JC, Kutluay E. Patterns of unclear significance. In: Schomer DL, Lopes da Silva FH, eds. *Niedermeyer's Electroencephalography: Basic Principles, Clinical Applications, and Related Fields*. 6th ed. Philadelphia, PA: Lippincott Williams & Wilkins; 2011:267–280.

Westmoreland BF. Benign electroencephalographic variants and patterns of uncertain clinical significance. In: Ebersole JS, Pedley TA, eds. *Current Practice of Clinical Electroencephalography*. 3rd ed. Philadelphia, PA: Lippincott Williams & Wilkins; 2003:235–245.

33. **C.** Epileptiform discharges typically have a steep ascending limb and a gradual (not steep) descending limb. They occur singly or in trains. They are often followed by aftergoing slow waves that disrupt the background. They are seen in all states, and they persist in deeper stages of sleep. Epileptiform discharges should be differentiated from the benign nonepileptiform variants, such as small sharp spikes (SSS). The latter have steep ascending and descending limbs, small (<50 mcV), and brief (<50 milliseconds). SSS typically occur in drowsiness or light sleep and tend to disappear in deeper stages of sleep. SSS may be accompanied by aftergoing slow waves that do not disrupt the background.

Edwards JC, Kutluay E. Patterns of unclear significance. In: Schomer DL, Lopes da Silva FH, eds. *Niedermeyer's Electroencephalography: Basic Principles, Clinical Applications, and Related Fields*. 6th ed. Philadelphia, PA: Lippincott Williams & Wilkins; 2011:267–280.

34. **A.** The EEG shows rhythmic sharp, high amplitude, beta activity over the right fronto-central region, consistent with breach rhythm. Given the history of brain tumor resection, the breach rhythm is most likely due to an underlying skull defect. There is no evolution of the rhythmic activity to suggest a seizure discharge. The figure also shows posterior dominant rhythm in the alpha range that appears with eye closure. Wicket rhythm consists of arciform waves occurring in the temporal region during drowsiness; this is unlikely because the rhythmic activity is in the fronto-central region and the patient is awake. SREDA is best seen in the temporo-parietal region; it is characterized by sudden buildup of rhythmic, monomorphic theta or delta activity that evolves and wanes, unlike the activity shown, which is in the beta frequency range.

Westmoreland BF. Benign electroencephalographic variants and patterns of uncertain clinical significance. In: Ebersole JS, Pedley TA, eds. *Current Practice of Clinical Electroencephalography*. 3rd ed. Philadelphia, PA: Lippincott Williams & Wilkins; 2003:235–245.

35. **A.** Unlike wicket spikes that occur in wakefulness, light sleep, and REM sleep, the epileptiform discharges persist or increase in deeper stages of sleep. Both epileptiform discharges and wicket spikes can occur singly or in short runs so this feature is not very useful in differentiating between the two. However, unlike wicket spikes, the epileptiform discharges usually have more complex morphology, are often associated with aftergoing slow waves, and tend to disrupt the underlying background.

Edwards JC, Kutluay E. Patterns of unclear significance. In: Schomer DL, Lopes da Silva FH, eds. *Niedermeyer's Electroencephalography: Basic Principles, Clinical Applications, and Related Fields*. 6th ed. Philadelphia, PA: Lippincott Williams & Wilkins; 2011:267–280.

36. **A.** A 12-Hz rhythmic discharge with notched appearance in the bifrontal region is consistent with frontal arousal rhythm (FAR). FAR is a nonspecific pattern, more commonly seen in children. It consists of 7- to 20-Hz rhythmic activity that could have a notched appearance. It occurs in runs, and can last as long as 20 seconds. It is typically seen upon arousal, but disappears during full wakefulness. A 12-Hz rhythmic discharge in the occipital region most likely represents a fast alpha variant pattern, and is seen during relaxed wakefulness, not upon arousal. It tends to occur concurrently with the normal posterior alpha rhythm. Similarly, a 6-Hz rhythmic discharge with notched appearance in the occipital region most likely represents a slow alpha variant pattern, and is seen during relaxed wakefulness, not upon arousal. The notched appearance suggests that it is a slow alpha variant, not a pathologically slow posterior dominant rhythm. A 6-Hz rhythmic discharge with a notched appearance in the temporal region most likely represents rhythmic temporal theta bursts of drowsiness (RTTBD). This pattern is seen during drowsiness, not upon arousal. It may have shifting asymmetry from side to side in the temporal regions.

Westmoreland BF. Benign electroencephalographic variants and patterns of uncertain clinical significance. In: Ebersole JS, Pedley TA, eds. *Current Practice of Clinical Electroencephalography*. 3rd ed. Philadelphia, PA: Lippincott Williams & Wilkins; 2003:235–245.

37. **D.** Spikes are generated by synchronous depolarization of neurons within 6 cm² (not mm²) of the cortex, whereas sharp waves result from synchronous depolarization of a small pool of neurons or neurons farther away from the recording electrode. IEDs tend to become more prominent during deeper stages of sleep, and are less likely to be seen in REM sleep. IEDs can be seen in individuals without seizures; for example, healthy siblings of

patients with benign rolandic epilepsy may show IEDs. Spike-and-wave complexes are felt to be strongly suggestive of underlying epilepsy because the slow wave represents inhibition caused by hyperpolarization of the cortical neurons after the initial synchronous depolarization.

Chang BS, Drislane FW. Epileptiform abnormalities. In: Blum AS, Rutkove SB, eds. *The Clinical Neurophysiology Primer*. Totowa, NJ: Humana Press; 2007:101–125.

38. **A.** The EEG shows photomyoclonic (i.e., photomyogenic) response, which consists of widespread muscle twitching time locked to the stimulus (the response corresponds to the 9-Hz stimulus frequency). Photomyoclonic response represents a heightened brainstem-mediated reflex. Photoparoxysmal response refers to generalized spike-wave discharges without clinical correlation; however, if there is any clinical change with it, the term photoconvulsive response would be appropriate. Both of these represent predisposition to generalized seizures. Photoelectric (photochemical) response occurs if there are changes in some channels (usually the anterior channels) that resolve with shielding the electrode from the photic light. Photoelectric response is caused by a reaction of the light with the sliver electrodes.

Dworetzky BA, Bromfield EB, Winslow NE. Activation of the EEG. In: Blum AS, Rutkove SB, eds. *The Clinical Neurophysiology Primer*. Totowa, NJ: Humana Press; 2007:73–82.

39. **B.** SSS may be accompanied by aftergoing slow waves that they do not disrupt the EEG background. However, they are considered benign variants, not associated with risk for seizures. The 6-Hz phantom spike-wave discharges consist of spikes that are rather small compared with the wave. They are divided into two types: wake, high-amplitude, anterior, male (WHAM) and female, occipital, low amplitude, drowsy (FOLD). The WHAM pattern is associated with seizures, whereas the FOLD pattern is associated with neuroautonomic disturbances. The association of WHAM with seizures is higher if the bursts are higher in amplitude, <6 Hz in frequency, and persist in deeper stages of sleep. Rudimentary spike-wave discharges (pseudo-petit mal discharges) are typically seen in drowsiness and consist of bursts of generalized, high voltage, 3- to 4-Hz waves with poorly developed spikes in the positive trough between the slow waves. This pattern is most prominent over the parietal areas, and can be seen in infants and children with hypnagogic hypersynchrony. These bursts may contain small spikes (i.e., rudimentary spike waves). They are not believed to transition into the classic spike-wave patterns associated with seizures.

Nordli DR, Jr, Riviello JJ, Jr, Niedermeyer E. Seizures and epilepsy in infants to adolescents. In: Schomer DL, Lopes da Silva FH, eds. *Niedermeyer's Electroencephalography: Basic Principles, Clinical Applications, and Related Fields*. 6th ed. Philadelphia, PA: Lippincott Williams & Wilkins; 2011:479–540.

40. **C.** The EEG shows 3 to 3.5 Hz, generalized spike-wave discharges. This is characteristic of typical absence seizures, which are predominantly associated with clinical absences. However, patients with juvenile absence epilepsy can have generalized tonic–clonic seizures (in 80%) as well as myoclonic seizures (in 15%–25%). Atonic and tonic seizures are typically seen in Lennox–Gastaut syndrome, which can be associated with atypical absence seizures with slow (<2.5 Hz) spike-wave discharges seen interictally and ictally. Myoclonic–atonic seizures (myoclonic astatic seizures) are characteristic of Doose syndrome, and are characterized by irregular, 2- to 3-Hz spike-wave and polyspike-wave

discharges interictally. Thus, among the given choices, myoclonic seizures would be more appropriate.

Panayiotopoulos CP. *A Clinical Guide to Epileptic Syndromes and Their Treatment*. Oxford, UK: Bladon Medical Publishing; 2002:114–160.

41. **C.** Generalized fast rhythmic discharge, consistent with generalized paroxysmal fast activity (GPFA), is characteristic of tonic seizures. All other patterns can be seen with atonic seizures.

Sperling MR, Clancy RR. Ictal electroencephalogram. In: Engel J, Jr, Pedley TA, eds. *Epilepsy: A Comprehensive Textbook*. 2nd ed. Philadelphia, PA: Lippincott Williams & Wilkins; 2008:825–854.

42. **C.** Generalized paroxysmal fast activity (GPFA), consisting of beta range activity, is seen with tonic seizures. Generalized slow spike-wave discharge (<3 Hz) suggests atypical absence seizure. Generalized, bifrontally predominant slow rhythmic discharge suggests atonic seizure. Generalized 4-Hz polyspike-wave discharge is seen in tonic–clonic seizures.

Sperling MR, Clancy RR. Ictal electroencephalogram. In: Engel J, Jr, Pedley TA, eds. *Epilepsy: A Comprehensive Textbook*. 2nd ed. Philadelphia, PA: Lippincott Williams & Wilkins; 2008:825–854.

43. **B.** On scalp EEG, temporal lobe seizures are typically characterized by rhythmic or semi-rhythmic sinusoidal activity in the theta frequency range at seizure onset. Delta range activity can be seen at onset, but it rapidly reaches 5 Hz or more within 30 seconds of onset. In depth electrodes located in the hippocampus, the ictal onset consists of 10- to 16-Hz rhythmic activity or 1- to 2-Hz periodic spike activity.

Sperling MR, Clancy RR. Ictal electroencephalogram. In: Engel J, Jr, Pedley TA, eds. *Epilepsy: A Comprehensive Textbook*. 2nd ed. Philadelphia, PA: Lippincott Williams & Wilkins; 2008:825–854.

44. **D.** Typical absence seizure starts with a 3.5- to 4-Hz spike-wave discharge, which slows down to 2.5 Hz toward the end. It is common to see an increase in spike amplitude soon after the onset. However, significant postictal slowing is not a feature of typical absence seizure.

Sperling MR, Clancy RR. Ictal electroencephalogram. In: Engel J, Jr, Pedley TA, eds. *Epilepsy: A Comprehensive Textbook*. 2nd ed. Philadelphia, PA: Lippincott Williams & Wilkins; 2008:825–854.

45. **C.** The figure shows a 2.5-Hz generalized spike-wave discharge. This is consistent with atypical absence seizures, which are typically seen in Lennox–Gastaut syndrome (LGS). Carbamazepine is not particularly efficacious in treating seizures associated with LGS, and, in fact, may worsen them. Lamotrigine, felbamate, and topiramate have been found to be effective in randomized clinical trials for treatment of LGS.

Fertig EJ, Mattson RH. Carbamazepine. In: Engel J, Jr, Pedley TA, eds. *Epilepsy: A Comprehensive Textbook*. 2nd ed. Philadelphia, PA: Lippincott Williams & Wilkins; 2008:1543–1555.

46. **C.** The figure shows a generalized, 3-Hz, polyspike-wave discharge lasting 4 seconds, consistent with an absence seizure. This ictal pattern is most compatible with a genetic (idiopathic) epilepsy syndrome. Blank stare and pause in activity are part of the semiology of an absence seizure. This EEG pattern can also be seen in the syndrome of eyelid myoclonia with absences (Jeavons syndrome), characterized by fast, rhythmic jerking

of eyelids, upward deviation of the eyeballs, and retropulsion of the head. Generalized seizures in patients with severe intellectual disability tend to be atypical absence seizures, which are <3 Hz in frequency, unlike the one shown in the figure.

Panayiotopoulos CP. *A Clinical Guide to Epileptic Syndromes and Their Treatment*. Oxford, UK: Bladon Medical Publishing; 2002:114–160.

47. **C.** The figure shows frontal intermittent rhythmic delta activity (FIRDA). FIRDA is thought to reflect acute or subacute, diffuse cortical or subcortical gray matter (rather than bifrontal) dysfunction. It is more common in patients with metabolic encephalopathy rather than structural abnormalities. FIRDA manifests as in-phase deflections in the frontopolar and infraorbital electrodes, whereas vertical eye blinks present as out-of-phase deflections in those sets of electrodes (not shown in the figure).

Zifkin BG, Cracco RQ. An orderly approach to the abnormal electroencephalogram. In: Ebersole JS, Pedley TA, eds. *Current Practice of Clinical Electroencephalography*. 3rd ed. Philadelphia, PA: Lippincott Williams & Wilkins; 2003:288–302.

48. **D.** According to the American Clinical Neurophysiology Society (ACNS) guideline, ECI recordings for suspected brain death should meet the following criteria: study duration of at least 30 minutes; use of a full set of conventional 10 to 20 scalp electrodes because the study may or may not be ECI; interelectrode impedances between 100 Ω and 10 kΩ; interelectrode distances of at least 10 cm; recording sensitivity of at least 2 mcV/mm for at least 30 minutes of the recording with inclusion of appropriate calibrations (i.e., use a 2- or 5-mcV calibration signal instead of a 50-mcV signal); low frequency filter no higher than 1 Hz; and high frequency filter no lower than 30 Hz. The integrity of the entire recording system should be tested (i.e., touching each electrode to create an artifact potential on the recording). Additional signals (e.g., EKG) can be monitored. If muscle artifact is significant, the use of a short-acting neuromuscular blocker may be necessary. Reactivity to intense stimulation (e.g., auditory, visual, and tactile) should be documented. Recording should be performed by a qualified technologist (not necessarily R.EEG.T. certified) working under the supervision of a qualified electroencephalographer. If there is any doubt, a repeat EEG should be obtained.

Anonymous. Guideline 3: Minimum technical standards for EEG recording in suspected cerebral death. *J Clin Neurophysiol* 2006; 23:97–104.

49. **D.** Focal slowing can be seen in association with tumors both in the white matter and cortex. Rapidly growing tumors are typically associated with very slow delta-range activity, whereas more slowly growing tumors are associated with arrhythmic theta-range activity with intermixed epileptiform abnormalities. Generalized slowing can be seen with tumors in the midbrain tegmentum or large tumors in the thalamus. Rhythmic delta activity suggests involvement of the thalamus or deep frontal white matter.

Hartman AL, Lesser RP. Brain tumors and other space-occupying lesions. In: Schomer DL, Lopes da Silva FH, eds. *Niedermeyer's Electroencephalography: Basic Principles, Clinical Applications, and Related Fields*. 6th ed. Philadelphia, PA: Lippincott Williams & Wilkins; 2011:321–330.

50. **A.** OIRDA is seen in children and adolescents <15 years of age. It consists of rhythmic, high voltage, delta activity in the occipital region. OIRDA is activated by HV, eye closure, and drowsiness. It attenuates with eye opening and disappears in stage 2 and deeper

stages of sleep. It can be seen in normal individuals as well as in children with absence epilepsy.

Bazil CW, Herman ST, Pedley TA. Focal electroencephalographic abnormalities. In: Ebersole JS, Pedley TA, eds. *Current Practice of Clinical Electroencephalography*. 3rd ed. Philadelphia, PA: Lippincott Williams & Wilkins; 2003:303–347.

51. **B.** The EEG shows hypnagogic hypersynchrony. This can be seen in infants, but is most common between the ages of 3 and 5 years. It is rare after age 11 years, with only 10% of the children exhibiting that pattern. The frequency is 3 to 4 Hz initially, increasing to 5 to 6 Hz later. Its amplitude can vary up to 200 mcV. At times, dramatic generalized bisynchronous bursts of rhythmic, 2 to 5 Hz, high-voltage waveforms (>350 mcV), can be seen. There may be superimposition of some background activity upon such bursts, with the appearance of generalized spike waves, leading to misinterpretation. These normal bursts disappear in moderate sleep, unlike spike-and-wave complexes, which persist or become more frequent in sleep. K complexes are characteristic of stage N2 sleep and consist of broad biphasic waveforms in the fronto-central region with vertex predominance; they are commonly seen in association with sleep spindles. GPFA consists of beta activity in a generalized distribution, and is associated with tonic seizures in patients with Lennox–Gastaut syndrome.

Kellaway P. Orderly approach to visual analysis: elements of the normal EEG and their characteristics in children and adults. In: Ebersole JS, Pedley TA, eds. *Current Practice of Clinical Electroencephalography*. 3rd ed. Philadelphia, PA: Lippincott Williams & Wilkins; 2003:100–159.

52. **C.** The EEG shows OIRDA, which is a normal response to HV in children. With HV, there is an accentuation of the posterior dominant rhythm, along with buildup of bisynchronous delta and theta activity. The buildup of slow activity tends to be predominant in the frontal region in adults (i.e., FIRDA) and in the occipital region in children (i.e., OIRDA, as seen in the figure). Although FIRDA and OIRDA indicate diffuse cerebral dysfunction when seen spontaneously, their isolated occurrence during HV is considered normal. Sometimes HV results in sharply contoured waveforms, particularly when the background has abundant beta and theta activity, leading to misinterpretation as generalized epileptiform abnormalities. The incidence of HV response is higher in children than in adults, particularly in children 8 to 12 years of age. The amount of slow-wave activity depends on the degree of hypocapnea and the blood sugar level (especially <80 mg/dL). In the given EEG, no clear spike-wave discharges are seen. The slow background may suggest onset of drowsiness, but the degree and distribution of slowing is uncharacteristic of drowsiness. Although the slowing is diffuse, the majority of slowing is posterior, consistent with OIRDA rather than FIRDA.

Fisch BJ, So EL. Activation methods. In: Ebersole JS, Pedley TA, eds. *Current Practice of Clinical Electroencephalography*. 3rd ed. Philadelphia, PA: Lippincott Williams & Wilkins; 2003:246–270.

53. **A.** The waveforms in the posterior head region are consistent with cone waves (also known as occipital sharply contoured waves or O waves), which are high-amplitude, diphasic waves that appear in sleep and increase as sleep deepens. They are seen in children up to 5 years of age. POSTS are surface-positive, triangular waves that appear in the occipital region during light and deeper stages of sleep, but not in REM sleep. They are usually symmetric and can occur in runs at a frequency of 4 to 5 Hz. POSTS are most

commonly seen in adults aged 15 to 35 years as a normal variant, but can be seen in children as young as 4 years. Shut eye waves are seen in the occipital region in the awake state, following eye blinks. They are seen in children <10 years of age. They occur singly as surface-negative, high-amplitude, monophasic or diphasic waves. OIRDA is seen in children and adolescents <15 years of age. It consists of rhythmic, high-amplitude delta activity in the occipital region. OIRDA is activated by hyperventilation, eye closure, and drowsiness; it attenuates with eye opening and disappears with stage 2 and deeper stages of sleep.

Bazil CW, Herman ST, Pedley TA. Focal electroencephalographic abnormalities. In: Ebersole JS, Pedley TA, eds. *Current Practice of Clinical Electroencephalography*. 3rd ed. Philadelphia, PA: Lippincott Williams & Wilkins; 2003:303–347.

Cervone RL, Blum AS. Normal variant EEG patterns. In: Blum AS, Rutkove SB, eds. *The Clinical Neurophysiology Primer*. Totowa, NJ: Humana Press; 2007:83–100.

54. **A.** Posterior slow waves of youth (or youth waves) are best seen with eyes closed, during relaxed wakefulness. They disappear with eye opening. They may be accentuated by HV. They appear around 3 to 4 years, are well developed between 8 and 14 years, and are rare after 21 years. They occur as sporadic single waves or as transient bursts interspersed by few seconds of normal background activity. Frequency of the waveform is 2.5 to 4.5 Hz. They are usually synchronous, but can have shifting asymmetry.

Kellaway P. Orderly approach to visual analysis: elements of the normal EEG and their characteristics in children and adults. In: Ebersole JS, Pedley TA, eds. *Current Practice of Clinical Electroencephalography*. 3rd ed. Philadelphia, PA: Lippincott Williams & Wilkins; 2003:100–159.

55. **A.** Paradoxically, neonates <30 weeks exhibit hypersynchrony of activity. However, by 31 to 32 weeks, only 70% of bursts are synchronous in quiet sleep; by 33 to 34 weeks, 80% of bursts are synchronous; after 37 weeks, 100% of bursts are synchronous. Initially, the EEG is discontinuous, with bursts of activity separated by flat IBIs. The median IBI is about 10 seconds at 24 weeks CA. Over time, with central nervous system (CNS) maturity and increased influence of deep gray structures, the EEG becomes more continuous, and the IBIs gradually decrease to 2 to 4 seconds. The discontinuous EEG pattern in quiet sleep during 30 to 34 weeks is called trace discontinue, in which the IBIs have a length of 5 to 8 seconds and an amplitude of <25 mcV. Around 35 to 36 weeks CA, trace discontinue pattern transitions into trace alternant pattern during quiet sleep, and this pattern persists until 40 weeks CA. Trace alternant pattern consists of IBIs having an amplitude >25 mcV, with the length of IBIs gradually shortening from 5 to 6 seconds to 2 to 4 seconds by 40 weeks CA.

Clancy RR, Bergqvist AGC, Dlugos DJ. Neonatal electroencephalography. In: Ebersole JS, Pedley TA, eds. *Current Practice of Clinical Electroencephalography*. 3rd ed. Philadelphia, PA: Lippincott Williams & Wilkins; 2003:160–234.

56. **D.** Delta brushes consist of an underlying 0.3- to 1.5-Hz delta waves of 50- to 250-mcV amplitude with superimposed 8- to 22-Hz (most commonly 18–22 Hz) faster frequencies. Delta brushes first appear at 26 weeks CA in the central head regions. They are prominent over the temporo-occipital regions in active sleep during 29 to 33 weeks. During 33 to 38 weeks, delta brushes are present only in quiet sleep in the temporo-occipital regions. Their disappearance during wakefulness around 36 to 37 weeks CA constitutes

a developmental milestone. By full term, they are rare and seen only in quiet sleep. They disappear completely by 48 weeks CA.

Mizrahi EM, Moshe SL, Jr, Hrachovy RA. Normal EEG and sleep: preterm and term neonates. In: Schomer DL, Lopes da Silva FH, eds. *Niedermeyer's Electroencephalography: Basic Principles, Clinical Applications, and Related Fields.* 6th ed. Philadelphia, PA: Lippincott Williams & Wilkins; 2011:153–162.

57. **B.** The EEG shows an initial diphasic vertex wave, which is followed by generalized 5- to 8-Hz rhythmic activity with a fronto-central maximum lasting a few seconds. This pattern is consistent with frontal arousal rhythm (FAR), which can be seen as an arousal pattern in children. Arousal in children can also be characterized by prolonged, diffuse, high-voltage 4- to 6-Hz activity with intermixed slower frequencies. Fast alpha variant, which consists of 16- to 20-Hz activity intermixed with the normal alpha rhythm in the posterior head region, is unlikely given the generalized distribution of the above activity. Ciganek rhythm (midline theta) is a normal variant, and consists of 5- to 7-Hz notched, arciform, or sinusoidal activity in the midline (Cz maximum) seen during wakefulness and drowsiness; this is unlikely as the activity is generalized. Electrographic seizure is unlikely as there is no clear evolution of the activity.

Kellaway P. Orderly approach to visual analysis: elements of the normal EEG and their characteristics in children and adults. In: Ebersole JS, Pedley TA, eds. *Current Practice of Clinical Electroencephalography.* 3rd ed. Philadelphia, PA: Lippincott Williams & Wilkins; 2003:100–159.

Westmoreland BF. Benign electroencephalographic variants and patterns of uncertain clinical significance. In: Ebersole JS, Pedley TA, eds. *Current Practice of Clinical Electroencephalography.* 3rd ed. Philadelphia, PA: Lippincott Williams & Wilkins; 2003:235–245.

58. **C.** Spindles are well developed by 3 to 4 months of age. They are most abundant over central and parietal regions, but may extend frontally. Mean spindle duration is 2.5 seconds at 3 months, but they can be prolonged, up to 4 seconds, during infancy (in the EEG, the spindle duration is approximately 3.5 seconds). Spindle frequency is 13 to 14 Hz from infancy to 6 years (as seen in the EEG) and decreases to 10 to 12 Hz thereafter. Interhemispheric asynchrony of spindles is not considered abnormal in children <2 years of age. The spindles of infants and young children may also be comb shaped, with sharp negative and rounded positive components.

Kellaway P. Orderly approach to visual analysis: elements of the normal EEG and their characteristics in children and adults. In: Ebersole JS, Pedley TA, eds. *Current Practice of Clinical Electroencephalography.* 3rd ed. Philadelphia, PA: Lippincott Williams & Wilkins; 2003:100–159.

Riviello JJ, Jr, Nordli DR, Jr, Niedermeyer E. Normal EEG and sleep: infants to adolescents. In: Schomer DL, Lopes da Silva FH, eds. *Niedermeyer's Electroencephalography: Basic Principles, Clinical Applications, and Related Fields.* 6th ed. Philadelphia, PA: Lippincott Williams & Wilkins; 2011:163–181.

59. **A.** Well-formed sleep spindles usually appear around 3 months of age. The spindles have a centro-parietal maximum during infancy and acquire a clear-cut midline (vertex) maximum around 2 to 3 years. They reach a frequency of 14 Hz by 2 to 3 years of age. Spindle bursts are 10 seconds long by 6 months, and shorten to <1 second by 6 to 12 years.

Riviello JJ, Jr, Nordli DR, Jr, Niedermeyer E. Normal EEG and sleep: infants to adolescents. In: Schomer DL, Lopes da Silva FH, eds. *Niedermeyer's Electroencephalography: Basic Principles, Clinical Applications, and Related Fields.* 6th ed. Philadelphia, PA: Lippincott Williams & Wilkins; 2011:163–181.

60. B. PDR becomes discernible with a frequency of 3 Hz at 3 months. It reaches 6 Hz by 12 months, 8 Hz by 3 years, 9 Hz by 9 years, and 10 Hz by 15 years of age. In older individuals (>58 years), the frequency of PDR decreases, but the mean frequency is maintained at or above 9 Hz. The age-related decrease in frequency is felt to be due to a decrease in cerebral perfusion. A toxic level of phenytoin and therapeutic level of carbamazepine in children can slow the PDR. In children, the PDR amplitude is typically >30 mcV, whereas in adults, it is 15 to 45 mcV with only 6% to 7% of healthy adults showing <15 mcV. PDR amplitude decreases with age, and is felt to be due to increase in skull bone density and increase in impedance of the scalp tissue. In 98% of children and 50% of adults, there is voltage asymmetry of PDR, with higher voltage on the right side. This does not correlate with handedness, but is felt to be related to greater skull thickness on the left side. Side-to-side amplitude difference of >50% is considered abnormal (as this is seen in none of healthy children and in only 1.5% of healthy adults). The regulation of PDR is good between 6 months and 3 years of age; after that, there is a continued decrease in the regulation of PDR with aging.

Kellaway P. Orderly approach to visual analysis: elements of the normal EEG and their characteristics in children and adults. In: Ebersole JS, Pedley TA, eds. *Current Practice of Clinical Electroencephalography*. 3rd ed. Philadelphia, PA: Lippincott Williams & Wilkins; 2003:100–159.

61. A. Epileptic seizures are most frequent in the neonatal period than any other time. Neonatal seizures are more often brief and recurrent with short interictal periods as opposed to a single prolonged seizure. Status epilepticus in neonates presents with brief, recurrent seizures from multiple foci. Compared with older children, the neonatal brain has immature dendritic growth, axonal-dendritic connections, synaptic stabilization, and myelination. This prevents rapid organized spread of seizure discharges, resulting in an erratic EEG evolution, shifting from one area to another. Electrical seizures without a clinical correlate (electroclinical dissociation) can be seen in 47% to 79% of neonatal seizures, which can also become more prominent after treatment with antiseizure medications such as phenobarbital and phenytoin.

Cilio MR. EEG and the newborn. *J Pediatr Neurol*. 2009;7:25–43.

62. A. Rhythmic temporal theta activity consists of 4.5- to 6-Hz activity that occurs synchronously or asynchronously in the temporal region, sometimes with a sharply-contoured morphology; they appear around 26 weeks, are most prominent during 30 to 32 weeks CA, and disappear after 33 weeks. Frontal sharp waves (encoches frontales) consist of >150 mcV, broad, biphasic, synchronous, and symmetric bifrontal sharp waves that occur during transition from active sleep to quiet sleep; they are often intermixed with an underlying 2- to 4-Hz rhythm called anterior dysrhythmia; they appear around 34 weeks CA and disappear around 44 weeks CA. Monorhythmic occipital delta activity consists of 0.5- to 1-Hz synchronous waves that occur in the occipital region in runs lasting 2 to 60 seconds; they appear around 23 to 24 weeks, are most prominent during 31 to 33 weeks, and disappear after 35 weeks. Delta brushes consist of 0.3- to 1.5-Hz delta waves with superimposed 18- to 22-Hz faster frequencies; they appear around 26 weeks CA, are prominent in active sleep during 29 to 33 weeks and in quiet sleep during 33 to 38 weeks, and disappear completely by 48 weeks CA.

Clancy RR, Bergqvist AGC, Dlugos DJ. Neonatal electroencephalography. In: Ebersole JS, Pedley TA, eds. *Current Practice of Clinical Electroencephalography*. 3rd ed. Philadelphia, PA: Lippincott Williams & Wilkins; 2003:160–234.

Mizrahi EM, Moshe SL, Jr, Hrachovy RA. Normal EEG and sleep: preterm and term neonates. In: Schomer DL, Lopes da Silva FH, eds. *Niedermeyer's Electroencephalography: Basic Principles, Clinical Applications, and Related Fields*. 6th ed. Philadelphia, PA: Lippincott Williams & Wilkins; 2011:153–162.

63. **C.** The EEG shows a discontinuous background consistent with trace discontinu pattern. Trace discontinu is the initial EEG pattern noted in premature infants, and consists of bursts of activity separated by flat interburst intervals (IBIs). The median IBI is about 10 seconds at 24 weeks CA. Over time, with central nervous system (CNS) maturity and increased influence of deep gray structures, the EEG becomes more continuous, and the IBIs gradually decrease to 2 to 4 seconds. The amplitude is typically <25 mcV. Around 35 to 36 weeks CA, trace discontinu pattern transitions into trace alternant pattern during quiet sleep, and the latter pattern persists until 40 weeks CA. Trace alternant pattern consists of IBIs with amplitude >25 mcV, with the length of IBIs gradually shortening from 5 to 6 seconds to 2 to 4 seconds by 40 weeks CA.

Clancy RR, Bergqvist AGC, Dlugos DJ. Neonatal electroencephalography. In: Ebersole JS, Pedley TA, eds. *Current Practice of Clinical Electroencephalography*. 3rd ed. Philadelphia, PA: Lippincott Williams & Wilkins; 2003:160–234.

64. **B.** BFNS is an autosomal-dominant focal epilepsy syndrome associated with mutations on KCNQ2 and KCNQ3 genes on chromosomes 20 and 8, respectively. Clinically, the seizures consist of apnea, tonic posturing, and focal or multifocal clonic twitching. EEG shows diffuse attenuation followed by repetitive bilateral sharp waves, which can shift between hemispheres from one seizure to the next. Seizures occur in clusters for a few days, and resolve after a few months. Family history is positive and neurological exam and developmental outcome are normal. OS and EME have onset in the first month of life with burst-suppression pattern on EEG. OS has predominant tonic spasms, whereas EME is associated with fragmentary myoclonus and focal seizures. Etiology is unknown, but nonketotic hyperglycinemia, pyridoxine or pyridoxal phosphate deficiency or dependency, and mitochondrial glutamate transporter deficiency are sometimes implicated. There is no effective treatment and prognosis is poor. Vigabatrin may be beneficial in OS, but not EME. MPSI is characterized by onset of epilepsy in infants <6 months of age. Seizures are nearly continuous with onset in different regions of both hemispheres; at times, seizures start from a second location before the prior seizure from the first location ends. Clinically, the seizures are characterized by focal motor activity, head or eye deviation, myoclonus, and autonomic manifestations (flushing, apnea, and drooling). Seizures do not respond to conventional antiepileptic drugs or the ketogenic diet. There may be some improvement with levetiracetam and potassium bromide. Its etiology is unknown, and the prognosis is poor, with intractable seizures, loss of cognitive and motor abilities, and decline in head circumference.

Cilio MR. EEG and the newborn. *J Pediatr Neurol*. 2009;7:25–43.

65. **C.** In an older individual with rapidly progressive dementia and myoclonus, the possibility of Creutzfeldt–Jakob disease (CJD) needs to be entertained. If so, bisynchronous GPEDs

occurring at a frequency of 0.5 to 2 Hz, can be pathognomonic of CJD. These discharges are present during wakefulness, but tend to disappear during sedation, sleep, and stimulation. GPEDs are not necessarily time locked to the clinical myoclonus. As a rule, GPEDs do not occur in variant CJD, but exceptions to this rule have been described. GPEDs may be localized to the occipital region in the Heidenhain variant of CJD. In the initial stages of the illness, the GPEDs can be seen in only one hemisphere. GPEDs have a sensitivity of 64%, specificity of 91%, positive predictive value of 95%, and negative predictive value of 49%. Triphasic waves can be seen in metabolic encephalopathies such as liver failure, renal failure, lithium toxicity, and Hashimoto's encephalitis. PLEDs can be seen in the setting of acute stroke, tumor, infection, abscess, or seizures (interictally and during the recovery phase of status epilepticus). Bitemporal, independent periodic discharges can be specific for limbic encephalitis and herpes simplex encephalitis. FIRDA is associated with metabolic encephalopathy, increased intracranial pressure, thalamic lesion, or deep frontal white matter abnormality. Thus, the latter three abnormalities are somewhat nonspecific, and the conditions associated with them do not lead to rapidly progressive dementia and myoclonus.

Wong MH, Fountain NB. Generalized periodic discharges. In: LaRoche SM, ed. *Handbook of ICU EEG Monitoring*. New York, NY: Demos Medical Publishing; 2013:149–155.

66. **C.** Focal periodic discharges (such as the left parieto-central discharges) tend to be nonspecific and can be seen in acute stroke, tumor, infection, abscess, or seizure disorders (interictally and during the recovery phase of status epilepticus). There are certain exceptions to this. Bitemporal, independent periodic discharges are specific for limbic encephalitis and herpes simplex virus (HSV) encephalitis. The interval of the periodic discharges can also be specific for neurological disorders. For example, in Creutzfeldt–Jakob disease, the discharges occur at a frequency of 1 to 2 Hz (interval of 0.5–1 seconds, considered "short interval"); in HSV encephalitis, the discharges occur at a frequency of 0.25 to 0.5 Hz (interval of 2–4 seconds); in subacute sclerosing panencephalitis, the discharges occur at a frequency of 0.06 to 0.25 Hz (interval of 4–15 seconds, considered "long interval").

LaRoche SM. The ictal-interictal continuum. In: LaRoche SM, ed. *Handbook of ICU EEG Monitoring*. New York, NY: Demos Medical Publishing; 2013:157–169.

Pollandt SW, Szaflarski JP. Encephalitis and other CNS infections. In: LaRoche SM, ed. *Handbook of ICU EEG Monitoring*. New York, NY: Demos Medical Publishing; 2013:61–68.

67. **C.** This EEG is discontinuous, and among the given options, it is most consistent with the trace alternant pattern. This pattern is characteristic of quiet sleep in neonates >35 to 36 weeks conceptional age (CA). It disappears around 44 weeks, to be replaced by a continuous background. Trace alternant pattern consists of discontinuous EEG with interburst intervals (IBIs) of >25-mcV amplitude, with the length of IBIs gradually shortening from 5 to 6 seconds to 2 to 4 seconds by 40 weeks CA. Normal sleep features such as frontal sharp transients, anterior slow dysrhythmia, and delta brushes (seen in this EEG) are seen during the bursts of trace alternant. Burst suppression is distinguished from trace alternant by the absence of normal age-related features, prolonged IBIs (approximately 30 seconds), and invariant background. Continuous slow-wave sleep pattern is characteristic of quiet sleep, and it replaces trace alternant. It appears around 36 weeks CA, but is maximally expressed around 44 weeks. It consists of continuous delta and theta activity

with amplitudes of 50 to 300 mcV. Activité moyenne is seen during wakefulness and active sleep in neonates >36 weeks CA; it consists of low amplitude (<25 mcV), predominantly theta and delta (4–7 Hz) activity.

Clancy RR, Bergqvist AGC, Dlugos DJ. Neonatal electroencephalography. In: Ebersole JS, Pedley TA, eds. *Current Practice of Clinical Electroencephalography*. 3rd ed. Philadelphia, PA: Lippincott Williams & Wilkins; 2003:160–234.

68. **B.** The EEG shows delta brushes in the bilateral temporo-occipital regions. Delta brushes consist of 0.3- to 1.5-Hz delta waves of 50- to 250-mcV amplitude with superimposed 18- to 22-Hz faster frequencies. Delta brushes first appear at 26 weeks conceptional age (CA) in the central head regions. They are prominent over the temporo-occipital regions in active sleep during 29 to 33 weeks. During 33 to 38 weeks, delta brushes are only present in quiet sleep in the temporo-occipital regions. They disappear completely by 48 weeks CA. Frontal sharp waves (encoches frontales) consist of >150 mcV, broad, biphasic, synchronous, and symmetric bifrontal sharp waves that occur during transition from active sleep to quiet sleep; they are often intermixed with an underlying 2- to 4-Hz rhythm called anterior dysrhythmia; none of these patterns is seen in this EEG. Rhythmic occipital delta activity consists of runs of 0.5- to 1-Hz synchronous activity in the occipital region; this is not seen in this EEG. Although not one of the options, this EEG shows rhythmic temporal theta/alpha activity on the left half of the tracing; it consists of 4.5- to >6-Hz activity that occurs synchronously or asynchronously in the temporal region, sometimes with a sharply contoured morphology; it appears around 26 weeks, is prominent during 30 to 32 weeks CA, and disappears after 33 weeks.

Clancy RR, Bergqvist AGC, Dlugos DJ. Neonatal electroencephalography. In: Ebersole JS, Pedley TA, eds. *Current Practice of Clinical Electroencephalography*. 3rd ed. Philadelphia, PA: Lippincott Williams & Wilkins; 2003:160–234.

Mizrahi EM, Moshe SL, Jr, Hrachovy RA. Normal EEG and sleep: preterm and term neonates. In: Schomer DL, Lopes da Silva FH, eds. *Niedermeyer's Electroencephalography: Basic Principles, Clinical Applications, and Related Fields*. 6th ed. Philadelphia, PA: Lippincott Williams & Wilkins; 2011:153–162.

69. **D.** The EEG shows a generalized periodic pattern with triphasic morphology, consistent with triphasic waves. This pattern can be seen in toxic-metabolic encephalopathies such as renal and liver failure, lithium toxicity, treatment with certain third-generation cephalosporins, and so on. Although a similar pattern can be seen in generalized status epilepticus, the bilateral nature of the waveforms makes focal status epilepticus unlikely. Stroke typically presents with slowing, voltage attenuation, or periodic lateralized (not generalized) discharges. HSV encephalitis usually presents with epileptiform and non-epileptiform changes unilaterally or bilaterally in the temporal region.

Hirsch LJ, Brenner RP. *Atlas of EEG in Critical Care*. Hoboken, NJ: Wiley-Blackwell; 2010:129–160.

70. **C.** TIRDA has been shown to correlate with temporal lobe epilepsy, and is felt to have similar implications as temporal interictal epileptiform discharges (IEDs). SSS (also known as benign epileptiform transients of sleep), SREDA, 6-Hz spike-and-wave complexes, wicket spikes, rhythmic midtemporal theta bursts of drowsiness (also known as psychomotor variant), positive occipital sharp transients of sleep (POSTS), 14- and 6-Hz positive spikes, and repetitive vertex waves in children are considered to be normal variants that are often misinterpreted as epileptiform patterns.

Moeller J, Haider HA, Hirsch LJ. Electroencephalography (EEG) in the diagnosis of seizures and epilepsy. *UpToDate*. Updated February 12, 2015. http://www.uptodate.com/contents/electroencephalography-eeg-in-the-diagnosis-of-seizures-and-epilepsy. Accessed December 30, 2015.

71. **C.** The EEG pattern shows intermittent rhythmic delta activity (IRDA). IRDA in the occipital region (i.e., OIRDA) in children can be associated with absence epilepsy. Temporal IRDA (i.e., TIRDA) is an interictal finding, and associated with increased risk for focal temporal lobe seizures. Frontal IDRA (i.e., FIRDA) and generalized IRDA (i.e., GIRDA) are nonspecific patterns, often associated with metabolic encephalopathy, and do not indicate poor prognosis. Of note, FIRDA can be a normal finding in children and during drowsiness in the elderly.

Friedman D. Encephalopathy and coma. In: LaRoche SM, ed. *Handbook of ICU EEG Monitoring.* New York, NY: Demos Medical Publishing; 2013:131–138.

72. **D.** It has been shown that the EEG changes during episodes of generalized convulsive status epilepticus (GCSE) follow five identifiable patterns, which occur in a predictable sequence: (a) discrete seizures, (b) merging seizures with waxing and waning of amplitude and frequency, (c) continuous ictal activity, (d) continuous ictal activity punctuated by low-voltage flat periods, and (e) periodic epileptiform discharges on a flat background. This sequence represents the natural history of EEG changes in untreated GCSE. The same sequence has also been seen in the EEGs of rats in which status epilepticus was induced by three different methods. Continuous background suppression is not an identifiable pattern of EEG progression during GCSE.

Treiman DM, Walton NY, Kendrick C. A progressive sequence of electroencephalographic changes during generalized convulsive status epilepticus. *Epilepsy Res.* 1990;5:49–60.

73. **B.** In patients with coma, etiology determines the prognosis. In addition, EEG reactivity has also been correlated with prognosis with reactive patterns being less ominous than nonreactive patterns. Normal sleep features such as spindles (along with vertex waves and K-complexes) seen with cyclic variability in comatose patients is referred to as spindle coma. Best outcomes occur when spindle coma is due to drugs, encephalopathy, or seizures; intermediate outcomes occur with trauma, hypoxia, and cardiopulmonary arrest; worst outcomes occur with brainstem and cerebral infarctions and tumors.

Bursts of high-amplitude, mixed-frequency activity alternating with low-voltage background (choice "A") are consistent with generalized burst suppression. Diffuse, monomorphic, nonreactive alpha activity (choice "C") is consistent with alpha coma. Anteriorly predominant, nonreactive, mixed theta and alpha frequencies (choice "D") are consistent with alpha-theta coma. Burst-suppression and nonreactive coma patterns are generally associated with unfavorable prognosis.

Kaplan PW, Bauer G. Anoxia, coma, and brain death. In: Schomer DL, Lopes da Silva FH, eds. *Niedermeyer's Electroencephalography: Basic Principles, Clinical Applications, and Related Fields.* 6th ed. Philadelphia, PA: Lippincott Williams & Wilkins; 2011:435–456.

Kaplan PW, Genoud D, Ho TW, Jallon P. Clinical correlates and prognosis in early spindle coma. *Clin Neurophysiol* 2000; 111:584–590.

74. **B.** The FFT spectrogram is a three-dimensional representation of EEG power (which is proportional to the square of the amplitude) over time with respect to the various frequencies.

Seizures are usually characterized by increasing power, evolving from lower to higher frequencies. On the FFT spectrogram, change in the color to red over both hemispheres indicates an increase in power at the corresponding frequencies. Amplitude-integrated EEG (aEEG) is a display of the minimum and maximum amplitudes of the EEG background over a preset time interval (typically, 1–2 seconds). Seizures and background suppression have specific appearances on aEEG, but other changes are nonspecific and often represent artifact. The peak envelope trend is a display of the median amplitude of the EEG background over a preset time interval (typically, 10–20 seconds). Peak envelope trend may be more specific than aEEG, but can miss seizures or other activity that are brief.

In this patient, the correct order of the scalp EEG patterns corresponding to the three blue vertical lines on the qEEG plot is P2; P1; and P3. In this case, the qEEG spectrogram shows a right hemispheric-onset seizure around 20:37 (see Panel 1 below) and a left hemispheric-onset seizure around 20:47 (see Panel 3 below). At the first vertical blue line, there is an increase in power across many frequencies (right greater than left and right preceding left), which supports a right hemispheric ictal discharge spreading to the left hemisphere. At the third vertical blue line, a similar pattern is seen, but with a left hemispheric ictal discharge spreading to the right hemisphere. Similar conclusions can be made from the aEEG trend, which shows an increase in baseline amplitude and the narrowing of the aEEG band, suggestive of a seizure discharge. Thus, the higher amplitude of the red band suggests that an asymmetric seizure discharge with right hemisphere predominance (first blue vertical line), whereas the higher amplitude of the blue band suggests an asymmetric seizure discharge with left hemisphere predominance (third blue vertical line). On the peak envelope trend, an upward deflection of the red tracing represents an increase in median amplitude over the right hemisphere that corresponds to an ictal discharge in that hemisphere (first blue vertical line). Similarly, an upward deflection of the blue tracing represents an ictal discharge in the left hemisphere (third blue vertical line). The delayed upward deflection of the blue tracing (first blue vertical line) represents contralateral spread of the seizure discharge.

Of note, there is a third area (see Panel 2 below) of increased power (around 20:43) in the middle of the other two, which is fairly lateralized to the left hemisphere. Although from the FFT, this could potentially represent an ictal discharge, the aEEG and peak envelope trends do not support this. Many artifacts (e.g., muscle or electrode) typically present with increased power on the FFT spectrogram, but the increase tends to be more abrupt, without evolution. In addition, many changes on the aEEG are nonspecific and often represent artifact. In this case, there is an electrode artifact at O1, which is likely contributing to the observed changes seen in Panel 2 below. This supports the notion that aEEG trends help to draw the focus where more detailed analysis is needed, but they cannot replace expert review of raw EEG.

Herman ST. Quantitative EEG for ischemia detection. In: LaRoche SM, ed. *Handbook of ICU EEG Monitoring*. New York, NY: Demos Medical Publishing; 2013:239–248.

LaRoche SM. Quantitative EEG for seizure detection. In: LaRoche SM, ed. *Handbook of ICU EEG Monitoring*. New York, NY: Demos Medical Publishing; 2013:229–238.

Sinha SR. Quantitative EEG basic principles. In: LaRoche SM, ed. *Handbook of ICU EEG Monitoring*. New York, NY: Demos Medical Publishing; 2013:221–227.

2. BASIC ELECTROENCEPHALOGRAPHY: Answers

Panel 1. Right hemispheric seizure.

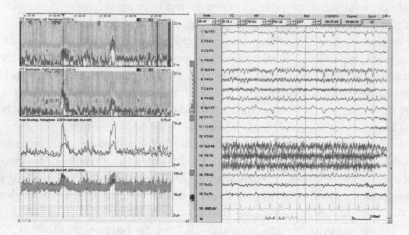

Panel 2. O1 artifact.

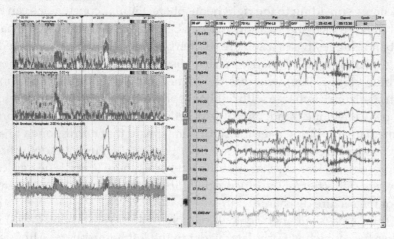

Panel 3. Left hemispheric seizure.

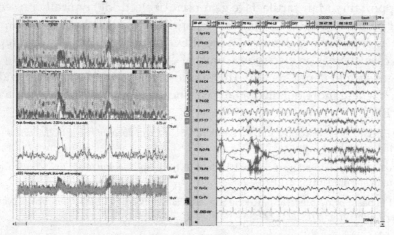

75. B. Sixteen channels of simultaneous EEG recording are considered the minimum number required to show the areas producing most normal and abnormal EEG patterns. Additional channels can be used for monitoring other physiologic parameters. In the usual clinical setting, electrical shielding of the patient and equipment is not necessary. Typical electrode impedance should not exceed 5,000 Ω (5 kΩ), but in neonates and young infants higher impedances may be allowed in order to avoid excessive manipulation or excessive abrasion of tender skin. The baseline record should contain at least 20 minutes of technically satisfactory recording. Longer recordings are often more informative. The addition of photic stimulation, hyperventilation, and sleep often requires an increase of recording time.

American Clinical Neurophysiology Society. Guideline One: Minimum Technical Requirements for Performing Clinical Electroencephalography. https://www.acns.org/pdf/guidelines/Guideline-1.pdf. Accessed December 28, 2015.

76. A. EEG changes vary depending on the subtype of SE. In absence SE, the EEG consists of continuous, rhythmic, bilaterally synchronous and symmetric, spike-wave or polyspike-wave discharges with a frequency of 1.5 to 3 Hz (not 4 to 6 Hz). In simple partial SE, the scalp EEG is often normal. If abnormal, there may be "tonic" discharges consisting of localized high-frequency activity, but more often, there are "clonic" discharges consisting of sharp waves with a frequency of 0.3 to 3 Hz (typically 1 Hz). Complex partial SE typically presents with variable ictal patterns including periodic lateralized discharges, 5- to 7-Hz rhythmic activity (seen in mesial temporal onsets), and asymmetric bilateral discharges (seen in frontal onsets). Myoclonic SE is divided into two forms: pure (primary; seen in patients with known generalized epilepsies) and symptomatic (secondary; seen in patients with degenerative encephalopathies). In the primary form, the jerks are usually associated with multiple, generalized synchronous, anteriorly predominant spikes on a normal background. In the secondary form, the EEG consists of arrhythmic spike-wave discharges separated by high amplitude, mixed delta and theta activity along with epileptic recruiting rhythms, on a slow background.

Ohtahara S, Ohtsuka Y. Myoclonic status spilepticus. In: Engel J, Jr, Pedley TA, eds. *Epilepsy: A Comprehensive Textbook.* 2nd ed. Philadelphia, PA: Lippincott Williams & Wilkins; 2008:725–729.

Thomas P, Snead OC III. Absence status epileptics. In: Engel J, Jr, Pedley TA, eds. *Epilepsy: A Comprehensive Textbook.* 2nd ed. Philadelphia, PA: Lippincott Williams & Wilkins; 2008:693–703.

Williamson PD. Complex partial status epilepticus. In: Engel J, Jr, Pedley TA, eds. *Epilepsy: A Comprehensive Textbook.* 2nd ed. Philadelphia, PA: Lippincott Williams & Wilkins; 2008:677–692.

Wiser HG, Chauvel P. Simple partial status epilepticus and epilepsia partialis continua of Kozhevnikov. In: Engel J, Jr, Pedley TA, eds. *Epilepsy: A Comprehensive Textbook.* 2nd ed. Philadelphia, PA: Lippincott Williams & Wilkins; 2008:705–723.

77. C. The FFT spectrogram is a three-dimensional representation of EEG power (which is proportional to the square of the amplitude) over time with respect to the various frequencies. Seizures are usually characterized by increasing power, evolving from lower to higher frequencies. On the FFT spectrogram, change in the color to red over both hemispheres indicates an increase in power at the corresponding frequencies. Many artifacts (e.g., related to muscle or electrode) present with an increased power on the FFT spectrogram as well, but the increase is more abrupt without evolution, unlike a seizure. Amplitude-integrated EEG (aEEG) is a display of the minimum and maximum amplitude of the EEG background over a preset time interval (typically, 1–2 seconds). Seizures and background suppression have specific appearances on aEEG, but other changes are non-specific and often represent artifact. The peak envelope trend is a display of the median amplitude of the EEG background over a preset time interval (typically, 10–20 seconds). Peak envelop trend may be more specific than aEEG, but can miss seizures or other activity that are brief. In general, qEEG trends help draw the focus to the periods where more detailed analysis is needed, but they are not intended to replace expert review of raw EEG.

The four panels in the following illustrate the qEEG and raw EEG in this patient: at baseline (panel A corresponds to choice A); during bradycardia (panel B corresponds to choice B); during asystole (panel C corresponds to choice C); and after spontaneous resumption of sinus rhythm (panel D corresponds to choice D). In this patient, the FFT spectrograms show a decrease in the alpha power, a transient increase in the theta power, subsequent decrease in the theta power, and an increase in the delta power. This is equivalent to a decrease in alpha–delta ratio (not shown). This occurred when the patient experienced bradycardia (see the EKG channel on the scalp EEG). Of note, there appears to be higher delta power in the right hemisphere (due to a prior right hemispheric tumor resection). At about 01:27, there was a sudden drop in power in both hemispheres as seen in the FFT, aEEG, and peak envelope trends. This suggests decreased or absent cerebral blood flow. This occurred when the patient was in asystole. The patient then remained in asystole for just over a minute before the spontaneous appearance of the sinus rhythm, at which point there is an incomplete reversal in the qEEG trends. After the event, there was decreased power overall, but an increase in delta activity, which lasted >30 minutes without any significant improvement, suggestive of diffuse infarction.

The most likely scenario is that the patient developed diffuse ischemia with subsequent infarction due to decreased cerebral blood flow that occurred in the setting of asystole. Although seizures can present with decreasing or increasing FFT power over time, the overall power tends to increase, but that is not seen here. Another possibility would be ictal bradycardia or asystole, which can present with an overall increase in power prior to rapid decrease in power, correlating with the decrease in cerebral blood flow, which is not seen here either. Also, disconnecting a patient from cVEEG may lead to an overall decrease in EEG power although the changes due to disconnecting and reconnecting the equipment would be more likely to occur abruptly rather than over several minutes. The pre- and postdisconnection trends would likely be similar, unless that patient had a clinical event while off cVEEG. Sleep transitions can also cause qEEG changes (e.g., decreasing alpha power and increasing delta power), but they would not typically lead to the overall suppression in power as seen here.

Herman ST. Quantitative EEG for ischemia detection. In: LaRoche SM, ed. *Handbook of ICU EEG Monitoring*. New York, NY: Demos Medical Publishing; 2013:239–248.

LaRoche SM. Quantitative EEG for seizure detection. In: LaRoche SM, ed. *Handbook of ICU EEG Monitoring*. New York, NY: Demos Medical Publishing; 2013:229–238.

Sinha SR. Quantitative EEG basic principles. In: LaRoche SM, ed. *Handbook of ICU EEG Monitoring*. New York, NY: Demos Medical Publishing; 2013:221–227.

Panel A. Baseline.

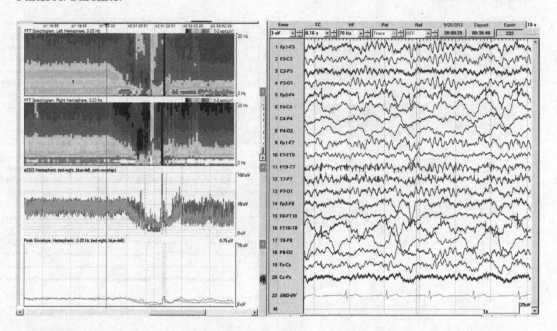

Panel B. Bradycardia.

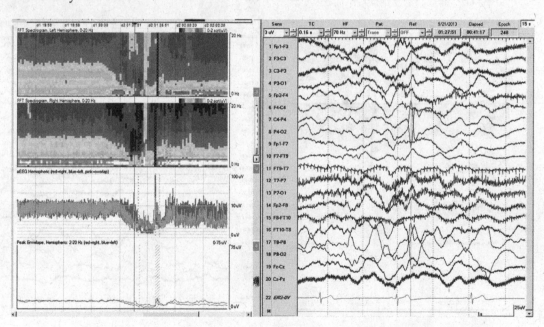

Panel C. Asystole.

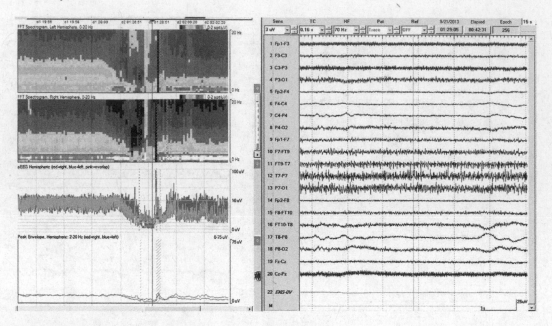

Panel D. Spontaneous resumption of sinus rhythm.

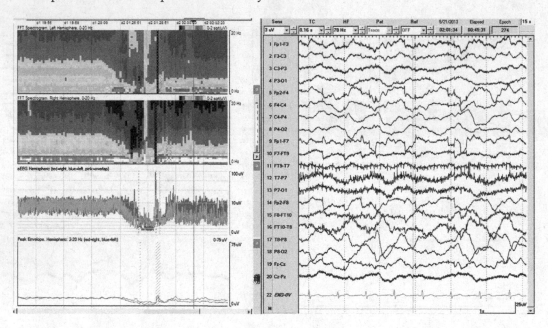

3

Diagnosis of Seizures and Epilepsy

QUESTIONS

1. Which of the following statements best describes the clinical significance of high-frequency oscillations (HFOs) in patients with epilepsy?

   A. Ripple oscillations are not pathologic
   B. Fast ripples (FRs) are generated over a smaller volume than ripples
   C. HFOs are absent in patients with MRI-negative epilepsy
   D. HFOs define a broader seizure onset zone than the conventional EEG frequencies

ANSWERS TO THIS SECTION CAN BE FOUND ON PAGE 131

2. A 3-month-old girl presented with episodes of flexion of her neck and extremities, right more than left, which occurred in clusters, most frequently upon awakening. On exam, she had macrocephaly and hypotonia in the axial musculature. EEG showed high amplitude, chaotic delta activity with intermixed multifocal spikes on the left side with relatively preserved normal background over the right. Her T2 MRI image is shown. What is the best treatment option for this child?

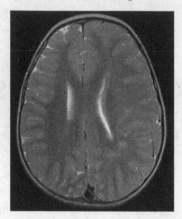

A. Adrenocorticotropic hormone (ACTH)
B. Vigabatrin
C. Functional hemispherectomy
D. Intravenous immunoglobulin

3. A 26-year-old male presents with a 9-year history of intractable epilepsy due to posttraumatic encephalomalacia in the left temporal lobe. As part of his presurgical evaluation, an MRI with diffusion tensor imaging (DTI) and tractography was done. All of the following regarding DTI/tractography are true EXCEPT:

A. DTI tracks movement of water in a three-dimensional space
B. DTI is sensitive for identifying disruption in white matter tracts
C. DTI abnormality is seen only when there is a corresponding MRI FLAIR abnormality
D. Tractography can identify patients at risk for visual field cuts after temporal lobectomy

4. A 40-year-old male with intractable temporal lobe epilepsy undergoes intracranial evaluation with depth electrodes. The EEG recording obtained from a depth electrode placed in the hippocampus at the onset of a seizure is shown. An average reference montage is used with low-frequency filter of 0.016 Hz and high-frequency filter of 30 Hz. Which of the following statements best describes the waveform in MT1 contact enclosed within the rectangle?

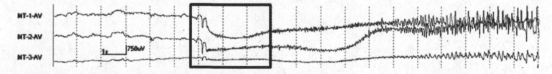

A. It is only recordable from the hippocampus in humans
B. It can be recorded routinely by using amplifiers with very short time constants
C. It is best recorded using amplifiers with very low input impedance
D. It is best recorded using platinum electrodes

5. A 1-year-old girl presents with intractable epilepsy. She was born at full term and was noted to have an extensive port wine stain over the right side of her face. At 6 weeks of age, she was diagnosed with epilepsy after she had focal motor seizures. Currently, she continues to have daily seizures despite treatment with four antiepileptic drugs (AEDs) and aspirin. On exam, she has moderate left upper extremity weakness and right gaze preference. An axial, postcontrast, T1 image of her MRI is shown. Which of the following statements describes her diagnosis and the best treatment option?

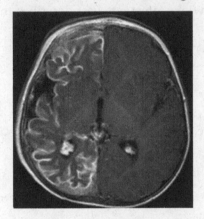

A. She has right occipital cavernoma and stereotactic thermal laser ablation is indicated
B. She has Sturge–Weber syndrome (SWS) and functional hemispherectomy is indicated
C. She has leptomeningeal carcinomatosis, and biopsy and chemotherapy are indicated
D. She has right occipital arteriovenous malformation (AVM) and radiosurgery is indicated

6. A 10-year-old girl with cognitive impairment presents with seizures since the age of 5 years. She has complex partial seizures characterized by staring, eye deviation to left, left arm posturing, and unresponsiveness lasting <1 minute followed by drowsiness. Axial FLAIR images of her brain MRI are shown. Which of the following findings is most likely to be seen on physical examination?

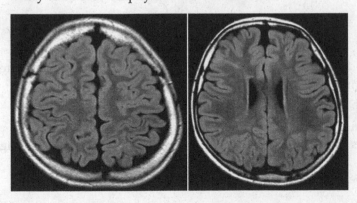

A. Café au lait spots
B. Ash leaf spots
C. Linear, raised hyperpigmented lesions
D. Nevus flammeus

7. A 38-year-old female is being evaluated for epilepsy surgery. She has history of a few febrile seizures at age 2. She remained seizure free until age 11, when the seizures recurred and became intractable. Her MRI showed right mesial temporal sclerosis. Video-EEG monitoring showed seizure onset distributed equally between right and left temporal regions. She undergoes invasive monitoring with standard clinical depth electrodes placed orthogonally in the anterior, middle, and posterior segments of both hippocampii. A sample of her interictal EEG obtained from the right middle segment of the hippocampus is shown (filter: 50–600 Hz). Which of the following statements best describes the highlighted waveforms?

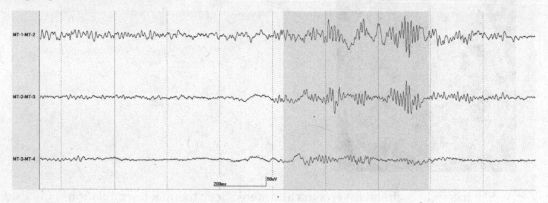

A. Similar waveforms can be seen at seizure onset
B. The waveforms are unique to the seizure focus
C. The waveforms are not seen outside the hippocampus
D. The waveforms carry no prognostic significance for surgical outcome

8. Which of the following agents needs to be administered as a continuous infusion to achieve successful anesthesia during the Wada test?

A. Sodium amytal
B. Methohexital
C. Etomidate
D. Propofol

9. Which of the following is true regarding the single-photon emission computed tomography (SPECT) scan in the presurgical evaluation of epilepsy?

A. SPECT measures increase in regional metabolism caused by the seizure
B. The test requires administration of a lipophilic radioisotope
C. The radioisotope leaves the tissue within a couple of minutes of first pass through the brain
D. Test sensitivity is independent of the radioisotope used

10. Which of the following statements best describes the multi-modality imaging findings in a patient with nonlesional epilepsy?

    A. Alpha methyl tryptophan (AMT) positron emission tomography (PET) has higher sensitivity and specificity than fluoro-deoxy glucose (FDG) PET for localizing the seizure onset zone

    B. Subtraction ictal SPECT coregistered to MRI (SISCOM) technique has high sensitivity in revealing an abnormality in nonlesional epilepsy

    C. Magnetic resonance spectroscopy (MRS) abnormality tends to be more restricted than the EEG seizure onset

    D. Magnetoencephalography (MEG) has higher yield in nonlesional mesial temporal lobe epilepsy than extratemporal epilepsy

11. A 9-month-old boy presented with hypotonia, seizures, developmental delay, failure to thrive, and hypopigmented skin and hair. MRI showed brain atrophy associated with left parietal subdural fluid collection. MR angiography showed coiling of the intracranial vessels. Which of the following tests is likely to confirm the diagnosis?

    A. Urine organic acids

    B. Fundoscopic exam

    C. Serum copper and ceruloplasmin

    D. Skeletal x-ray survey

12. A 30-year-old man with intractable epilepsy has a normal MRI. His video-EEG showed interictal epileptiform discharges and seizure onset in the right temporal region. Which of the following findings on his magnetoencephalography (MEG) is most consistent with a lateral temporal seizure focus?

    A. Right anterior temporal horizontal anterior–posterior dipoles

    B. Right anterior temporal vertical dipoles

    C. Right posterior temporal vertical dipoles

    D. Right inferior frontal vertical dipoles

13. A 21-year-old male with history of mild developmental delay presents with intractable epilepsy. His MRI shows right mesial temporal sclerosis (MTS) and slight T2 hyperintensity of the left hippocampus. He undergoes intracranial monitoring with bilateral depth electrodes inserted by a parasagittal approach via occipital burr holes. Contacts RD1 and LD1 are in the anterior part of the right and left hippocampii, respectively. RT is a subdural strip placed over the right middle temporal gyrus such that RT1 is anterior and RT6 is posterior. The activity in RD in the EEG segment (filter: 1.6–70 Hz) can be described by all of the following statements EXCEPT:

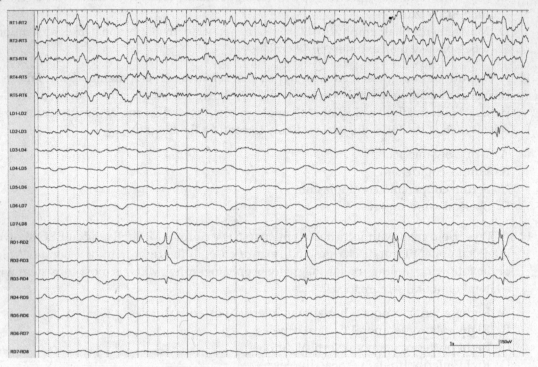

A. It is compatible with seizure onset
B. It is more likely to spread to LD first before spreading to RT
C. It is known to occur exclusively in the hippocampus
D. It correlates with hippocampal atrophy

14. Which of the following factors is NOT likely to increase the complication rate of intracranial monitoring with subdural grids?

A. Use of platinum–iridium electrodes
B. More than 100 implanted electrode contacts
C. Monitoring for more than 2 weeks
D. Two or more cable exits from the skull

15. A 30-year-old right-handed male presents with intractable left temporal lobe epilepsy. As part of presurgical workup, he undergoes fMRI as shown in the following during a verb generation task (left image) and in the resting state (right image). Which of the following is the best interpretation of the fMRI findings?

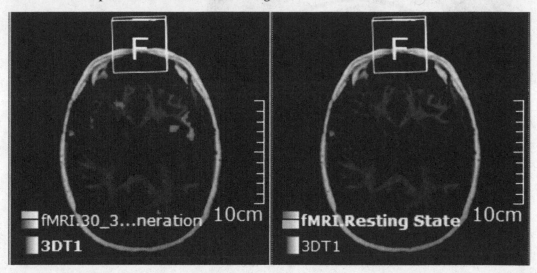

A. Broca's area is localized to the left frontal lobe
B. There is atypical language dominance
C. Wernicke's area is localized to the left temporal lobe
D. Verbal memory is localized as expected

16. Which of the following is true regarding the utility of single-photon emission computed tomography (SPECT) scan in the presurgical evaluation of epilepsy?

A. Sensitivity of ictal SPECT in temporal lobe epilepsy (TLE) is significantly superior to that of extratemporal epilepsy
B. Sensitivity of ictal SPECT is similar to that of postictal SPECT in TLE
C. Sensitivity of interictal SPECT is <50% regardless of temporal or extratemporal seizure focus
D. Resection of the focus defined by subtraction ictal SPECT coregistered to MRI (SISCOM) is associated with a favorable outcome in 90% of patients

17. The utility of long-term EEG monitoring in comatose patients can be described by all of the following statements EXCEPT:

A. EEG changes follow ischemic injury
B. EEG can predict neurologic outcome in postanoxic coma
C. EEG changes correlate with blood pressure changes after acute ischemic stroke
D. EEG can predict vasospasm after subarachnoid hemorrhage

18. A 39-year-old male with history of remote head trauma presents with intractable epilepsy. His coronal FLAIR MRI image is shown. Which of the following is LEAST likely to be part of his semiology at seizure onset?

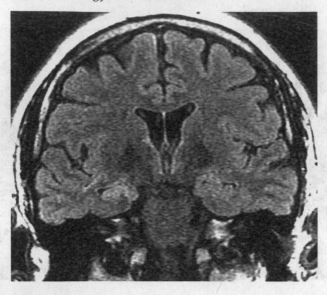

A. Lip smacking
B. Screaming and kicking
C. Rhythmic clenching and unclenching movements of the left hand
D. Looking to the right side

19. All of the following statements regarding waveform frequencies recorded on electrocorticography are correct EXCEPT:

A. Gamma activity refers to 30- to 70-Hz activity
B. Ripple oscillations refer to 80- to 200-Hz activity
C. Fast ripple oscillations refer to 600- to 1,000-Hz activity
D. High-frequency oscillations (HFOs) refer to 70 Hz or higher activity

20. A 21-year-old male with moderate intellectual disability and intractable epilepsy is evaluated by video-EEG monitoring. The EEG during one of his seizures is shown (filter: 1–70 Hz). He was noted to have elevation of both arms and subtle elevation of head off the pillow. This is most consistent with:

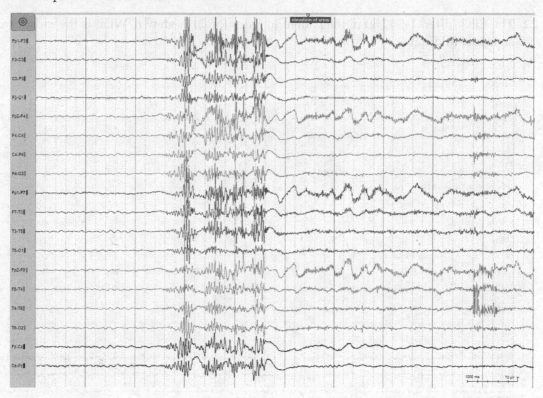

A. Atonic seizure

B. Tonic seizure

C. Atypical absence seizure

D. Myoclonic seizure

21. A 52-year-old male was admitted to the hospital with a 1-week history of nervousness and olfactory hallucinations. He was afebrile. His general and neurologic examinations were unremarkable. His MRI images without (left) and with (right) contrast are shown. What is the most likely diagnosis?

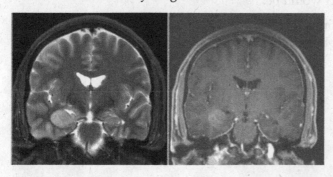

A. Mesial temporal sclerosis (MTS)
B. Hippocampal dysplasia
C. Glioma
D. Herpes simplex virus (HSV) encephalitis

22. The EEG (filter: 1–70 Hz) of the patient in Question 21 is shown. What is the most characteristic finding?

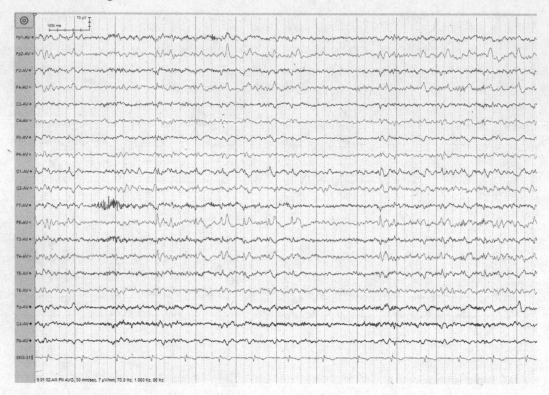

A. Right temporal sharp waves
B. Right fronto-temporal sharp waves
C. Right temporal intermittent rhythmic delta activity (TIRDA)
D. Right fronto-temporal periodic lateralized epileptiform discharges (PLEDs)

23. Based on the available evidence, the next most appropriate step in the workup of the patient described in Question 21 would be:

A. Inpatient video-EEG monitoring
B. Positron emission tomography (PET) scan
C. Lumbar puncture
D. Biopsy of the lesion

24. A 12-year-old girl presents with seizures since the age of 6 years. Seizures consist of tingling in the mouth and tongue followed by generalized convulsions. She was developmentally normal. An axial T2 image of her brain MRI is shown. What is the most likely diagnosis?

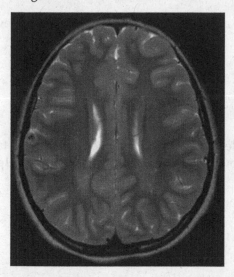

A. Cavernoma
B. Ganglioglioma
C. Meningioma
D. Pilocytic astrocytoma

25. A 14-year-old boy presents with medically intractable epilepsy with seizures characterized by an aura of headache followed by staring, unresponsiveness, nonsensical speech, left-hand automatisms, versive head turning to right, and postictal confusion and aggression. Occasionally, he has secondary generalized tonic–clonic seizures. EEG showed left temporal interictal spikes and left temporal seizure onset. Neuropsychologic testing showed deficits in verbal memory and fine motor dexterity on the right side. Coronal T2 image of his MRI is shown. Assuming that he undergoes invasive monitoring for seizure localization and language mapping, what would be his prognosis for favorable postoperative seizure outcome if the seizure onset localizes >2 cm away from the language area?

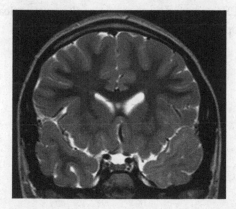

A. <10%
B. 20% to 40%
C. 50% to 60%
D. 70% to 80%

26. During intraoperative electrocorticography, the epileptic spikes can be activated by low doses of all of the following agents EXCEPT:

A. Propofol
B. Etomidate
C. Remifentanyl
D. Methohexital

27. A 25-year-old male with a 15-year history of epilepsy was found to have bilateral parietal calcification on neuroimaging. Which of the following features is LEAST likely to be helpful in establishing the diagnosis in this patient?

A. Facial angioma
B. Evidence of neuropathy
C. Antigliadin antibody
D. Anti-GAD65 antibody

28. Abnormalities on magnetoencephalography (MEG) in mesial temporal lobe epilepsy (MTLE) can include of the following EXCEPT:

A. Anterior temporal vertical (ATV) dipoles suggest medial basal temporal epileptogenic focus
B. ATV dipoles can be associated with bitemporal seizure onsets
C. Anterior temporal horizontal (ATH) dipoles suggest temporal pole epileptogenic focus
D. ATH dipoles suggest lateral temporal epileptogenic focus

29. A 37-year-old male has a 15-year history of medically refractory epilepsy, currently on two antiepileptic drugs (AEDs) after having failed four other AEDs. Scalp video-EEG monitoring showed left temporal interictal spikes, left temporal ictal semiology, and left anterior temporal ictal onset. The brain MRI was normal. Wada test showed left hemispheric language lateralization and right hemispheric memory dominance. Neuropsychometric testing showed below-average verbal memory and average nonverbal memory. A 2-deoxy-2-[18F]fluoro-D-glucose (FDG) positron emission tomography (PET) scan, done as part of the presurgical workup, is shown. What would be the most appropriate therapy at this point?

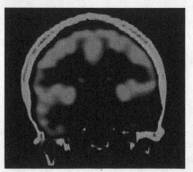

   A. Left temporal lobectomy
   B. Invasive monitoring with bilateral depth electrodes
   C. Vagus nerve stimulation (VNS) implant
   D. Continued medical therapy

30. Bilateral language representation during the Wada test can be described by all of the following statements EXCEPT:

   A. It can be seen in up to 50% of individuals regardless of handedness
   B. It can be seen in individuals with left hemisphere lesions found before age 6
   C. It can manifest as prolonged speech arrest after each injection
   D. It can manifest as no speech arrest after either injection

31. A 15-year-old boy presents to the emergency department after a witnessed seizure an hour ago. On examination, he is back to baseline, but feels sleepy as he had stayed up all night studying for a test. Head CT shows right temporal calcification. The patient agrees to start levetiracetam, but wants to be discharged and get an EEG a few weeks later. Which of the following statements would be most relevant in counseling the patient regarding the yield of detecting interictal epileptiform discharges (IEDs) on the EEG?

   A. The EEG can be delayed because the yield will be low at <10% regardless of the timing of the test
   B. The EEG can be delayed because the yield is not related to the timing of the last known seizure
   C. The EEG should be done now because the yield can be higher as the medication has not been started yet
   D. The EEG can be delayed because the yield will be low for detecting temporal lobe IEDs regardless of the timing of the test

32. Which of the following is true regarding the sensitivity of finding interictal epileptiform discharges (IEDs) on a routine EEG?

   A. The first routine EEG has a sensitivity of 70%
   B. Serial EEGs increase the sensitivity to 100%
   C. Antiepileptic drugs (AEDs) do not affect the sensitivity
   D. More frequent seizures increase the sensitivity

33. Which of the following genotype and adverse effect combinations shows an association with carbamazepine (CBZ) exposure in people of Asian descent?

   A. HLA-A*3101 and skin rash
   B. HLA-B*1502 and serious skin reaction
   C. Both A and B
   D. Neither A or B

34. A 6-year-old, right-handed boy with mild developmental delay and sensory integration disorder presents with intractable epilepsy. His seizures consist of throat clearing, unprovoked laughter, and postictal confusion. Neurological examination was nonfocal. MRI was normal. Ictal EEG showed initial, rhythmic, left frontotemporal fast activity with rapid spread to bilateral fronto-central regions. An ictal single photon emission computer tomography (SPECT) scan was performed as shown in the following, with the injection administered within 10 seconds of seizure onset. Which of the following best localizes the seizure focus?

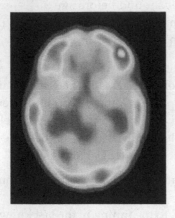

A. Left frontal lobe
B. Left parietal lobe
C. Left occipital lobe
D. Right frontal lobe

35. A 23-year-old male presents after a single seizure during sleep. The semiology by history was suggestive of a frontal lobe seizure with secondary generalization, but a routine EEG was interpreted as showing generalized discharges. Which of the following features of the interictal epileptiform discharges (IEDs) best supports a focal seizure rather than a generalized seizure?

A. Variable morphology
B. Bilateral synchrony
C. Shifting predominance
D. Consistent unilateral lead-in

36. Depth electrode recording of medial temporal lobe seizures can be characterized by all of the following statements EXCEPT:

A. Seizure onset can present as 1-Hz periodic spikes
B. Seizure onset can present as rhythmic alpha activity
C. Prolonged propagation time to the contralateral hippocampus correlates with poor postoperative seizure outcome
D. Prolonged interhippocampal propagation time suggests CA4 cell loss

37. A 35-year-old female with medically intractable epilepsy was admitted to the epilepsy monitoring unit for characterization of spells. Two events were captured with similar but nonstereotyped features consisting of onset in sleep, waxing and waning symptomatology, pelvic thrusting, eye closure with opposition to opening, ictal crying, asymmetric tonic posturing of extremities, and lack of tongue biting. Unfortunately, the EEG file was corrupted and the diagnosis had to be made on clinical features alone. Although this semiology is strongly suggestive of psychogenic nonepileptic seizures (PNES), which of the following features most likely supports the diagnosis of epileptic seizure?

    A. Onset in sleep
    B. Waxing and waning symptomatology
    C. Asymmetric tonic posturing of extremities
    D. Pelvic thrusting

38. A 30-year-old male with MRI-negative temporal lobe epilepsy undergoes ictal single photon emission computed tomography (SPECT) scan as part of presurgical evaluation. A complex partial seizure, consisting of behavioral arrest, left-hand automatisms, head turning to the left, lip smacking, and unresponsiveness, was seen. It lasted 65 seconds. The seizure onset on the EEG was nonlateralized, but the ictal changes were predominantly seen in the left temporal region. Because the seizure was not recognized in time by the staff, the radioisotope was injected 15 seconds after the seizure ended. Which of the following findings is likely to be seen on the scan?

    A. Marked hyperperfusion in the left mesial and anterolateral temporal regions
    B. Marked hypoperfusion in the left lateral temporal region
    C. Diffuse hypoperfusion in both the left medial and lateral temporal regions
    D. Hyperperfusion in the left inferior frontal region

39. Interictal epileptiform discharges (IEDs) are rare, but can be seen in healthy individuals. In which of the following scenarios are IEDs considered specific for epilepsy?

    A. Spikes and sharp waves during quiet sleep in a healthy neonate
    B. Photoparoxysmal response in a 12-year-old boy
    C. Anterior/midtemporal spikes in a 30-year-old woman
    D. Occipital spikes in an 8-year-old boy with congenital blindness

40. A 16-year-old girl presents with a 3-week history of headache, vomiting, confusion, memory impairment, and seizures. There was no fever. Her seizures are characterized by staring, lip puckering, and bilateral hand automatisms. Seizures have been intractable to three antiepileptic drugs and a course of IV methylprednisolone. Cerebro spinal fluid (CSF) analysis showed four lymphocytes, slightly elevated protein, and normal glucose. CSF culture and viral polymerase chain reaction (PCR) (for herpes simplex virus [HSV], Epstein-Barr virus [EBV], cytomegalovirus [CMV], and human herpes virus 6 [HHV6]) were negative. A FLAIR image of her brain MRI is shown. What further testing would be most appropriate to establish diagnosis?

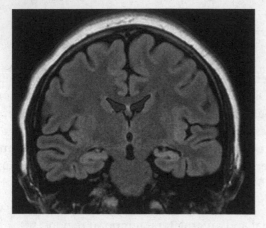

A. Brain biopsy
B. Genetic testing
C. Paraneoplastic antibody panel
D. Antithyroid antibodies

41. A 9-year-old girl presents with intractable seizures characterized by tingling in the left hand, drooling, and inability to talk but with retained ability to nod and comprehend, followed by postictal slurred speech and left hand weakness for a few minutes. A noncontrast, coronal T2 image of her MRI is shown. Which of the following statements correctly matches the lesion and associated outcome of its surgical resection?

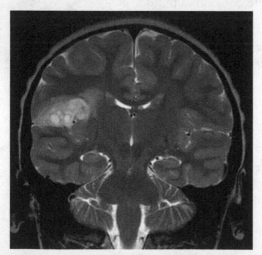

A. Ganglioglioma, associated with approximately 90% Engel class I/II outcome
B. Dysembryoplastic neuroepithelial tumor (DNET), associated with approximately 70% Engel class I/II outcome
C. Ganglioglioma, associated with approximately 50% Engel class I/II outcome
D. DNET, associated with approximately 10% Engel class I/II outcome

42. A 40-year-old male presents with intractable seizures starting around age 15. A coronal FLAIR image of his MRI is shown. Which of the following scalp ictal EEG patterns is most concordant with the MRI finding?

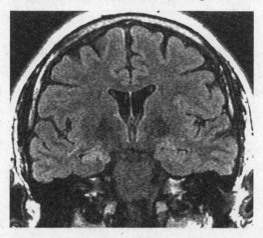

A. 3-Hz irregular discharge in the right fronto-temporal region
B. 20-Hz rhythmic discharge in the right temporal region
C. 4-Hz nonlateralized irregular discharge in the bitemporal region
D. 7-Hz rhythmic discharge in the right temporal region

43. A 30-year-old woman with nonlesional left temporal lobe epilepsy (TLE) is evaluated for resective epilepsy surgery. In addition to the assessment of temporal lobe cognitive function, which of the following neuropsychological tests would be most specific for assessing coexisting frontal lobe function?

A. Minnesota Multiphasic Personality Inventory
B. Stroop Color Word Test
C. Visual Reproduction subset of the Wechsler Memory Scale
D. Buschke Selective Reminding Test

44. A 14-year-old boy is brought to the emergency department (ED) for a generalized tonic–clonic seizure (GTCS) that occurred at 7 a.m., upon awakening. He went to bed late the previous night as he was playing video games. Which of the following is most relevant for making a syndromic diagnosis?

A. Presence of jerks in his extremities, especially in the mornings
B. Presence of staring spells and behavioral arrest
C. Positive family history of convulsive seizures occurring exclusively upon awakening
D. Presence of body jerks or staring spells while playing video games

45. The seizure shown in the following EEG (filter: 1–70 Hz) most likely originates in:

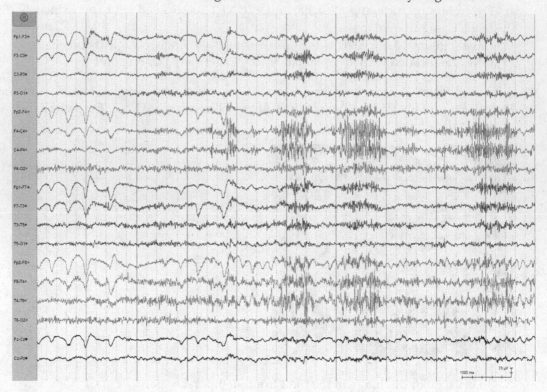

A. Mesial temporal region
B. Neocortical temporal cortex
C. Lateral frontal lobe
D. Medial frontal lobe

46. Visual-induced seizures can be characterized by all of the following features EXCEPT:

A. Seizures can be provoked by flickering lights or striped patterns
B. Polarized glasses are beneficial in preventing photosensitive seizures
C. Focal seizures can be provoked by visual stimuli
D. Watching TV from close distances is protective against seizures

47. A 32-year-old female is being evaluated for epilepsy surgery. She suffered from a single febrile seizure at age 1 year, then remained seizure free for 12 years before developing intractable epilepsy at age 13. Her seizures are characterized by a sensation of heart pounding, right-hand automatisms, left-hand stiffness, impaired responsiveness, left facial twitching, and mild postictal confusion. Her ictal EEG is shown (filter: 1.6–70 Hz; the annotation "comment" corresponds to the occurrence of right-hand automatisms). Which of the following is most likely to be her epileptogenic zone?

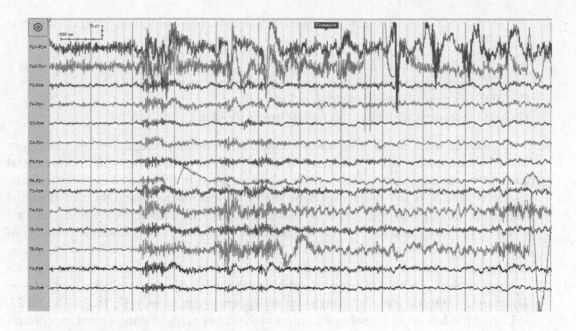

A. Right hippocampus
B. Right lateral temporal cortex
C. Right insula
D. Right lateral frontal cortex

48. Fast ripples (FR):

A. Are best recorded with depth electrodes with larger surface area
B. Decrease in slow-wave sleep
C. Are exclusive to hippocampus
D. Can be seen independent of spikes

49. A 22-year-old male with a cystic lesion in the left occipital region was admitted to the epilepsy monitoring unit for presurgical evaluation. Which of the following features suggests seizure onset in close proximity to the lesion?

A. Asymmetric tonic posturing
B. Eye blinking
C. Impaired consciousness
D. Speech arrest

50. Epilepsy patients often complain about impaired memory. Which of the following is the best predictor of memory complaint?

A. Mood
B. Age
C. Gender
D. Seizure localization

51. All of the following statements regarding magnetoencephalography (MEG) are true EXCEPT:

A. MEG reflects pyramidal cell activity
B. MEG consists of signals that are less likely to be attenuated by the skull
C. MEG has a more compact field than EEG
D. MEG measures tangential and radial current dipoles

52. A 42-year-old male has suspected nonlesional right frontal lobe epilepsy. He undergoes invasive monitoring with a 32-contact subdural grid placed over the right fronto-parietal convexity and a 2 × 8 dual-sided subdural strip placed in the interhemispheric fissure. Contacts 17 to 32 of the interhemispheric strip were located over the right medial frontal region such that the bottom row consisted of contacts 17 to 24 and the top row consisted of contacts 25 to 32 (contact 17 was antero-inferior, contact 25 was antero-superior, contact 24 was postero-inferior, and contact 32 was postero-superior). The following figure, consisting of a subset of the right medial frontal contacts, shows the lower limb somatosensory evoked potential obtained by stimulating the left tibial nerve. Seizure onset was noted in the anterior contacts of the interhemispheric strip, namely, 17, 18, 25, 26, and 27. Which of the following semiologic features at the onset of his seizure is most concordant with the data presented?

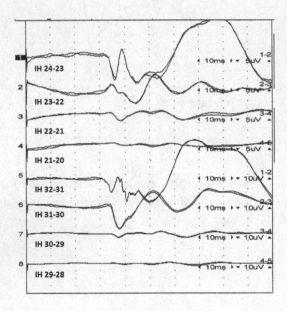

A. Throat discomfort
B. Lip smacking
C. Left arm extension with slight flexion of the right arm
D. Fumbling with the right hand

53. Which of the following is NOT likely to be associated with a clear ictal discharge on the scalp EEG?

A. Typical absence seizure associated with staring

B. Simple partial seizure of supplementary motor area onset associated with bilateral movements

C. Complex partial seizure of temporal lobe onset associated with staring and lip smacking

D. Frontal lobe seizure associated with contralateral head and eye deviation

54. A 40-year-old man with epilepsy has a history of seizures between the ages of 3 and 8 years, characterized by prolonged periods of clonic twitching of the right side of the body with preserved consciousness. These seizures were followed by prolonged periods of postictal right hemiplegia. He remained seizure free from ages 8 to 19 years, and then started having focal seizures with temporal lobe semiology. Which of the following features is LEAST likely to be found in his history and examination?

A. Initial seizure onset in the context of a febrile illness

B. Family history of febrile seizures

C. Nonfocal neurologic examination

D. History of learning difficulty

55. A 24-year-old male has MRI-negative left temporal lobe epilepsy. The waveforms shown in the following EEG segment were obtained during bipolar cortical stimulation of the subdural contacts PH5 and PH6 located near the posterior aspect of the hippocampus using biphasic pulses (filter: 1–300 Hz). The arrow indicates the end of the 5-second stimulus. Which of the following statements best describes the activity appearing after the arrow?

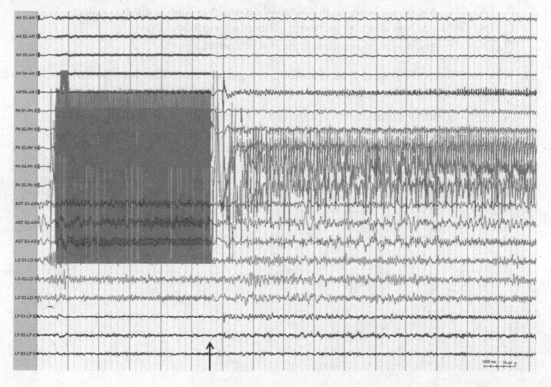

A. It can be abolished by application of cold Ringer solution to the cortex
B. Its occurrence supports the results obtained from functional mapping
C. It suggests propensity to the occurrence of a clinical seizure with repeat stimulation regardless of the current intensity
D. It localizes the seizure onset zone to the contacts generating them

56. The utility of long-term ambulatory EEG monitoring can be described by all of the following statements EXCEPT:

A. Detailed visual analysis of behavior is not available
B. Temporal correlation of EEG findings and behavior is accurate
C. It provides preliminary data that can minimize inpatient monitoring
D. Events can be easily missed

57. Which of the following is true regarding postoperative memory in patients who have had temporal lobectomy?

A. Postoperative memory deficits, if present, are consistently material specific
B. Presence of mesial temporal sclerosis predicts postoperative memory impairment
C. Impaired memory performance after contralateral injection during the Wada test predicts better postoperative memory outcome
D. Worse preoperative memory predicts worse postoperative memory

58. All of the following statements regarding the utility of direct current (DC) shifts in clinical practice are true EXCEPT:

A. DC shifts can be recorded using an amplifier with a long time constant
B. DC shifts are better seen on intracranial recordings than scalp recordings
C. DC shifts are best seen by increasing the low-frequency filter
D. DC shifts are useful in localizing the seizure onset zone

59. Which of the following is true regarding the performance and interpretation of cortical stimulation for localizing the eloquent cortex?

A. Biphasic pulse stimulation is preferred over monophasic stimulation
B. The pathological cortex has a lower threshold for generating afterdischarges
C. Longer pulse trains are needed for stimulation of the motor cortex
D. Postoperative language deficit can occur if the resection margin is within 4 cm of the language area

60. A 30-year-old right-handed female is being evaluated for possible reoperation after failed right frontal resection for nonlesional frontal lobe epilepsy. The video-EEG semiology of her seizures suggested right supplementary motor area onset. However, the ictal and interictal EEG findings predominantly localized to the midline centro-parietal region. The magnetic source imaging findings on her magnetoencephalography (MEG) scan are shown. The utility of MEG in presurgical evaluation, as illustrated in this example, includes all of the following EXCEPT:

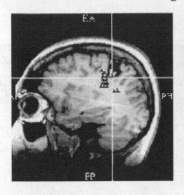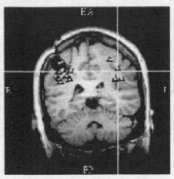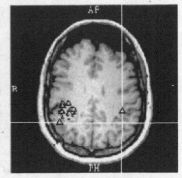

A. MEG is more sensitive than EEG for detecting epileptogenic foci in the superficial cortex

B. MEG-defined epileptogenic focus has no prognostic value for surgical outcome

C. MEG can provide unique information that is not obtained from EEG

D. MEG dipole clusters are anatomically more restricted than the EEG dipole clusters

61. The neuropsychological profile of patients with temporal lobe epilepsy (TLE) can be described by all of the following statements EXCEPT:

A. The predominant impairment is in declarative memory

B. Lower IQ is associated with earlier age of seizure onset

C. Material-specific memory impairment is associated with earlier age of seizure onset

D. Cognitive deficits often involve frontal lobes

62. Which of the following results obtained during the Wada test is expected to be associated with the least risk of memory decline postoperatively?

A. High memory score after injection of the surgical hemisphere versus the nonsurgical hemisphere

B. Low memory score after injection of the surgical hemisphere versus the nonsurgical hemisphere

C. High memory scores after bilateral injections

D. Low memory scores after bilateral injections

63. A 6-month-old boy presents with clusters of events of flexion of arms and legs lasting 4 to 5 minutes. His skin examination reveals hypopigmented macules on the trunk and extremities. Which of the following prenatal history and diagnosis combinations is likely in this patient?

    A. Cardiac rhabdomyoma and tuberous sclerosis
    B. Intrauterine hiccups and nonketotic hyperglycinemia (NKH)
    C. Polyhydramnios and tuberous sclerosis
    D. Hydrocephalus and hypomelanosis of Ito

64. A 4-year-old girl presents with complex partial and secondary generalized seizures after nonspecific cold symptoms, which then progressed to severe aphasia, upper limb dyskinesia, agitation, aggressive behavior, fluctuation in consciousness, and inability to walk. The brain MRI was normal. Which of the following tests should be included in her evaluation?

    A. Cerebrospinal fluid (CSF) oligoclonal bands and IgG synthesis index
    B. CSF Epstein–Barr virus (EBV) titers
    C. CSF N-methyl-D-aspartate (NMDAR) antibodies
    D. CSF lactate

65. A 45-year-old female with nonlesional (MRI-negative) epilepsy undergoes subdural grid evaluation for seizure localization. Her seizures are characterized by repetitive bilateral eye blinking, occurrence of bright white spots in the right visual field, followed several seconds later by generalized tonic–clonic activity. The following figure shows EEG recordings from a 20-contact subdural grid (LP) placed over the left temporo-occipital junction and a 16-contact subdural strip (LT) placed over the left superior and middle temporal gyri (filter: 1.6–70 Hz). The activity in the LP grid was noted on the day of implantation and persisted throughout the 7-day monitoring period. The activity in the LP grid can be attributed to all of the following EXCEPT:

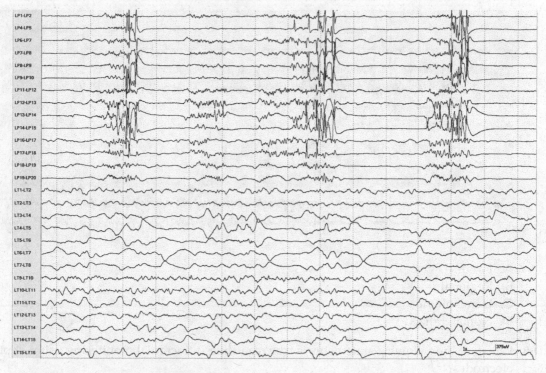

A. Underlying cortical dysplasia
B. Underlying postimplantation hemorrhage
C. Interictal abnormality
D. Impending ictal discharge

66. Ictal onset patterns on intracranial EEG can be characterized by all of the following EXCEPT:

A. EEG frequency at extratemporal seizure onset is usually slower than the temporal onset
B. Periodic spiking at seizure onset correlates with better outcome after temporal lobectomy
C. Faster frequency at seizure onset correlates with better postoperative seizure outcome
D. Slower frequency at seizure onset suggests propagated activity

67. The seizure onset shown in the following EEG (filter: 1.6–70 Hz) is:

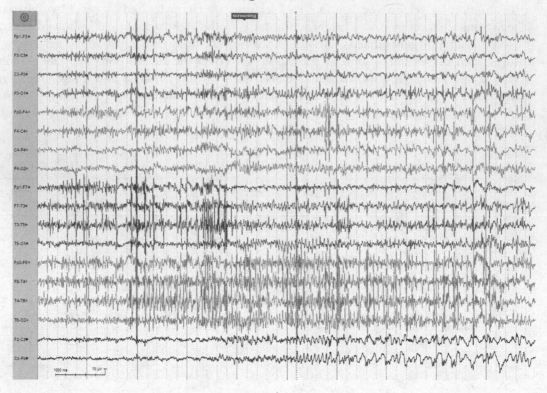

A. Focal
B. Regional
C. Hemispheric
D. Nonlateralized

68. Which of the following statements is true regarding intracranial monitoring using depth electrodes?

A. Depth electrodes are best suited for recording from the hippocampus, insula, and cortical surface
B. There is a 10% risk of intracerebral hemorrhage after depth electrode placement
C. Localized attenuation in a depth electrode contact almost always suggests hemorrhage
D. Prolonged seizure freedom can occur after a depth electrode study without resection

69. Memory impairment in patients with temporal lobe epilepsy (TLE) is characterized by all of the following EXCEPT:

A. Impaired verbal memory is consistently seen in left TLE
B. Impaired nonverbal memory is consistently seen in right TLE
C. Verbal memory correlates with degree of neuronal loss in left TLE
D. Impaired delayed recall suggests left mesial temporal lobe dysfunction

70. Antiepileptic drug (AED) withdrawal in the epilepsy monitoring unit to record seizures can be expected to result in all of the following EXCEPT:

    A. Increase in seizures
    B. Similar seizure semiology as habitual seizures
    C. Increased predisposition toward secondary generalized seizures
    D. Increase in interictal spiking even in the absence of seizures

71. A 52-year-old woman with intractable epilepsy was found to have an abnormal MRI as shown in the axial FLAIR image. The clinical profile of the condition shown in the MRI includes:

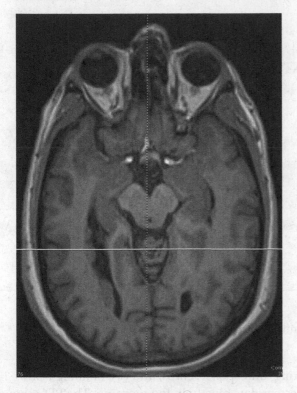

    A. Female preponderance
    B. Rare occurrence of epilepsy
    C. Seizure onset in infancy
    D. Severe intellectual disability

72. The EEG recording at the onset of the seizure for the patient described in Question 71 (filter: 1.6–70 Hz). Which of the following features is LEAST likely to be seen at seizure onset?

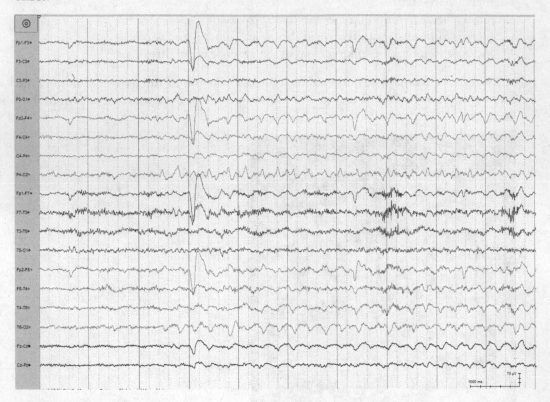

A. Eye blinking
B. Left-hand posturing
C. Asymmetric bilateral upper extremity posturing
D. Right-hand fumbling

73. A 12-month-old boy has events of staring, unresponsiveness, and eye blinking lasting 10 to 25 seconds that occur multiple times per day, mostly in the morning. The EEG shows 3-Hz spike-wave discharges correlating with the episodes of staring. He has mild developmental delay and his exam is normal. Ethosuximide, valproic acid, and lamotrigine were not beneficial. What would be the most appropriate next step in establishing the diagnosis?

A. Cerebrospinal fluid (CSF) analysis and SLC2A1 gene test
B. Positron emission tomography (PET) scan
C. ARX gene test
D. Karyotype for ring chromosome 20

74. Which of the following requirements is NOT absolutely necessary to evaluate high-frequency oscillations (HFOs) in epilepsy patients?

A. Sampling rate of >1,000 Hz
B. Microelectrode recordings
C. High setting for low-frequency filter (LFF)
D. High setting for high-frequency filter (HFF)

75. Which of the following findings on proton magnetic resonance spectroscopy (MRS) can be seen in the epileptogenic temporal lobe foci?

A. Elevation of N-acetylaspartate (NAA)
B. Reduction of choline and creatine (CR)
C. Reduction of NAA/(choline+CR) ratio
D. Postictal reduction of lactate

76. A 17-year-old right-handed boy started to have episodes of stuttering and myoclonic movements of the jaw and mouth after reading aloud for a few minutes. Which of the following features is likely to be present as part of his clinical profile?

A. Resolution of symptoms with continued reading aloud
B. Resolution of symptoms with continued reading silently
C. Lack of response to conventional antiepileptic drugs
D. Positive family history

77. A 5-year-old boy presents with seizures, developmental delay, speech impairment, ataxia, and jerky extremity movements. On examination, he is noted to be playful and smiling, but has hypotonia and a prominent jaw. Prior brain MRI was normal and the EEG showed frequent bursts of high-amplitude, slow spike-wave discharges. Which of the following genetic tests would most likely confirm the diagnosis?

A. Deletion in chromosome 15
B. MECP2 mutation
C. CDKL5 mutation
D. ARX mutation

78. Based on electrical stimulation of the cortex, resection in which of the following locations in the language-dominant hemisphere is LEAST likely to result in permanent language deficit?

A. Supplementary motor area
B. Basal temporal area
C. Superior perisylvian region
D. Inferior perisylvian region

79. Which of the following features is inconsistent with a diagnosis of Panayiotopoulos syndrome?

A. Autonomic status epilepticus
B. Seizure occurrence predominantly during sleep
C. Age at onset of 16 years
D. Multifocal spikes with posterior predominance activated by sleep

80. Which of the following statements is true regarding the utility of interictal 2-deoxy-2-[18F] fluoro-D-glucose (FDG) positron emission tomography (PET) in mesial temporal lobe epilepsy (MTLE)?

A. It has a sensitivity of about 50% at best
B. Hypometabolism is greater in the lateral temporal than mesial temporal structures
C. The contralateral thalamus is the most common extratemporal site to show hypometabolism
D. Bilateral but asymmetric changes in the temporal lobes can be seen even with unilateral MTLE

3

DIAGNOSIS OF SEIZURES AND EPILEPSY

ANSWERS

1. **B.** Initial microelectrode studies on interictal HFOs concluded that only the FRs, but not ripples, were pathologic and epileptogenic. However, subsequent observations showed that ripples in the dentate gyrus could be pathologic and epileptogenic as well. Further, macroelectrode studies supported the notion that both ripples and FRs were pathologic and epileptogenic and probably represented the same phenomenon. Microelectrode studies have shown that FRs are generated over a smaller volume than ripples in humans; in animals, the FR generator appeared to be less than 1 mm^3. HFOs occur in both lesional and nonlesional (MRI-negative) epilepsy. The interictal HFOs are tightly linked to the seizure onset zone rather than the underlying lesion. Although both interictal and ictal HFOs have widespread spatial distribution, studies have shown distinct spatial differences between HFO-defined and conventional EEG frequency-defined seizure onset zones, with the former more spatially restricted than the latter.

   Gotman J, Crone NE. High-frequency EEG activity. In: Schomer DL, Lopes da Silva FH, eds. *Niedermeyer's Electroencephalography: Basic Principles, Clinical Applications, and Related Fields*. 6th ed. Philadelphia, PA: Lippincott Williams & Wilkins; 2011:749–766.

   Modur PN. High frequency oscillations and infraslow activity in epilepsy. *Ann Indian Acad Neurol*. 2014; 17(suppl 1):S99-S106.

2. **C.** The MRI shows hemimegalencephaly (HME), which is a rare congenital disorder of cortical formation with hamartomatous overgrowth of all or part of a cerebral hemisphere. The majority (90%) of patients present with focal and generalized infantile spasms. Developmental delay, hemiparesis, and hemianopia are usually present as well. HME may occur as an isolated or sporadic brain malformation or in association with other neurodevelopmental syndromes such as Proteus syndrome, neurofibromatosis, and linear sebaceous nevus syndrome. Microscopic features may include polymicrogyria, heterotopic gray matter, cortical dysplasia, blurring of the gray–white junction, and an increase in the number of neurons and astrocytes. Neither antiseizure medications nor immunoglobulins are effective in controlling seizures in HME, and therefore surgery is often recommended. It is believed that if the affected side is surgically removed (i.e., anatomic hemispherectomy) or disconnected from the other brain structures (i.e., functional hemispherectomy),

the unaffected side may gradually take over the functions normally performed by the affected side.

Mirzaa G, Kuzniecky R, Geurrini R. Malformations of cortical development and epilepsy. In: Wyllie E, ed. *Wyllie's Treatment of Epilepsy: Principles and Practice*. 5th ed. Philadelphia, PA: Lippincott Williams & Wilkins; 2011:339–351.

Rowland LP, ed. *Merritt's Neurology*. 10th ed. Philadelphia, PA: Lippincott Williams & Wilkins; 2000:487.

3. **C.** DTI is based on tracking the movement of water molecules in a three-dimensional space. It is sensitive for identifying disruptions in the integrity of white matter tracts based on the principle of fractional anisotropy. Abnormalities on DTI can be seen without corresponding MRI FLAIR hyperintensities. Tractography is used for reconstructing the three-dimensional trajectories of the white matter tracts by following the continuous path of greatest diffusivity. This is typically accomplished by line-propagation algorithms, where the lines (representing the axons) are terminated based on their anisotropy value and angle of curvature. Tractography is useful in delineating regions of interest based on fiber orientation and integrity. DTI/tractography is being explored in epilepsy surgery workup, including identifying axonal degeneration in the fornix and cingulum in patients with mesial temporal sclerosis. Tractography has also been used to identify patients at risk for postoperative visual field defects due to disruption of Meyer's loop after anterior temporal lobectomy.

Lin JJ, Mazziotta JC. Computational anatomy. In: Engel J Jr, Pedley TA, eds. *Epilepsy: A Comprehensive Textbook*. 2nd ed. Philadelphia, PA: Lippincott Williams & Wilkins; 2008:999–1009.

4. **D.** The figure shows a direct current (DC) shift (also known as ictal baseline shift [IBS]) at the onset of a focal seizure in the hippocampal contacts of a depth electrode. DC shifts are not unique to the hippocampus; they can be recorded in the neocortex as well. They can be routinely recorded using an alternating current (AC) amplifier with a long time constant. Therefore, the term IBS may be more appropriate than DC shift. Successful recording of IBSs is facilitated by the use of platinum electrodes (as opposed to gold or stainless steel), larger surface area of the electrodes (e.g., subdural as opposed to depth electrodes), and higher input impedance of the amplifier (usually >50 MΩ). For display, a low-frequency filter of 0.016 Hz and a time scale of 30 seconds per page are usually employed. The origin of ictal DC shifts appears to be multifactorial. The proposed mechanisms of its generation include neuronal activity, glial activity, and blood–brain barrier alteration.

Ikeda A, Luder HO, Shibasaki H. Ictal direct-current shifts. In: Luders HO, Noachtar S, eds. *Epileptic Seizures: Pathophysiology and Clinical Semiology*. Philadelphia, PA: Churchill Livingstone; 2000:53–62.

Modur PN. High frequency oscillations and infraslow activity in epilepsy. *Ann Indian Acad Neurol*. 2014; 17(suppl 1):S99–S106.

5. **B.** The MRI shows marked leptomeningeal enhancement in the right hemisphere, most prominent in the occipital region. This suggests SWS or leptomeningeal carcinomatosis. The clinical presentation, along with the facial port wine stain ipsilaterally, suggests SWS rather than leptomeningeal carcinomatosis. A CT scan shows subcortical calcification (tram track calcification). Neither cavernoma nor AVM is associated with such prominent leptomeningeal enhancement. SWS is a neurocutaneous disorder that occurs sporadically in both males and females. It presents at birth with a capillary malformation on the face (port wine stain, hemangioma, or nevus flammeus). The underlying somatic mosaic

mutation causing both SWS and isolated port wine birthmarks is an activating mutation in GNAQ on chromosome 9q21. A newborn with a facial port wine stain on the upper face has a 15% to 50% risk of developing SWS. Epilepsy develops within 2 years in 90% of patients with brain involvement. Although many patients will obtain reasonable seizure control on conventional AEDs and low-dose aspirin, some children remain intractable. Many of these children also develop significant hemiparesis, visual field deficits, and developmental and learning impairment. For these patients, hemispherectomy (or focal or multilobar resection) would be a reasonable option. A survey-based study showed that 81% achieve seizure freedom after hemispherectomy, with many patients successfully coming off AEDs.

Comi AM. Sturge-Weber syndrome. *Handb Clin Neurol.* 2015;132:157–168.

Kossoff EH, Buck C, Freeman JM. Outcomes of 32 hemispherectomies for Sturge–Weber syndrome worldwide. *Neurology* 2002;59:1735–1738.

6. **B.** The MRI shows hyperintense lesions on FLAIR imaging, in the left parieto-occipital region (left image) and right frontal region (right image). There is also a thin streak of hyperintense signal in the white matter in the right frontal region extending up to the ventricle (right image). These findings are consistent with tuberous sclerosis (TS). Among the options given, only the ash leaf spots are characteristic of TS. Ash leaf spots are hypopigmented macules that are best seen with a Wood's lamp. Café au lait spots are irregular, light-brown, hypopigmented lesions seen in neurofibromatosis type 1 (NF-1). MRI in NF-1 shows hyperintense hamartomas in the deep white matter. Linear, raised hyperpigmented lesions are seen in epidermal nevus syndrome, which is characterized by dysplastic lesions and hemimegalencephaly on MRI. Nevus flammeus is a facial capillary angioma seen in the distribution of trigeminal nerve, characteristic of Sturge–Weber syndrome (SWS). The MRI in SWS shows a calcified lesion (hypointense signal) in the posterior head region.

Gupta A. Epilepsy in the setting of neurocutaneous syndromes. In: Wyllie E, ed. *Wyllie's Treatment of Epilepsy: Principles and Practice.* 5th ed. Philadelphia, PA: Lippincott Williams & Wilkins; 2011:375–384.

7. **A.** The highlighted waveforms are high-frequency oscillations (HFOs). Clues to the recognition of these waveforms include the appropriate filter settings (50–600 Hz), expanded time base, and high display gain. In patients with epilepsy, initial studies focused on the interictal HFOs, but more recent studies have shown that HFOs occur at seizure onset as well, and such ictal HFOs can be helpful in localizing the seizure onset zone. Interictal HFOs generally tend to be prominent inside the seizure focus (i.e., the seizure onset zone), but they are shown to occur outside the seizure focus and even at a remote distance from the seizure focus. HFOs have been recorded from mesial temporal as well as neocortical structures. Recently, several studies have shown that the resection of the tissue containing the interictal HFOs is associated with favorable postoperative seizure outcome, suggesting that the HFOs can serve as electrophysiological biomarkers of epilepsy.

Modur PN, Zhang S, Vitaz TW. Ictal high-frequency oscillations in neocortical epilepsy: implications for seizure localization and surgical resection. *Epilepsia* 2011;52:1792–1801.

Zijlmans M, Jiruska P, Zelmann R, et al. High-frequency oscillations as a new biomarker in epilepsy. *Ann Neurol.* 2012;71:169–178.

8. **C.** The effect of sodium amytal is about 6 to 8 minutes, allowing for a single-dose administration with waning effect to achieve successful anesthesia. Methohexital is so short acting that it usually has to be reinjected within a test, leading to waxing and waning of the anesthetic effect during critical testing time. This lack of control over the level of anesthesia limits presentation of new memory items with methohexital. With etomidate, the level of anesthesia is maintained with an infusion following the initial bolus injection. However, a shiver-like tremor can occur with etomidate infusion. Propofol is similar to sodium amytal in that it is given as a single injection as it has a subsequent waning of the effect. However, propofol must be injected in a lipid carrier.

Jones-Gotman M, Smith ML, Weiser HG. Intraarterial amobarbital procedures. In: Engel J Jr, Pedley TA, eds. *Epilepsy: A Comprehensive Textbook.* 2nd ed. Philadelphia, PA: Lippincott Williams & Wilkins; 2008:1833–1842.

9. **B.** Brain SPECT scan measures regional cerebral blood flow (rCBF) using lipophilic radioisotopes, which are transported from the vascular compartment to the normal brain tissue compartment by diffusion. These agents are distributed in proportion to the regional tissue blood flow. During the first pass through the brain, the radioisotope is irreversibly trapped in the tissue compartment and does not change its relative distribution over time. As the radioisotope is essentially trapped during the first few seconds after injection and maintains that distribution for hours, the emission of photons still reflects the radioisotope's distribution pattern postinjection. The two commonly used agents for brain SPECT imaging are technetium-99m hexamethyl-propylene-amine-oxime (Tc-99m HMPAO) and Tc-99m ethyl cysteinate dimer (Tc-99m ECD). Tc-99m HMPAO and Tc-99m ECD have similar localization rates in patients with TLE (82% vs. 71%). In patients with neocortical epilepsy, the localization rate is higher for Tc-99m HMPAO (70%) versus Tc-99m ECD (29%); the degree of hyperperfusion is also higher in the former. Overall, the Tc-99m HMPAO ictal SPECT is better than Tc-99m ECD ictal SPECT in terms of diagnostic performance and the contrast of hyperperfused areas.

Kim S, Mountz JM. SPECT imaging of epilepsy: an overview and comparison with F-18 FDG PET. *Int J Mol Imaging* 2011;2011:813028.

10. **B.** Comparison of AMT-PET and FDG-PET in patients with normal MRI has shown that the sensitivity of AMT-PET in terms of agreement with intracranial seizure onset was lower than that of FDG-PET (39% vs. 73%), but the specificity of AMT-PET was better than that of FDG-PET (100% vs. 63%). In patients with nonlesional temporal or extratemporal epilepsy, the sensitivity of SISCOM in showing a hyperperfusion focus is 91%. The predictive value of SISCOM for surgical outcome is independent of MRI. Excellent postsurgical outcome is seen in approximately 70% of patients when the SISCOM focus is resected as opposed to only 20% when the focus is excluded from the resection. In 27% to 92% of nonlesional temporal lobe epilepsy patients, the MRS abnormality lateralizes to the ictal EEG focus. In nonlesional temporal and extratemporal epilepsy patients, MRS-detected abnormal focus is concordant with localization by seizure semiology and EEG in 60%. There is no evidence that MRS abnormality independently predicts seizure control after surgical resection in nonlesional temporal lobe epilepsy. MRS abnormalities often extend well beyond the seizure onset zone in 35% of patients with either temporal or extratemporal epilepsy. Interictal spikes restricted to the mesial temporal region are

not as easily detected by MEG as those in the neocortical region. Accordingly, the yield of MEG in extratemporal neocortical epilepsy is higher than mesial temporal lobe epilepsy. The extent of the magnetic source imaging (MSI) resection is associated with surgical outcome in nonlesional extratemporal epilepsy, with 80% seizure freedom after complete MSI focus resection versus 10% after partial resection or nonresection.

So EL. Nonlesional cases. In: Wyllie E, ed. *Wyllie's Treatment of Epilepsy: Principles and Practice*. 5th ed. Philadelphia, PA: Lippincott Williams & Wilkins; 2011:964–972.

11. **C.** Based on the information given, the most likely diagnosis is Menkes disease (MD), which is an infantile-onset, X-linked recessive neurodegenerative disorder. It is attributed to an abnormality involving the ATP7A gene on chromosome Xq21.1 resulting in disturbed copper transport and connective tissue disturbance. Variable phenotypes are related to abnormal collagen and elastin formation, resulting in skin and hair ("kinky hair") alterations, tortuous and elongated intracranial vessels, bladder diverticula, and bony abnormalities. MR angiography can show the abnormalities in the intracranial vessels. Skeletal x-rays often show femoral and tibial metaphyseal spurs, but no fractures. Three successive periods in the course of epilepsy have been observed: early focal status, infantile spasms, and myoclonic and multifocal epilepsy after age 2 years. When clinical features and imaging suggest MD, low serum copper and ceruloplasmin help confirm the diagnosis. Early treatment with daily copper injections is felt to improve outcome for this rare disease.

Papetti L, Parisi P, Leuzzi V, et al. Metabolic epilepsy: an update. *Brain Dev*. 2013;35:827–841.

12. **C.** In nonlesional temporal lobe epilepsy, anterior temporal horizontal anterior–posterior dipoles correlate well with mesial temporal seizure onset; anterior temporal vertical dipoles correlate with anterior temporal, and perhaps medial temporal, seizure onset; posterior temporal vertical dipoles correlate with lateral or nonlocalized seizure onset. Thus, MEG can be helpful in differentiating mesial temporal from lateral neocortical temporal epileptogenic foci in patients with nonlesional temporal lobe epilepsy.

Ebersole JS, Stefan H, Baumgartner C. Electroencephalographic and magnetoencephalographic source modeling. In: Engel J, Jr, Pedley TA, eds. *Epilepsy: A Comprehensive Textbook*. 2nd ed. Philadelphia, PA: Lippincott Williams & Wilkins; 2008:895–916.

13. **B.** Depth electrode recordings of medial temporal lobe epilepsy often show a 1- to 2-Hz periodic discharges at seizure onset, as shown in contacts RD1, RD2, and RD3. This pattern subsequently evolves into continuous rhythmic activity. This distinct periodic pattern is reported to be seen exclusively in the hippocampus and correlates with CA1 cell loss (i.e., hippocampal atrophy). Most of the medial temporal seizures initially propagate to the ipsilateral temporal neocortex (RT in the figure) or frontal lobe; <25% of such seizures propagate first to the contralateral hippocampus (LD in the figure).

Spencer SS, Sperling MR, Shewmon DA, et al. Intracranial electrodes. In: Engel J, Jr, Pedley TA, eds. *Epilepsy: A Comprehensive Textbook*. 2nd ed. Philadelphia, PA: Lippincott Williams & Wilkins; 2008:1791–1815.

14. **A.** Studies have shown that the use of >100 electrodes, longer monitoring sessions (>2 weeks), and two or more cable exits are associated with an increase in the complication rate of intracranial monitoring. The intracranial electrodes are made of platinum–iridium

or nickel–chrome alloys, and neither of them increases the morbidity by itself. Platinum electrodes may be advantageous as they are compatible with MR imaging.

Seeck M, Schomer DL, Niedermeyer E. Intracranial monitoring: depth, subdural, and foramen ovale electrodes. In: Schomer DL, Lopes da Silva FH, eds. *Niedermeyer's Electroencephalography: Basic Principles, Clinical Applications, and Related Fields.* 6th ed. Philadelphia, PA: Lippincott Williams & Wilkins; 2011:677–713.

15. **A.** The ability of fMRI to detect brain activity relies on the correlation that an increase in synaptic activity (e.g., during a task) is followed by localized increase in blood flow. fMRI shows all regions associated by a task, identifying the areas that may be involved but not critical to a task as well as other possible redundant areas that may compensate after resection. In the given case, the task is focused on speech production, and, therefore, only conclusions regarding the language areas can be made. The figure shows clear activation in the left frontal lobe during the verb generation task, consistent with the location of the Broca's area. There is no posterior temporal activation in the given image to indicate localization of the Wernicke's area. There is some signal in the right frontal region, but this does not suggest atypical language dominance in this right-handed person with very prominent activation in the left frontal region. The given task does not allow localization of memory.

Cohen MS, Bookheimer SY. Functional magnetic resonance imaging. In: Engel J, Jr, Pedley TA, eds. *Epilepsy: A Comprehensive Textbook.* 2nd ed. Philadelphia, PA: Lippincott Williams & Wilkins; 2008:989–998.

Harrington GS, Buonocorea MH, Farias ST. Intrasubject reproducibility of functional MR imaging activation in language tasks. *AJNR* 2006;27:938–944.

16. **C.** In TLE, the sensitivity of ictal SPECT is 75% to 97% and the specificity is 71% to 100%. In extratemporal epilepsy, the sensitivity of SPECT is 81% to 95% and the specificity is 93%. Thus, the value of ictal SPECT is similar regardless of temporal or extratemporal seizure focus. However, the sensitivity of postictal SPECT is somewhat lower (approximately 75%), with a false-positive rate of 1.5% in TLE. Sensitivity of interictal SPECT in TLE is 44% and the FPR is 7.5%; its sensitivity is about 20% to 47% in nonlesional TLE. Because of this low sensitivity, the interictal SPECT images are generally used as baseline images for comparison with the ictal SPECT images. In lesional and nonlesional extratemporal epilepsy, the presence of a SISCOM focus that is subsequently resected has a better probability for postsurgical seizure control than when it is unresected or absent (58% vs. 18%).

Kazemi NJ, O'Brien TJ, Cascino GD, et al. Single photon emission computed tomography. In: Engel J, Jr, Pedley TA, eds. *Epilepsy: A Comprehensive Textbook.* 2nd ed. Philadelphia, PA: Lippincott Williams & Wilkins; 2008:965–973.

17. **A.** EEG changes occur at cerebral blood flow (CBF) levels less than 18 to 25 mL/100 g/min, whereas ischemic injury occurs at lower CBF levels of 12 to 18 mL/100 g/min. Thus, the EEG changes may slightly precede ischemic injury, and serve as a useful tool in monitoring for brain perfusion. The initial EEG change after ischemia consists of loss of fast activity; this is followed by occurrence of polymorphic delta activity and eventually suppression. In postanoxic and posttraumatic comatose patients, a slow monotonous EEG pattern is associated with unfavorable outcome in 95% of patients, whereas variable or sleep–wake cycle EEG patterns are associated with unfavorable outcome in only 30%. EEG changes have been shown to correlate with clinical control of hypertension and

hypotension, with EEG improvement during periods of hypertension and EEG worsening during periods of hypotension. In one study, EEG was 100% sensitive for angiographically defined vasospasm after subarachnoid hemorrhage. Several EEG patterns (e.g., total power trends, relative alpha variability, and poststimulation alpha/delta ratio) have been reported to herald the onset of vasospasm.

Gotman J, Nuwer M, Emerson RG. Principles and techniques for long-term EEG recording (EMU, ICU, Ambulatory). In: Schomer DL, Lopes da Silva FH, eds. *Niedermeyer's Electroencephalography: Basic Principles, Clinical Applications, and Related Fields*. 6th ed. Philadelphia, PA: Lippincott Williams & Wilkins; 2011:725–740.

18. **B.** The MRI shows increased FLAIR signal in the right hippocampus, suggestive of right mesial temporal sclerosis (MTS). Additional T2 and T1 images would be important in confirming the diagnosis. Assuming that he has right temporal lobe seizures, lip smacking and initial head turning to the ipsilateral side (i.e., right side) can be expected. Rhythmic clenching and unclenching movements of left hand can also be seen; these fall under the category of rhythmic ictal nonclonic hand (RINCH) movements, which are felt to be automatisms that typically lateralize the seizure onset to the contralateral side (i.e., left side in this patient). Although agitation with screaming and kicking behavior can be seen in temporal lobe seizures, it is the least likely among the given options.

Foldvary N. Ictal electroencephalography in neocortical epilepsy. In: Luders HO, Comair YG, eds. *Epilepsy Surgery*. 2nd ed. Philadelphia, PA: Lippincott Williams & Wilkins; 2001:431-439.

Lee GR, Arain A, Lim N, et al. Rhythmic ictal nonclonic hand (RINCH) motions: a distinct contralateral sign in temporal lobe epilepsy. *Epilepsia* 2006; 47:2189–2192.

19. **C.** Gamma band usually refers to activity in the 30- to 70-Hz range. Activity >70 Hz is considered to be in the range of high-frequency oscillations although some authors consider activity in the range of 50 to 80 Hz as "high gamma." In addition to these, microelectrode studies have shown two named high-frequency bands: ripples in the range of 80 to 200 Hz and fast ripples in the range of 250 to 500 Hz.

Gotman J, Crone NE. High-frequency EEG activity. In: Schomer DL, Lopes da Silva FH, eds. *Niedermeyer's Electroencephalography: Basic Principles, Clinical Applications, and Related Fields*. 6th ed. Philadelphia, PA: Lippincott Williams & Wilkins; 2011:749–766.

20. **B.** The EEG shows generalized fast activity (approximately 20 Hz), which precedes elevation of arms and head, consistent with a tonic seizure. Atonic seizures are characterized by loss of tone, involving the body or head, and are typically associated with generalized slow spike-wave discharges, polyspike-wave discharges, or fast activity. Atypical absence seizures are characterized by impaired consciousness and pause in activity, and are typically associated with generalized slow spike-wave discharges. Myoclonic seizures are characterized by sudden myoclonic jerks of the axial or limb muscles and are typically associated with generalized slow polyspike-wave discharges. All of these seizures types can be seen in Lennox–Gastaut syndrome, which is the most likely diagnosis in this patient.

Panayiotopoulos CP. *A Clinical Guide to Epileptic Syndromes and Their Treatment*. Oxford, UK: Bladon Medical Publishing; 2002:70–80.

21. **C.** The MRI shows an enhancing lesion, suggesting a neoplastic or an infectious/inflammatory process. Lack of fever and mental status changes, and an otherwise normal

examination makes HSV encephalitis unlikely. Thus, a glioma is the most likely diagnosis in this patient. Neither MTS nor dysplasia is associated with enhancement.

22. **B.** The EEG shows sharp waves in a wider spatial distribution involving the right fronto-temporal region (Fp2, F4, F8, and T4). The sharp waves occur singly or in series, but not in a periodic manner. Some of the sharp waves have an aftergoing slow wave, but there is no rhythmic delta activity.

23. **C.** Lumbar puncture would be the most appropriate next step for workup. Cerebrospinal fluid (CSF) analysis will be helpful in ruling out infectious or inflammatory causes, and in looking for malignant cells. If lumbar puncture is nondiagnostic, biopsy of the lesion can be considered. The history and EEG are consistent with temporal lobe seizures, so video-EEG monitoring will not provide additional information. Similarly, the PET scan will not provide additional information either because the MRI shows a clear lesion.

24. **A.** The MRI shows a circumscribed, hypointense, intra-axial lesion on T2 involving the cortex of the right anterior parietal lobe surrounded by mild edema. Among the options given, a cavernoma is most likely because the low T2 signal could correspond to hemosiderin. A gradient-echo sequence would be more sensitive in identifying a cavernoma, especially when they are small. Meningioma is an extra-axial lesion and appears isointense or hyperintense on T2 imaging. Both ganglioglioma and pilocytic astrocytoma are hyperintense on T2 imaging.

Duncan JS. Imaging and epilepsy. *Brain* 1997;120:339–377.

25. **C.** The MRI shows left temporal focal cortical dysplasia (FCD). Typical MRI findings of FCD include thickened cortex, blurring of gray–white junction, and abnormal signal in the deep white matter. FCD is highly epileptogenic and is found in 18% to 40% of focal epilepsy. Recent clinico-pathologic classification of FCD includes three types: type I is associated with abnormal radial, tangential, or mixed cortical lamination; type II is associated with dysmorphic neurons (type IIa) or dysmorphic neurons and balloon cells (type IIb); and type III is associated with another principal lesion such as hippocampal sclerosis, tumors, vascular malformations, trauma, ischemia, or encephalitis. Favorable postoperative outcome for FCD is typically around 50% to 60%. The EEG and histopathological abnormalities typically exceed the limits of the visible MRI abnormalities.

Blümcke I, Thom M, Aronica E, et al. The clinico-pathological spectrum of focal cortical dysplasias: a consensus classification proposed by an ad hoc Task Force of the ILAE Diagnostic Methods Commission. *Epilepsia* 2011;52:158-174.

Wang VY, Chang EF, Barbaro NM. Focal cortical dysplasia: a review of pathological features, genetics, and surgical outcome. *Neurosurg Focus.* 2006;20:1-7.

26. **C.** At low doses, propofol, etomidate, and methohexital can activate epileptic spikes. Methohexital is sometimes used to activate spikes prior to resection. Continuous infusion of low-dose remifentanyl does not activate spikes, whereas a high-dose infusion does.

Nuwer M. Electrocorticography. In: Schomer DL, Lopes da Silva FH, eds. *Niedermeyer's Electroencephalography: Basic Principles, Clinical Applications, and Related Fields.* 6th ed. Philadelphia, PA: Lippincott Williams & Wilkins; 2011:715-724.

27. **D.** Epilepsy in the setting of bilateral parietal calcification suggests Sturge–Weber syndrome and celiac disease. Sturge–Weber syndrome is characterized by seizures, leptomeningeal angiomatosis, facial angioma (typically of the ophthalmic division of the trigeminal nerve), and intracranial calcifications ("tram-track" sign). Celiac disease is characterized by focal seizures of occipital or temporal onset and bilateral parieto-occipital calcifications, which are thought to consist of patchy pial angiomas, fibrosed veins, and large microcalcifications containing calcium and silica. Celiac disease can lead to multiple vitamin deficiencies, including B and E, which can lead to neuropathy, ataxia, myelopathy, ophthalmoplegia, and dementia. It is associated with the antigliadin antibody. Anti-GAD65 antibody is associated with limbic encephalitis, stiff-person syndrome, and diabetes, and is not likely to be helpful in establishing the diagnosis in this patient.

Freeman HJ. Neurological disorders in adult celiac disease. *Can J Gastroenterol.* 2008;22:909-911.

28. **B.** In MTLE, the ATV dipoles indicate epileptic activity in the medial basal temporal region. In patients with the ATV dipoles, the interictal and ictal EEG changes localize consistently to the ipsilateral temporal lobe. On the other hand, the ATH dipoles indicate epileptic activity in the temporal pole and adjacent parts of the lateral temporal cortex. About 50% of patients with ATH dipoles exhibit bitemporal spikes and/or seizure onsets.

Ebersole JS, Stefan H, Baumgartner C. Electroencephalographic and magnetoencephalographic source modeling. In: Engel J, Jr, Pedley TA, eds. *Epilepsy: A Comprehensive Textbook.* 2nd ed. Philadelphia, PA: Lippincott Williams & Wilkins; 2008:895-916.

29. **A.** The FDG PET scan shows hypometabolism in the left mesial, basal, and lateral temporal regions; there is also subtle hypometabolism in the right medial temporal region. Prior to the PET scan, the patient could be described as having medically intractable nonlesional (MRI-negative), left temporal lobe epilepsy. However, PET abnormality can be considered to be supportive of a lesion. All of the findings on his presurgical workup are concordant, and support left temporal lobe epilepsy. Thus, the most appropriate therapy at this point would be to proceed to surgical resection. Invasive monitoring would be reasonable in the context of discordant data or widespread ictal onset. Vagus nerve stimulator (VNS) implant is typically an option if the patient is not a candidate for resective surgery. The patient can be considered to have already failed six AEDs, so another agent would not be beneficial.

LoPinto-Khoury C, Sperling MR, Skidmore C, et al. Surgical outcome in PET-positive, MRI-negative patients with temporal lobe epilepsy. *Epilepsia* 2012;53(2):342-348.

30. **A.** Bilateral language representation has been reported in 0% to 30% of right-handed and 0% to 38% of left-handed individuals based on Wada test results. In the presence of a left hemisphere lesion before age 6, the incidence of atypical language representation in the right or bilateral hemispheres in right-handed individuals increases significantly. An intrahemispheric shift of language from the posterior to the anterior region has also been described in patients with early onset of temporal lobe epilepsy in the dominant hemisphere. Patients with bilateral language representation can have prolonged speech arrest after each injection as each hemisphere appears to depend on the other to support language ("bilateral dependent") or have no speech arrest after either injection because each

hemisphere appears capable of supporting language independently of the opposite side ("bilateral autonomous").

Benbadis SR. Intracarotid amobarbital test to define language lateralization. In: Luders HO, Comair YG, eds. *Epilepsy Surgery*. 2nd ed. Philadelphia, PA: Lippincott Williams & Wilkins; 2001:525-529.

31. **C.** An EEG is not needed to diagnose epilepsy in most cases. However, EEGs can help in certain situations, especially in cases that are medically intractable. The sensitivity of a single EEG is limited (about 20%–55%). Sensitivity is influenced by a number of factors: number of EEG studies (sensitivity plateaus to 80%–90% with four or more EEGs); EEG duration (the yield can increase to 90% with continuous monitoring for days); seizure frequency; timing in regard to recent seizure (higher yield within 24 hours of a seizure); antiepileptic drug therapy (valproate, levetiracetam, and ethosuximide reduce generalized IEDs, whereas diazepam and phenobarbital suppress IEDs after acute administration); epilepsy syndrome (higher yield with infantile spasms, Landau–Kleffner syndrome, and benign rolandic epilepsy; yield is also higher with temporal versus frontal lobe seizures); and the use of activation procedures.

Moeller J, Haider HA, Hirsch LJ. Electroencephalography (EEG) in the diagnosis of seizures and epilepsy. *UpToDate*. Updated February 12, 2015. http://www.uptodate.com/contents/electroencephalography-eeg-in-the-diagnosis-of-seizures-and-epilepsy. Accessed December 30, 2015.

32. **D.** More frequent seizures have been associated with a higher frequency of IEDs on an EEG. The first routine EEG is felt to have a sensitivity of 20% to 55%. Sensitivity is influenced by a number of factors: number of EEG studies (sensitivity plateaus to 80%–90% with four or more EEGs); EEG duration (the yield can increase to 90% with continuous monitoring for days); seizure frequency; timing in regard to recent seizure (higher yield within 24 hours of a seizure); antiepileptic drug (AED) therapy (valproate, levetiracetam, and ethosuximide reduce generalized IEDs, whereas diazepam and phenobarbital suppress IEDs after acute administration); epilepsy syndrome (higher yield with infantile spasms, Landau–Kleffner syndrome, and benign rolandic epilepsy; yield is also higher with temporal than frontal lobe seizures); and the use of activation procedures.

Moeller J, Haider HA, Hirsch LJ. Electroencephalography (EEG) in the diagnosis of seizures and epilepsy. *UpToDate*. Updated February 12, 2015. http://www.uptodate.com/contents/electroencephalography-eeg-in-the-diagnosis-of-seizures-and-epilepsy. Accessed December 30, 2015.

33. **C.** The HLA-B*1502 allele is strongly associated with an increased risk for CBZ-induced Stevens–Johnson syndrome (SJS) and toxic epidermal necrolysis (TEN), but not CBZ-induced hypersensitivity syndrome (HSS) or maculopapular exanthema (MPE). HLA-B*1502–positive patients have been reported in people of Asian descent only (including China, Thailand, Malaysia, and India). HLA-B*1502 is rare among Caucasians or Japanese. In contrast, HLA-A*3101 allele is associated with a risk of CBZ-induced HSS and MPE, and possibly SJS/TEN. HLA-A*3101 association has been shown in Caucasian, Japanese, Korean, Chinese, and patients of mixed origin. It should be noted that not all patients carrying either risk variant develop a hypersensitivity reaction, resulting in a relatively low positive predictive value for these genetic markers.

Amstutz U, Shear NH, Rieder MJ, et al. Recommendations for HLA-B*15:02 and HLA-A*31:01 genetic testing to reduce the risk of carbamazepine-induced hypersensitivity reactions. *Epilepsia* 2014; 55:496-506.

34. **A.** In a SPECT scan, gamma-ray detectors are used to image the distribution of the injected radiotracer in the brain. The commonly used radiotracers are hexamethyl-propylene-amine-oxime (HMPAO) or ethylene cysteine dimer (ECD) labeled with technetium-99 (99mTc). These radiotracers cross the blood–brain barrier and are about 80% extracted by brain during first pass. Inside the brain, they are metabolized to nondiffusible compounds, which accumulate in the brain 1 to 2 minutes after injection. Therefore, early radiotracer injection is imperative to capture the blood flow changes in the seizure focus during a seizure. Blood flow during the ictal phase can increase up to 300% in the seizure focus, which appears as an area of hyperperfusion in the ictal SPECT scan. An interictal SPECT scan, on the other hand, shows baseline perfusion and allows for a comparison to the ictal scan either visually or quantitatively. In the figure, there is an area of hyperperfusion (pinkish-white) in the left frontal region, consistent with the seizure focus. There is diffuse hypoperfusion in the left parietal region, which may indicate underlying widespread dysfunction. There is normal perfusion in the right hemisphere and in the occipital lobes.

Kumar A, Chugani HT. Application of PET and SPECT in pediatric epilepsy surgery. In: Cataltepe O, Jallo GI, eds. *Pediatric Epilepsy Surgery: Preoperative Assessment and Surgical Treatment.* New York, NY: Thieme; 2010:82-92.

35. **D.** Of the options listed, consistent unilateral lead-in as part of secondary bilateral synchrony best supports a focal seizure focus. Generalized IEDs tend to have primary bilateral synchrony with no consistent asymmetry or focal lead-in. Distinguishing between generalized and focal IEDs with secondary bilateral synchrony can sometimes be difficult, especially when the discharges are frontal. Generalized IEDs may show variable morphology such as spikes, polyspikes, spike waves, or sharp waves. The morphology could change between individual discharges. Focal IEDs too exhibit morphological variability, sometimes more so than the generalized IEDs. Generalized IEDs may present as focal fragments or show shifting predominance. When they occur as focal fragments, the generalized discharges tend to have variable locations, unlike focal IEDs, which tend to occur persistently in one area.

Pedley TA, Mendiratta A, Walczak TS. Seziures and epilepsy. In: Ebersole JS, Pedley TA, eds. *Current Practice of Clinical Electroencephalography.* 3rd ed. Philadelphia, PA: Lippincott Williams & Wilkins; 2003:506-587.

36. **C.** Depth electrode recordings of medial temporal lobe epilepsy (MTLE) often show a 1- to 2-Hz periodic spike pattern at seizure onset. This pattern can last for over a minute before evolving into continuous rhythmic activity. The periodic pattern is reported to be seen exclusively in the hippocampus and correlates with CA1 cell loss. In addition, a 10- to 16-Hz rhythmic pattern can be seen at seizure onset in MTLE. Prolonged interhippocampal propagation time (>20 seconds) has been correlated with excellent outcome after temporal lobectomy. Furthermore, interhippocampal propagation time has been shown to correlate inversely with CA4 cell counts. Because CA4 is the origin of the interhippocampal commissural connection, it is believed that CA4 cell loss results in prolongation of the seizure propagation process.

Spencer SS, Sperling MR, Shewmon DA, et al. Intracranial electrodes. In: Engel J, Jr, Pedley TA, eds. *Epilepsy: A Comprehensive Textbook.* 2nd ed. Philadelphia, PA: Lippincott Williams & Wilkins; 2008:1791-1815.

37. C. It is possible that patients with epilepsy are misdiagnosed with PNES. Based on video-EEG findings, it has been reported that the referring physician could wrongly label 57% of patients as PNES. Such a misdiagnosis is likely in patients with mesial frontal or parietal seizure onset. PNES always arise out of wakefulness. However, PNES can arise out of "preictal pseudosleep," where the patient appears to be asleep behaviorally but is actually awake. Waxing and waning behavior are characteristic of PNES. Although pelvic thrusting is typically seen with PNES, it has also been reported with frontal lobe seizures, and therefore, not very helpful in differentiating between the two. On the other hand, postictal weeping has been reported with both epileptic and nonepileptic seizures. Asynchronous shaking of extremities is common in PNES, but asymmetric tonic posturing of extremities is a feature of frontal lobe seizures, especially those that involve the supplementary sensorimotor area in the mesial frontal lobe. Of the given choices, this is most likely to support the diagnosis of an epileptic seizure.

Kanner AM, Lafrance WC, Jr, Betts T. Psychogenic non-epileptic seizures. In: Engel J, Jr, Pedley TA, eds. *Epilepsy: A Comprehensive Textbook*. 2nd ed. Philadelphia, PA: Lippincott Williams & Wilkins; 2008:2795-2810.

38. B. In temporal lobe seizures, ictal injection of SPECT radioisotope results in focal hyperperfusion in the mesial and anterolateral regions of the temporal lobe (at times, it may be seen only in the lateral temporal region in mesial temporal seizures). Within 1 to 5 minutes after the termination of the seizure, the lateral temporal region becomes intensely hypoperfused, whereas the mesial temporal region remains slightly hyperperfused. Over the next few minutes, the hypoperfusion becomes more diffuse in both the lateral and the mesial temporal regions. This pattern of conversion from ictal hyperperfusion to postictal hypoperfusion is called postictal switch. The degree of this hypoperfusion gradually decreases over the next 15 minutes until it reaches the interictal state of mild hypoperfusion. Late ictal or postictal injection may result in hyperperfusion in a region that is remote from the actual seizure focus, or hypoperfusion instead of hyperperfusion. If both intense hypoperfusion and hyperperfusion areas are seen in the same scan, it is likely that the hypoperfusion area represents the actual seizure focus and the hyperperfusion area represents propagated seizure activity. Based on this, it is likely that the scan will show marked hypoperfusion in the left lateral temporal region. If there had been seizure propagation, it is possible to see hyperperfusion remote from the temporal site (e.g., frontal lobe), but the seizure in this case did not show propagation outside the left temporal region based on the ictal EEG finding.

Kazemi NJ, O'Brien TJ, Cascino GD, et al. Single photon emission computed tomography. In: Engel J, Jr, Pedley TA, eds. *Epilepsy: A Comprehensive Textbook*. 2nd ed. Philadelphia, PA: Lippincott Williams & Wilkins; 2008:965-973.

39. C. Anterior/midtemporal spikes have >90% probability of being associated with seizures. Although IEDs are rare in healthy individuals (0.5% of healthy flight personnel), a higher rate has been seen in other populations (3.5%–6.5% of healthy children and 2%–2.6% of hospitalized adults with neurologic or psychiatric illness). The rate could be higher with inexperienced EEG readers who may be unaware of benign variants. Spikes and sharp waves seen during quiet sleep in a neonate are typically normal. In addition, central/midtemporal IEDs, generalized spike-wave discharges, and photoparoxysmal responses can be seen in individuals with genetic predisposition but no clinical seizures. Occipital spikes can be seen in blind individuals, especially those with congenital blindness.

Moeller J, Haider HA, Hirsch LJ. Electroencephalography (EEG) in the diagnosis of seizures and epilepsy. *UpToDate*. Updated February 12, 2015. Available at: http://www.uptodate.com/contents/electroencephalography-eeg-in-the-diagnosis-of-seizures-and-epilepsy. Accessed December 30, 2015.

40. **C.** The MRI shows increased FLAIR signal in bilateral hippocampii and left insula. These findings, along with the clinical presentation, suggest HSV encephalitis or limbic encephalitis. The absence of fever and negative HSV PCR are inconsistent with HSV encephalitis. Limbic encephalitis is more likely, and therefore, a paraneoplastic antibody panel would be the most appropriate test at this stage. Late onset of seizures and lack of family history argue against familial epilepsy syndromes, so genetic testing will not be helpful. Antithyroid antibodies (e.g., antithyroid peroxidase and antithyroglobulin antibodies) are seen in Hashimoto's encephalopathy, which is not likely in this case given the lack of response to steroids and the medial temporal abnormalities on the MRI. Brain biopsy may be necessary if other tests are unrevealing, but not at this stage.

Mocellin R, Walterfang M, Velakoulis D. Hashimoto's encephalopathy: epidemiology, pathogenesis and management. *CNS Drugs* 2007;21:799-811.

Toledano M, Pittock SJ. Autoimmune epilepsy. *Semin Neurol*. 2015;35:245-258.

41. **B.** The MRI shows a T2 hyperintense lesion with a cystic appearance in the right insula and posterior frontal region, consistent with a DNET. The lesion is located above the sylvian fissure. The seizure semiology is concordant with location of the lesion. DNET predominantly affects temporal and frontal lobes. They are characterized by low T1 and high T2 signal on the MRI, and have a bubbly, multicystic, and multinodular appearance. Contrast enhancement is seen in approximately 20% to 30% of patients. Tumor may be wedge shaped and extend to the ventricle. Surgical resection of DNET is associated with favorable outcome, with 70% of patients achieving Engel class I/II outcome. Long-term follow-up shows reduced seizure-free outcome, likely due to incomplete resection or the presence of cortical dysplasia beyond the resection area. On the other hand, gangliogliomas are 10 times more common in children, and mostly located in the temporal lobes. They are associated with epilepsy in 85% of cases. They appear as a solid mass (43%), cyst (5%), or mixed lesion (52%). They do not have the multicystic, bubbly appearance of the DNET. Contrast enhancement is seen in up to 60% of patients. Surgical resection is associated with the best outcome compared with other epilepsy-associated tumors, with 92% of patients achieving Engel class I/II outcome.

Raybaud C, Widjaja E. Structural brain imaging in epilepsy. In: Cataltepe O, Jallo GI (Eds). *Pediatric Epilepsy Surgery: Preoperative Assessment and Surgical Treatment*. New York, NY: Thieme; 2010:59-73.

42. **D.** The MRI shows increased FLAIR signal in the right hippocampus, which raises the possibility of right mesial temporal sclerosis (MTS). Increased T2 signal and hippocampal atrophy would be confirmatory. Based on the given MRI, this patient is most likely

to have seizures of mesial temporal lobe onset. Such seizures are typically characterized by rhythmic theta activity at onset so a 7-Hz rhythmic discharge in the right temporal region would be most concordant with the MRI finding. Widespread or nonlateralized irregular discharges (choices A and C) can be seen with neocortical temporal lobe seizures. Although right neocortical seizure onset is possible in this patient, the ictal patterns described in choices A and C are not concordant with the MRI finding. Ictal onset in the beta frequency range (choice B) is not seen on scalp recordings of temporal lobe seizures, but can be seen in depth electrode recordings.

Ebersole JS, Pacia SV. Localization of temporal lobe foci by ictal EEG patterns. *Epilepsia* 1996;37:386-399.

43. B. TLE predominantly affects verbal and nonverbal memories, which are tested by the logical memory and visual reproduction subsets of the Wechsler Memory Scale, Rey–Osterrieth Figure Test, California Verbal Learning Test, and Buschke Selective Reminding Test. Frontal lobe epilepsy predominantly causes executive dysfunction, which includes impairment in attention, problem solving, language, and psychomotor speed. The Stroop Color Word Test is a measure of attention, and therefore, it is the most appropriate test to evaluate frontal lobe function among the choices given. Other tests to assess frontal lobe function include the Wisconsin Card Sorting Test (for problem solving), Animal Fluency Test (for language), and Grooved Pegboard Test (for motor speed). Minnesota Multiphasic Personality Inventory is a broad measure of emotional distress and personality, and is not specific to frontal lobe function.

Renteria L, Pliskin NH. Neuropsychological evaluation in adults with epilepsy. In: Ettinger AB, Kanner AM, eds. *Psychiatric Issues in Epilepsy: A Practical Guide to Diagnosis and Treatment*. 2nd ed. Philadelphia, PA: Lippincott Williams & Wilkins; 2007:160-172.

44. A. Juvenile myoclonic epilepsy (JME) is one of the most common forms of epilepsy seen in adolescents. Age of onset is 12 to 18 years in 80% patients. Seizures occur predominantly on awakening, often in clusters, and are very sensitive to sleep deprivation, stress, fatigue, and alcohol. JME begins as sporadic myoclonic jerks before the patient develops GTCS. Therefore, obtaining a history of myoclonic jerks, especially in the mornings, is essential to establishing a syndromic diagnosis of JME. Typical absence seizures are reported to occur in 10% to 30% of patients with JME and are not a constant feature of this syndrome. Photosensitivity is present in 30% to 45% of patients during EEG, however, the prevalence of clinical photosensitivity in JME is lower. The EEG pattern consists of high amplitude generalized 4- to 6-Hz polyspike-wave complexes. Presence of staring spells and behavioral arrest indicate absence seizures and are more consistent with juvenile absence epilepsy. Positive family history of convulsive seizures upon awakening is suggestive of the syndrome of epilepsy with grand mal seizures on awakening. This syndrome is characterized by onset in the second decade with GTCS occurring exclusively or predominantly on awakening. Genetic predisposition is relatively frequent. Presence of body jerks or staring spells while playing video games is suggestive of photosensitive epilepsy, which can be seen in approximately 40% of JME patients and is a feature of other idiopathic generalized epilepsy syndromes and idiopathic occipital epilepsy syndrome as well.

Genton P, Gonzales-Sanchez M, Thomas P. Epilepsy with grand mal on awakening. In: Roger J, Bureau M, Dravet C, et al., eds. *Epileptic Syndromes in Infancy, Childhood and Adolescence*. 4th ed. Montrouge, France: John Libbey Eurotext; 2005:389-394.

Thomas P, Genton P, Gelisse P, et al. Juvenile myoclonic epilepsy. In: Roger J, Bureau M, Dravet C, et al., eds. *Epileptic Syndromes in Infancy, Childhood and Adolescence*. 4th ed. Montrouge, France: John Libbey Eurotext; 2005:367-388.

45. **A.** The figure shows seizure onset with a 5- to 6-Hz rhythmic discharge in the right temporal region, evolving into a slightly higher frequency activity within a few seconds. Such a lateralized, rhythmic activity on scalp EEG appearing within 30 seconds of clinical or electrographic seizures onset is seen in 80% of mesial temporal seizures. This pattern correctly predicts ipsilateral temporal seizure onset confirmed by depth electrodes. It has been reported that the presence of such a pattern requires synchronous recruitment of the adjacent inferolateral temporal neocortex. On the other hand, neocortical temporal seizures start with irregular, polymorphic 2- to 5-Hz lateralized or nonlateralized activity on scalp recordings, which is not the case in the figure. No ictal discharge is seen in the frontal or midline region to suggest extratemporal seizure onset.

Foldvary N. Ictal electroencephalography in neocortical epilepsy. In: Luders HO, Comair YG, eds. *Epilepsy Surgery*. 2nd ed. Philadelphia, PA: Lippincott Williams & Wilkins; 2001:431-439.

46. **D.** Visual-induced seizures are genetically determined. Seizures can be provoked by flickering lights or striped patterns. Only the generalized epileptiform discharges triggered by intermittent photic stimulation (IPS) are clearly linked to epilepsy. Such discharges are described in about 5% of patients with epilepsy. Pattern sensitivity is seen in about 70% of photosensitive patients tested with patterned IPS, but sensitivity to stationary striped patterns is seen in only about 30%. There are three types of sensitivity to IPS: patients with light-induced seizures only (pure photosensitivity); patients with photosensitivity and other seizure types; and asymptomatic individuals with isolated photosensitivity. In patients with photosensitivity, the seizures are generalized tonic–clonic in 55% to 84%, absences in 6% to 20%, focal in 2.5%, and myoclonic in 2% to 8% of patients. Nonpharmacologic measures for seizure prevention include monocular viewing, use of polarized glasses, and longer viewing distance (from the TV).

Panayiotopoulos CP. *A Clinical Guide to Epileptic Syndromes and Their Treatment*. Oxford, UK: Bladon Medical Publishing; 2002:214-239.

Zifkin B, Andermann F. Epilepsy with reflex seizures. In: Wyllie E, ed. *Wyllie's Treatment of Epilepsy: Principles and Practice*. 5th ed. Philadelphia, PA: Lippincott Williams & Wilkins; 2011:305-316.

47. **A.** The semiology of her seizure suggests right temporal onset with spread to the right frontal region (ipsilateral hand automatisms and contralateral hand stiffening, followed by contralateral facial twitching). Ictal EEG shows a theta-range (5 Hz) rhythmic discharge in the right anterior/midtemporal region. These findings are most consistent with a right mesial temporal (hippocampal) seizure onset. Neocortical temporal seizures usually have irregular delta activity at onset. Insular or lateral frontal onset is not likely based on semiology or EEG.

Foldvary N. Ictal electroencephalography in neocortical epilepsy. In: Luders HO, Comair YG, eds. *Epilepsy Surgery*. 2nd ed. Philadelphia, PA: Lippincott Williams & Wilkins; 2001:431-439.

48. D. Combined microelectrode and macroelectrode studies have shown that FRs are most likely to be recorded by single microelectrodes, but only rarely recorded by the adjacent macroelectrodes. This is felt to be due to spatial averaging of local field potentials by the relatively large surface area of the macroelectrodes leading to spatial undersampling of the focal high-frequency oscillations (HFOs). FRs increase in slow-wave sleep. Although the initial studies described FRs in the hippocampus, subsequent studies have shown that FRs occur in all brain regions. FRs occur independent of or are superimposed on the spikes.

Gotman J, Crone NE. High-frequency EEG activity. In: Schomer DL, Lopes da Silva FH, eds. *Niedermeyer's Electroencephalography: Basic Principles, Clinical Applications, and Related Fields.* 6th ed. Philadelphia, PA: Lippincott Williams & Wilkins; 2011:749-766.

49. B. Eye blinking is a feature of occipital lobe seizures, and therefore, suggests seizure onset in close proximity to the lesion (i.e., the occipital lobe) in this patient. Impaired consciousness and speech arrest suggest involvement of the temporal lobe, probably by infrasylvian spread, but they do not necessarily suggest seizure onset in the occipital lobe. Similarly, asymmetric tonic posturing suggests medial frontal involvement, probably by suprasylvian spread, but not necessarily seizure onset in the occipital lobe.

Foldvary N. Ictal electroencephalography in neocortical epilepsy. In: Luders HO, Comair YG, eds. *Epilepsy Surgery.* 2nd ed. Philadelphia, PA: Lippincott Williams & Wilkins; 2001:431-439.

50. A. Subjective memory impairment correlates best with mood. No significant relationship has been found between subjective memory and clinical factors such as age, gender, age of seizure onset, seizure type, seizure frequency, seizure localization, and number of anti-epileptic drugs.

Loring DW, Barr WB, Hamberger M, et al. Neuropsychology evaluation—adults. In: Engel J, Jr, Pedley TA, eds. *Epilepsy: A Comprehensive Textbook.* 2nd ed. Philadelphia, PA: Lippincott Williams & Wilkins; 2008:1057-1066.

51. D. MEG signals, like EEG, are produced mainly by pyramidal cells oriented perpendicular to the surface of the cortex. Unlike EEG, MEG signals are not attenuated or smeared by the skull, which is advantageous because this allows the use of the single-shell head model. The MEG field is more compact than the EEG field. MEG is sensitive to the component of the magnetic field that is perpendicular to the head surface. Such a field is generated by tangentially oriented current dipoles. In contrast, EEG measures both radial and tangential current dipoles.

Ebersole JS, Stefan H, Baumgartner C. Electroencephalographic and magnetoencephalographic source modeling. In: Engel J, Jr, Pedley TA, eds. *Epilepsy: A Comprehensive Textbook.* 2nd ed. Philadelphia, PA: Lippincott Williams & Wilkins; 2008:895-916.

52. C. The lower limb somatosensory evoked potential in the figure shows phase reversal of the cortical potential (P37) at contacts 23 and 31. Thus, these two contacts correspond to the primary sensory area, which is localized to the posterior aspect of the interhemispheric strip. However, from the information given, the seizure onset was noted in the anterior aspect of the strip, suggesting that the seizure onset zone might be in the primary motor area of the leg or in the supplementary motor area. Among the semiology options given, option C (left arm extension with slight flexion of the right arm) is concordant with supplementary motor area seizure onset. Throat discomfort suggests insular onset, whereas lip smacking and fumbling suggest temporal lobe onset.

Foldvary N. Ictal electroencephalography in neocortical epilepsy. In: Luders HO, Comair YG, eds. *Epilepsy Surgery*. 2nd ed. Philadelphia, PA: Lippincott Williams & Wilkins; 2001:431-439.

53. B. Seizures arising in the medial, basal, and interhemispheric cortical areas may not have an ictal EEG electrical discharge on the scalp. Thus, simple partial seizures of supplementary motor area onset that originate in the mesial frontal region may not have an ictal EEG correlate even if they may be associated with bilateral movements. Frontal lobe seizures associated with contralateral head and eye deviation have a lateral frontal localization, and are likely to be associated with an ictal discharge on the scalp. Clinical absence seizures are associated with generalized spike-wave discharges. Temporal lobe complex partial seizures are usually associated with clear ictal discharges although the ictal onset may not be well lateralized.

Sperling MR, Clancy RR. Ictal electroencephalogram. In: Engel J, Jr, Pedley TA, eds. *Epilepsy: A Comprehensive Textbook*. 2nd ed. Philadelphia, PA: Lippincott Williams & Wilkins; 2008:825-854.

54. C. History is an important part of establishing the diagnosis of epilepsy. In this patient, a history of seizures, characterized by prolonged hemiconvulsions followed by prolonged hemiplegia, raises the possibility of hemiconvulsions-hemiplegia epilepsy syndrome (HHES). This is characterized by onset in early childhood (5 months to 4 years) of prolonged hemiconvulsions followed by ipsilateral hemiplegia lasting more than 7 days. In 80% of patients, the hemiplegia becomes permanent. The initial episode usually occurs in the context of a febrile illness. There is high incidence of family history of febrile seizures. In 80% of patients, focal seizures of temporal, extratemporal, or multifocal origin appear within 1 to 5 years. Learning difficulties are common in these patients. Exam shows evidence of hemiplegia. MRI and CT scans show unilateral or bilateral edema initially followed by uniform hemiatrophy with recurrent seizures. Seizures are intractable to conventional drugs. Prevention and rapid acute treatment of febrile convulsions have resulted in a reduction in incidence of this syndrome.

Panayiotopoulos CP. *A Clinical Guide to Epileptic Syndromes and Their Treatment*. Oxford, UK: Bladon Medical Publishing; 2002:50-69.

55. A. The activity occurring after the arrow in the figure is the afterdischarge, which is an epileptic-like discharge that outlasts the stimulation. Afterdischarges consist of rhythmic, repetitive, high-amplitude spikes or spike-waves. They are usually subclinical, but may be associated with subtle clinical manifestations. Presence of an afterdischarge indicates spread of stimulation to surrounding cortical regions. Because of this, the results of stimulation are not reliable. Further stimulation at the site of afterdischarge may lead to a clinical seizure. In some cases, repeat stimulation at a reduced stimulus current may result in no further afterdischarges. Application of cold Ringer's lactate solution directly to the cortex can stop the seizure provoked by afterdischarge, which can be helpful during intraoperative mapping. Afterdischarges can be elicited from cortical regions that are not necessarily involved in seizure onset.

Nuwer M. Electrocorticography. In: Schomer DL, Lopes da Silva FH, eds. *Niedermeyer's Electroencephalography: Basic Principles, Clinical Applications, and Related Fields*. 6th ed. Philadelphia, PA: Lippincott Williams & Wilkins; 2011:715-724.

56. **B.** Ambulatory EEG monitoring provides preliminary data that can minimize inpatient monitoring. The monitoring can be done in the home surroundings, which are more natural. It is less expensive and does not involve inpatient hospitalization. However, detailed visual analysis of the behavior is not available. Temporal correlation of EEG findings and behavior is inaccurate, even when the event marker is used. Trained personnel cannot assess mental function and neurologic deficits during the events and the event description is reported by the observer. Events can be missed if observers are not constantly watching the patient, especially with young children or cognitively impaired patients who cannot self-report. Events can also be missed if the patient has no warning or memory of them.

American Clinical Neurophysiology Society. Guideline twelve: guidelines for long-term monitoring for epilepsy. http://www.acns.org/pdf/guidelines/Guideline-12.pdf. Accessed December 28, 2015.

57. **C.** Postoperative memory deficits are not consistently material-specific; while verbal memory deficits are strongly associated with dominant temporal lobe resections, visual memory deficits are inconsistent after nondominant temporal resections. Presence of mesial temporal sclerosis in the surgical hemisphere predicts a better memory outcome (not memory impairment) after temporal lobectomy. Impaired memory performance after contralateral injection during the Wada test also predicts a better memory outcome after temporal lobectomy. Better (not worse) preoperative memory correlates with worse memory after surgery regardless of the side of surgery.

Naugle RI. Subjective evaluation of postsurgical neuropsychological deficits. In: Luders HO, Comair YG, eds. *Epilepsy Surgery*. 2nd edition. Philadelphia, PA: Lippincott Williams & Wilkins; 2001:865-872.

58. **C.** The term DC EEG refers to a frequency response of the EEG with a minimum at 0 Hz. Although DC shifts are typically recorded using dedicated DC-coupled amplifiers, the routine alternating current (AC) amplifiers with long time constants (e.g., 10 seconds) can adequately record the DC shifts as well. DC shifts are best seen on intracranial recordings as they are relatively artifact free unlike scalp recordings. DC shifts are ultraslow fluctuations of the EEG signal. Therefore, they are best seen by decreasing the low-frequency filter (high pass filter) to significantly low values (e.g., 0.016 Hz). Several studies have shown that DC shifts occurring at seizure onset are useful in localizing the seizure onset zone.

Modur PN. High frequency oscillations and infraslow activity in epilepsy. *Ann Indian Acad Neurol*. 2014; 17(suppl 1):S99-S106.

Vanhatalo S, Voipio J, Kaila K. Infraslow EEG activity. In: Schomer DL, Lopes da Silva FH, eds. *Niedermeyer's Electroencephalography: Basic Principles, Clinical Applications, and Related Fields*. 6th ed. Philadelphia, PA: Lippincott Williams & Wilkins; 2011:741-747.

59. **A.** A biphasic pulse switches polarity at the midpoint of the pulse cycle. Biphasic stimulation is preferred for cortical stimulation in order to avoid a net electrical polarization at the electrode–cortex interface, which could alter the electrical sensitivity of the underlying cortex to subsequent pulses. Sites of afterdischarge occurrence during cortical stimulation do not correlate with pathology. Afterdischarges can arise from normal cortex. Stimulation threshold is higher in pathological cortex such that those regions are less likely to generate afterdischarges. Longer pulse trains are generally employed for

stimulation of the language cortex, whereas shorter trains are adequate for motor cortex mapping. Cortical stimulation typically localizes the language function to a 1- to 2-cm^2 area. Postoperative language deficits have been reported when the resection margins are within 2 cm of the language area.

Nuwer M. Electrocorticography. In: Schomer DL, Lopes da Silva FH, eds. *Niedermeyer's Electroencephalography: Basic Principles, Clinical Applications, and Related Fields*. 6th ed. Philadelphia, PA: Lippincott Williams & Wilkins; 2011:715-724.

60. **B.** MEG is more sensitive than EEG for the detection and delineation of the irritative zone in neocortical epilepsy involving superficial cortex. MEG is helpful in localizing the irritative zone in nonlesional epilepsy and in determining the relationship of epileptic activity with respect to large lesions. Thus, MEG can guide the placement of invasive electrodes. MEG can also provide unique information for reoperation as in this case. Here, the MEG dipoles suggest residual epileptic activity inferior to the prior resection cavity, whereas the EEG suggests a more distant and widespread epileptic focus probably involving the medial frontal region. MEG dipoles form tighter, anatomically more restricted clusters then EEG dipoles. Resection of the MEG-defined irritative zone has been shown to have prognostic implications for postoperative seizure control. Successful surgical outcome correlates with MEG dipoles being included in the surgical resection; small distance separating the center of the MEG dipole ellipsoid and the center of the resection volume; and homogeneous distribution of MEG dipole localizations.

Ebersole JS, Stefan H, Baumgartner C. Electroencephalographic and magnetoencephalographic source modeling. In: Engel J, Jr, Pedley TA, eds. *Epilepsy: A Comprehensive Textbook*. 2nd ed. Philadelphia, PA: Lippincott Williams & Wilkins; 2008:895-916.

61. **C.** TLE is characterized by impaired declarative memory, affecting both verbal and nonverbal components. Earlier age of seizure onset is associated with lower IQ and reduction of total brain volume. Furthermore, earlier age of seizure onset is associated with global memory impairment, whereas later age of seizure onset is associated with more focal and material-specific memory impairment. The neuropsychological deficits in TLE often extend beyond the temporal lobes, and involve the frontal lobes. This is attributed to the "nociferous cortex" effects, in which the ongoing seizures impair function at sites remote from the seizure focus.

Loring DW, Barr WB, Hamberger M, et al. Neuropsychology evaluation—adults. In: Engel J, Jr, Pedley TA, eds. *Epilepsy: A Comprehensive Textbook*. 2nd ed. Philadelphia, PA: Lippincott Williams & Wilkins; 2008:1057-1066.

62. **A.** Patients with high Wada memory scores after injection of the surgical hemisphere compared with injection of the nonsurgical hemisphere (i.e., correct asymmetry) demonstrate the least amount of memory decline postoperatively. Patients with low Wada memory scores after injection of the surgical hemisphere compared with injection of the nonsurgical hemisphere (i.e., reverse asymmetry) are considered to be at greatest risk of memory decline postoperatively. Equivalent memory scores after bilateral injections can also be associated with greater risk of memory decline postoperatively. If high memory scores are obtained after bilateral injections, the postoperative memory decline would be predicted based upon the memory performance of the surgical hemisphere (i.e., functional

adequacy). On the other hand, if low memory scores are obtained after bilateral injections, the postoperative memory decline would be predicted based upon the memory performance of the nonsurgical hemisphere (i.e., functional reserve). Thus, among the options given, option A has the least risk of postoperative memory decline.

Loring DW, Meador KJ. Wada testing to define hippocampal function. In: Luders HO, Comair YG, eds. *Epilepsy Surgery*. 2nd ed. Philadelphia, PA: Lippincott Williams & Wilkins; 2001:531-535.

63. **A.** The events described in this child are infantile spasms. There is high incidence (40%) of infantile spasms and hypsarrhythmia in tuberous sclerosis complex (TSC). About 50% to 85% of cardiac rhabdomyomas are associated with TSC and can be detected during routine prenatal ultrasound. More than 80% of TSC patients with cardiac rhabdomyomas are asymptomatic and often the tumors regress during infancy. Polyhydramnios is not specifically associated with tuberous sclerosis. Intrauterine hiccups are reported retrospectively by mothers of children diagnosed with NKH, which is an autosomal recessive disorder of glycine cleavage leading to abnormally high levels of glycine in the body fluids and tissues. Classic neonatal presentation of NKH is with hypotonia, apnea, myoclonic seizures, and lethargy. EEG often shows a burst-suppression pattern. Mortality in the neonatal period is high and survivors have mental retardation and neurological disability. Hypopigmented skin lesions are not a typical feature of NKH. Hypomelanosis of Ito is characterized by hypopigmented streaks or whorls of skin associated with seizures, learning disability, and scoliosis. Hydrocephalus detected prenatally is not a known feature of hypomelanosis of Ito, but white matter signal abnormalities may be seen.

Lyon G, Kolodny EH, Pastores GM. *Neurology of Hereditary Metabolic Diseases of Childhood*. 3rd ed. New York, NY: McGraw-Hill; 2006:9-64.

Olson L, Maria B. Hypomelanosis of Ito. In: Maria BL, ed. *Current Management in Child Neurology*. 3rd ed. Shelton, CT: BC Decker; 2005:476-478.

Tuberous sclerosis 1. http://www.omim.org/entry/191100. Accessed January 22, 2016.

64. **C.** Anti-NMDAR encephalitis has been well characterized in adults in whom the well-defined sequential clinical phases of the disease include the prodromal phase, psychotic phase, dysautonomic/central hypoventilation phase, and extrapyramidal dysfunction phase followed by recovery, which can be delayed or incomplete. The disease may occur either as an idiopathic form or as a paraneoplastic syndrome, the latter being commonly associated with ovarian teratomas (in about 60% of women). Pediatric cases are somewhat ill-defined and behave differently from adults. Younger patients present with speech problems, seizures, behavioral issues, and abnormal movements. The probability of finding a tumor is low. Antibodies against the NR1 subunit of NMDAR are thought to be pathogenic for this condition. CSF oligoclonal bands and IgG synthesis index are indicated in a demyelinating illness such as acute demyelinating encephalomyelitis, but this patient had a normal MRI, which is not consistent with a demyelinating illness. Viral encephalitis is often considered as an early presumptive diagnosis in patients with autoimmune and NMDAR encephalitis and CSF viral studies such as EBV titers are obtained. However, the evolution in this patient, with movement disorder and psychiatric symptoms, should raise the suspicion for autoimmune encephalitis such as NMDAR encephalitis. CSF and serum lactate are elevated in mitochondrial encephalomyelopathies that present with progressive central nervous system (CNS) and peripheral nervous system

signs, ophthalmoplegia, retinal degeneration, myoclonus and myoclonic epilepsy, ataxia, muscle weakness, MRI findings of basal ganglia abnormalities, white matter abnormalities, recurrent stroke-like episodes, and muscle biopsy findings of ragger red fibers.

Dalmau J, Lancaster E, Martinez-Hernandez E, et al. Clinical experience and laboratory investigations in patients with anti-NMDAR encephalitis. *Lancet Neurol.* 2011;10:63-74.

Lyon G, Kolodny EH, Pastores GM. *Neurology of Hereditary Metabolic Diseases of Childhood.* 3rd ed. New York, NY: McGraw-Hill; 2006:243-372.

65. **B.** The figure shows a train of polyspike-wave complexes occurring in a widespread manner in the LP grid in the 15-second segment. Such a pattern is described as a characteristic interictal finding in cortical dysplasia. The same pattern may become more continuous or be replaced by a more regular pattern at ictal onset, suggesting that it can be an ictal pattern as well. Postimplantation hemorrhage typically results in focal flattening or slowing of the EEG, which is not seen in the figure.

Spencer SS, Sperling MR, Shewmon DA, et al. Intracranial electrodes. In: Engel J, Jr, Pedley TA, eds. *Epilepsy: A Comprehensive Textbook.* 2nd ed. Philadelphia, PA: Lippincott Williams & Wilkins; 2008:1791-1815.

66. **A.** Extratemporal onset is faster (usually gamma) compared with temporal onset (usually beta). The initial fast EEG patterns tend to have focal distribution, and therefore, are felt to be closer to the seizure onset zone. On the other hand, slower EEG frequencies at onset (delta and theta) suggest propagation from a remote focus. Faster EEG onset frequencies (in the beta or gamma range) have been shown to correlate with class I and II outcomes. Periodic spiking at seizure onset has been correlated with the presence of hippocampal sclerosis and CA1 neuronal loss, which by itself suggests favorable postoperative outcome.

Seeck M, Schomer DL, Niedermeyer E. Intracranial monitoring: depth, subdural, and foramen ovale electrodes. In: Schomer DL, Lopes da Silva FH, eds. *Niedermeyer's Electroencephalography: Basic Principles, Clinical Applications, and Related Fields.* 6th ed. Philadelphia, PA: Lippincott Williams & Wilkins; 2011:677-713.

67. **D.** Ictal discharge is seen in the left hemisphere and midline leads. It is unclear if there is an ictal discharge in the right hemisphere because of prominent muscle artifact. Therefore, this seizure can be best regarded as nonlateralized. Focal onset refers to seizures that are confined to a single scalp electrode or to 1 to 2 intracranial electrode contacts. Regional onset refers to ictal onset confined to a single lobe with a spatial extent of several centimeters. Hemispheric onset is more widespread but lateralized, involving two or more lobes.

Sperling MR, Clancy RR. Ictal electroencephalogram. In: Engel J, Jr, Pedley TA, eds. *Epilepsy: A Comprehensive Textbook.* 2nd ed. Philadelphia, PA: Lippincott Williams & Wilkins; 2008:825-854.

68. **D.** Depth electrodes are indicated for recording from deep structures such as the amygdala and hippocampus, insula, sulcal cortex, and in the proximity of deep-seated lesions; they are not ideal for recording from the cortical surface even though some contacts may lie on the cortical surface. In contrast, subdural electrodes are best suited for recording from the cortical surface, including the dorsal, basal, and interhemispheric regions. Depth electrode placement is associated with a 1% to 4% risk of intracerebral hemorrhage. In one study, punctate hyperintensities along the electrode track were found in 41% of cases. It is common to see localized attenuation or slowing in depth

electrode contacts. This is often due to location of the electrode contact in the white matter. However, other causes such as hemorrhage, fiuid collection, and infection may need to be ruled out. There are reports of prolonged seizure freedom ("cure" of epilepsy) after a depth electrode study done under general anesthesia. The reason for this remains unclear.

Spencer SS, Sperling MR, Shewmon DA, et al. Intracranial electrodes. In: Engel J, Jr, Pedley TA, eds. *Epilepsy: A Comprehensive Textbook*. 2nd ed. Philadelphia, PA: Lippincott Williams & Wilkins; 2008:1791-1815.

69. **B.** Association of material-specific impairment of verbal memory is consistent in left TLE. Verbal memory correlates with the degree of neuronal loss and MRI-determined hippocampal volume. Impaired delayed recall suggests left mesial rather than neocortical temporal lobe dysfunction because mesial structures subserve consolidation and retrieval, whereas neocortical structures subserve content processing. Association of material-specific impairment of nonverbal (figural) memory is less consistent in right TLE. This is attributed to many factors including the bilateral distribution of nonverbal memory networks, covert verbalization of nonverbal stimuli during task performance, and the type of nonverbal testing employed. Because of this, using figural memory tests to infer right mesial temporal dysfunction can lead to false lateralization of seizure focus to the left side.

Loring DW, Barr WB, Hamberger M, et al. Neuropsychology evaluation—adults. In: Engel J, Jr, Pedley TA, eds. *Epilepsy: A Comprehensive Textbook*. 2nd ed. Philadelphia, PA: Lippincott Williams & Wilkins; 2008:1057-1066.

70. **D.** It has been shown that the seizure semiology and the EEG pattern at onset are similar after AED withdrawal. Secondary generalized seizures are more likely to occur after AED withdrawal, which needs to be kept in mind to provide appropriate and timely intervention, if necessary. Studies have shown that AED withdrawal results in occurrence of seizures, and that spiking increases as a result of increased seizures; however, spiking does not increase following AED withdrawal per se. In the absence of seizures, interictal spiking does not change. In fact, spiking could even decrease as a result of AED withdrawal in the absence of seizures.

Gotman J, Nuwer M, Emerson RG. Principles and techniques for long-term EEG recording (EMU, ICU, Ambulatory). In: Schomer DL, Lopes da Silva FH, eds. *Niedermeyer's Electroencephalography: Basic Principles, Clinical Applications, and Related Fields*. 6th ed. Philadelphia, PA: Lippincott Williams & Wilkins; 2011:725-740.

71. **A.** The MRI shows periventricular nodular heterotopia (PNH), also known as subependymal nodular heterotopia, which is most prominently seen along the right lateral ventricle in the figure. PNH is caused by the failure of neurons to migrate toward the cortical surface along the radial glia. Epilepsy occurs in nearly 80% of patients, with seizures starting in adolescence. Patients with PNH usually have normal neurologic development, and normal intellectual function or only mild intellectual disability. PNH can be associated with FILA (Filamin) mutation on chromosome Xq28. Because of the X-linked mutation, most pregnancies with male fetuses terminate in spontaneous abortions, making this condition to be preponderant in women.

Kuzniecky RI, Jackson GD. Malformations of cortical development. In: Engel J, Jr, Pedley TA, eds. *Epilepsy: A Comprehensive Textbook*. 2nd ed. Philadelphia, PA: Lippincott Williams & Wilkins; 2008:2575-2588.

72. **C.** In PNH, the seizures typically have temporal, temporo-occipital, or parieto-occipital semiology. In the given EEG, the seizure onset is rather widespread, involving the right parieto-occipito-temporal region. Accordingly, the semiology at seizure onset can include motionless staring, eye blinking, lip smacking, left-hand posturing, and right-hand automatisms (fumbling). Asymmetric bilateral upper extremity posturing at seizure onset suggests onset in the medial frontal lobe (i.e., supplementary motor area), which is not supported by the findings in the given EEG, and therefore, least likely to be seen.

Kuzniecky RI, Jackson GD. Malformations of cortical development. In: Engel J, Jr, Pedley TA, eds. *Epilepsy: A Comprehensive Textbook.* 2nd ed. Philadelphia, PA: Lippincott Williams & Wilkins; 2008:2575-2588.

73. **A.** This child has features of absence seizures along with mild developmental delay and failure to respond to the common medications to treat absence seizures. This raises the suspicion for Glut1 deficiency syndrome. This is an autosomal-dominant disorder, which results from a defect in the Glut1 glucose transporter causing decreased glucose concentration in the central nervous system. Ninety percent of cases result from a de novo mutation in the SLC2A1 gene on chromosome 1. Hypoglycorrhachia (CSF glucose <40 mg/dL) and low CSF lactate are diagnostic of the disorder. The most severe "classic" phenotype comprises infantile-onset epileptic encephalopathy associated with delayed development, acquired microcephaly, motor incoordination, and spasticity. Onset of seizures, usually characterized by apneic episodes, staring, and episodic eye movements, occurs within the first 4 months of life. Other paroxysmal findings include intermittent ataxia, confusion, lethargy, sleep disturbance, and headache. Varying degrees of cognitive impairment are seen, ranging from learning disabilities to severe mental retardation. Ten percent of early-onset absence epilepsy, before age 4 years, could be due to Glut1 deficiency syndrome. Although PET scan can show distinctive findings of diffuse hypometabolism of the cerebral cortex and regional hypometabolism of the cerebellum and thalamus in patients with Glut1 deficiency, its sensitivity and specificity are not established. Mutations in the ARX gene can cause X-linked infantile spasm syndrome, which begins in the first year of life. This syndrome is also associated with intellectual disability. ARX mutations are also associated with focal dystonia (Partington syndrome) and X-linked lissencephaly with abnormal genitalia. Ring chromosome 20 syndrome is characterized by cognitive impairment, behavior disorders, and epilepsy, without specific dysmorphic features. Another characteristic feature is frequent episodes of nonconvulsive status epilepticus associated with diffuse low rhythmic discharges. The clinical features in this child are not consistent with the latter two conditions.

Gobbi G, Genton P, Pini A, et al. Epilepsies and chromosomal disorders. In: Roger J, Bureau M, Dravet C, et al., eds. *Epileptic Syndromes in Infancy, Childhood and Adolescence.* 4th ed. Montrouge, France: John Libbey Eurotext; 2005:467-492.

Sherr EH. The ARX story (epilepsy, mental retardation, autism, and cerebral malformations): one gene leads to many phenotypes. *Curr Opin Pediatr.* 2003;15:567-571.

Wang D, Pascual JM, De Vivo D. Glucose transporter type 1 deficiency syndrome. In: Pagon RA, Adam MP, Ardinger HH, et al., eds. *GeneReviews* [Internet]. Seattle, WA: University of Washington; 2015. http://www.ncbi.nlm.nih.gov/books/NBK1430. Accessed December 14, 2015.

74. **B.** The term HFOs refers to EEG activity >70 Hz. The 80- to 200-Hz activity is often referred to as ripples, whereas the 250- to 500-Hz activity is referred to as fast ripples. The sampling rate determines the recording of high frequencies. Theoretically, the maximum frequency of the oscillations that can be evaluated corresponds to one half of the sampling rate. However, because of the limitations of the amplifiers used in the EEG systems, the maximum frequency that can be clearly evaluated tends to be roughly one third of the sampling rate such that a sampling rate of 1,000 Hz allows evaluation of activity up to 333 Hz. Accordingly, a sampling rate of 1,000 Hz (preferably 2,000 Hz) is recommended for recording the HFOs. To evaluate the HFOs, both the LFF and HFF should be set to values higher than usual, that is, LFF >50 Hz and HFF ≥600 Hz. Although the initial studies recorded HFOs using microelectrodes, more recent studies have shown that HFOs can be recorded using clinical depth and subdural electrodes; so microelectrode recordings are not absolutely necessary for evaluating the HFOs.

Gotman J, Crone NE. High-frequency EEG activity. In: Schomer DL, Lopes da Silva FH, eds. *Niedermeyer's Electroencephalography: Basic Principles, Clinical Applications, and Related Fields*. 6th ed. Philadelphia, PA: Lippincott Williams & Wilkins; 2011:749-766.

Modur PN. High frequency oscillations and infraslow activity in epilepsy. *Ann Indian Acad Neurol.* 2014;17(suppl 1):S99-S106.

75. **C.** MRS is a noninvasive method of measuring cerebral metabolites and some neurotransmitters using proton imaging. Patients with epilepsy show reduction of NAA, elevation of choline, elevation of CR, and reduction of NAA/(choline+CR) ratio in the epileptogenic foci in the temporal lobe. Reduction of NAA/(choline+CR) ratio can be seen bilaterally in patients with unilateral temporal lobe foci. NAA is located primarily within the neurons and precursor cells, and therefore, a reduction of the NAA signal is usually regarded as indicating loss or dysfunction of neurons. The concentrations of CR, phosphocreatine, and choline are much higher in oligodendrocytes and astrocytes than in neurons, and therefore, the increased signal from these compounds may reflect gliosis. Postictal rise (not reduction) in lactate has been noted in the ipsilateral temporal lobe for up to 6.5 hours in patients with unilateral temporal lobe epilepsy, and this may be useful for lateralizing seizure foci.

Duncan JS. Imaging and epilepsy. *Brain.* 1997;120:339-377.

76. **D.** Based on the brief history given, this boy seems to have primary reading epilepsy (PRE), which is an idiopathic reflex epilepsy syndrome preferentially related to abnormalities in the dominant temporo-parietal region or other regions functionally involved in reading. It starts around 12 to 19 years of age and has male preponderance. In PRE, the seizures are triggered by reading aloud or silently. Seizure semiology consists of myoclonic jerks of jaw and mouth muscles. They are described as clicking sensations that occur a few minutes or hours after reading. Reading aloud and reading difficult material are particularly provocative. Continued reading results in spread of the activity to the trunk and limb muscles, and eventually, a generalized tonic–clonic seizure occurs. In 25% of patients, seizures can be triggered by talking (especially when fast or argumentative), writing, reading music, or chewing. Ictal EEG consists of bursts of bilateral sharp waves with left temporo-parietal predominance. Positive family history is noted, with similar

symptoms in identical twins and first-degree relatives. Prognosis is good with favorable response to antiepileptic drugs.

Panayiotopoulos CP. *A Clinical Guide to Epileptic Syndromes and Their Treatment.* Oxford, UK: Bladon Medical Publishing; 2002:214-239.

77. **A.** Based on the information given, Angelman syndrome (AS) needs to be considered as a diagnostic possibility. AS is caused by deletion in chromosome 15q11.2-q13: in about 70% of affected patients, this is due to de novo maternal deletions; in 2%, there is paternal uniparental disomy; in 3%, there is an imprinting defect; and in a subset of the remaining 25%, there are UBE3A mutations. AS is characterized by severe developmental delay, microcephaly, prominent jaw, open mouth, speech impairment, ataxia, jerky limb movements, and inappropriate happy demeanor, with laughing, smiling, and excitability. Epilepsy, often severe and refractory, is present in 85% of patients within the first 3 years of life. Most frequent types are atypical absences, generalized tonic–clonic, atonic, or myoclonic seizures. EEG findings include high-amplitude, slow spike-wave discharges. Both MECP2 and CDKL5 mutations on X chromosome cause Rett syndrome, with the majority of cases resulting from MECP2 mutation. Rett syndrome is seen in females as the mutation is lethal in hemizygous males. Rett syndrome is characterized by normal development and head circumference until 6 months of age, followed by loss of speech and purposeful hand use, along with microcephaly, autism, ataxia, stereotypic hand movements, seizures, and breathing irregularities. ARX mutation causes multiple phenotypes including X-linked early infantile encephalopathy and X-linked lissencephaly, both associated with seizures; the former is characterized by infantile spasms, whereas the latter has abnormal findings on MRI, none of which is described in this patient.

OMIM Entry #105830. Angelman syndrome [updated 8/4/2015]. http://www.omim.org/entry/105830 Accessed December 28, 2015.

OMIM Entry #300382. Aristaless-related homeobox, X-linked [updated 10/30/2013]. http://www.omim.org/entry/300382. Accessed December 28, 2015.

Weaving LS, Ellaway CJ, Gecz J, et al. Rett syndrome: clinical review and genetic update. *J Med Genet.* 2005;42:1-7.

78. **B.** Cortical resection in the perisylvian region, within 2 cm of the stimulation-defined language area, is likely to result in permanent language deficit. Resection of the dominant supplementary motor area can result in acute profound speech and language deficit, but it resolves without permanent deficit. Resection of the language area localized to the basal temporal region has not been shown to result in permanent language deficits.

Jayakar P, Lesser RP. Extraoperative functional mapping. In: Engel J, Jr, Pedley TA, eds. *Epilepsy: A Comprehensive Textbook.* 2nd ed. Philadelphia, PA: Lippincott Williams & Wilkins; 2008:1851-1858.

Nuwer M. Electrocorticography. In: Schomer DL, Lopes da Silva FH, eds. *Niedermeyer's Electroencephalography: Basic Principles, Clinical Applications, and Related Fields.* 6th ed. Philadelphia, PA: Lippincott Williams & Wilkins; 2011:715-724.

79. **C.** Most cases of Panayiotopoulos syndrome begin around 3 to 6 years of age, but the range of onset is 1 to 14 years. Panayiotopoulos syndrome is frequently mistaken for nonepileptic disorders due to unusual ictal manifestations that are prolonged, with recurrent vomiting, pallor, pupillary changes, flaccidity, and unresponsiveness. Seizures may end in hemiconvulsion or generalized convulsion. Although occurrence of long trains of

occipital sharp waves, which are abolished by central fixation, has been emphasized in the past, the presence of multifocal spike foci, activated by sleep, is a characteristic finding. Prognosis is favorable, with one-third of the patients having a single seizure and 5% to 10% of patients having >10 seizures. Duration of active seizures is short and remission occurs within 1 to 2 years from onset. Thus, prophylactic medication is best reserved for children whose seizures are frequent and disabling.

Covanis A, Ferrie CD, Koutromanidis M, et al. Panayiotopoulos syndrome and Gastaut type idiopathic childhood occipital epilepsy. In: Roger J, Bureau M, Dravet C, et al., eds. *Epileptic Syndromes in Infancy, Childhood and Adolescence*. 4th ed. Montrouge, France: John Libbey Eurotext; 2005:227-253.

80. **D.** Interictal FDG-PET usually demonstrates hypometabolism of one or both temporal lobes. When both lobes are affected, one lobe tends to show more severe hypometabolism. This asymmetric hypometabolism is seen in unilateral MTLE, in >70% of patients with visual qualitative analysis, and in >90% of patients with quantitative analysis. Hypometabolism typically represents an area of cerebral dysfunction and is usually seen interictally. A single seizure could lead to relative hypermetabolism, but this is not a typical finding. Modern scans show greater mesial temporal than lateral temporal hypometabolism of the affected temporal lobe. The opposite finding was noted in older PET scans, and this is felt to be caused by partial volume averaging of the severely hypometabolic amygdala and hippocampus together with the less hypometabolic basal temporal cortex. Hypometabolism tends to be diffuse, and often involves the ipsilateral frontal, parietal, thalamic, or basal ganglia, but occipital hypometabolism is rare. Among the extratemporal sites, the ipsilateral thalamus is most likely to demonstrate hypometabolism in MTLE.

Henry TR, Chugani HT. Positron emission tomography. In: Engel J, Jr, Pedley TA, eds. *Epilepsy: A Comprehensive Textbook*. 2nd ed. Philadelphia, PA: Lippincott Williams & Wilkins; 2008:945-964.

4

Treatment of Seizures and Epilepsy

QUESTIONS

1. A 20-year-old female with no risk factors for epilepsy presents with a 6-year history of refractory epilepsy, suspected to be of left temporal onset based on noninvasive evaluation. She undergoes invasive monitoring with a combined left hippocampal depth electrode inserted via a parasagittal approach along with left convexity subdural grid and strips. The following figure shows EEG recording at seizure onset (filter: 1.6–70 Hz). The marker "CO" corresponds to clinical onset. Subdural contacts are as follows: LT41–LT48 are on the superior temporal gyrus (LT41 anterior, LT48 posterior); ST1–ST8 are on the middle temporal gyrus (ST1 anterior, ST8 posterior); ST9–ST16 are on the inferior temporal gyrus (ST9 anterior, ST16 posterior); LD is placed in the hippocampus (LD1 is in the amygdala, LD6 is in the posterior hippocampus). Which of the following statements best describes the seizure onset?

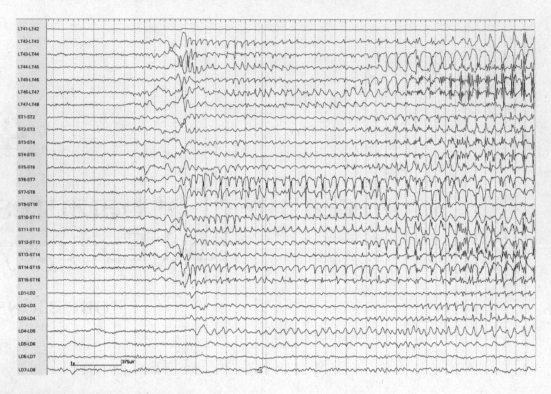

A. Focal in the hippocampus
B. Focal in the parahippocampal gyrus
C. Regional in the temporal neocortex
D. Nonlocalized

2. The localization of electrical seizure onset shown in the figure in Question 1 is LEAST likely to include which of the following features as part of the semiology at seizure onset?

A. Cold sensation all over the body
B. Oroalimentary automatisms
C. Right facial twitching
D. Well-formed speech

3. The patient described in Question 1 has normal MRI and positron emission tomography (PET) scans. The neuropsychological testing was nonlateralizing. The Wada test showed left hemispheric language and memory dominance. Functional stimulation mapping showed impaired naming and reading 1-cm posterior to LT48. Which of the following surgical interventions would be most appropriate in this patient?

A. Standard anteromedial temporal resection
B. Selective amygdalo-hippocampectomy
C. Neocortical temporal resection (corticectomy)
D. Multiple subpial transections

4. A 10-year-old boy presents with history of seizures since age 3 years. They are characterized by a visual aura of geometric shapes, followed by tonic eye and head deviation to the right, with occasional secondary generalization. He also has atonic and absence seizures. His seizures have been intractable to multiple antiepileptic drugs. Interictal scalp EEG showed multifocal spikes in the bilateral temporal and midline/centro-parietal regions. There were generalized polyspikes during sleep. Ictal EEG showed seizure onset in the bilateral frontal and midline/centro-parietal regions. An axial T2 image of his MRI is seen in the following figure. All of the following are appropriate evaluations at this stage EXCEPT:

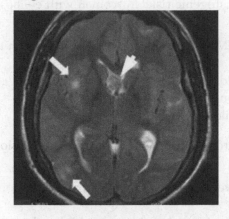

A. Wood's lamp examination
B. Genetic testing
C. Magnetoencephalography (MEG)
D. Biopsy of the lesion

5. The patient in Question 4 undergoes an ictal SPECT scan, as shown in the following figure. Which of the following decisions is most appropriate at this stage?

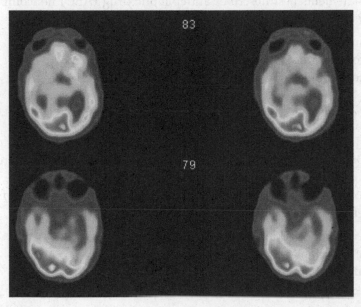

A. Proceed with intracranial EEG monitoring with subdural strips over bilateral lateral fronto-temporal regions, and medial frontal regions, and a subdural grid over the right parieto-occipital region

B. Proceed with intracranial EEG monitoring with subdural grid placement over the right parieto-occipital region

C. The patient is not an epilepsy surgery candidate due to multifocal spikes and poly-spikes interictally

D. The patient is not an epilepsy surgery candidate due to multiple tubers

6. Which of the following is true regarding the teratogenic risks in women with epilepsy (WWE)?

A. Risk of major congenital malformations (MCM) is 10 times higher in infants born to WWE compared with those without epilepsy

B. Risk of MCM is about 17% with antiepileptic drug (AED) polytherapy

C. Risk of MCM is highest for phenobarbital monotherapy

D. The most common MCM is spina bifida in children born to WWE

7. Which of the following statements is true regarding folic acid supplementation during pregnancy?

A. Benefits of folic acid supplementation in preventing major congenital malformations (MCMs) has been proven in studies

B. Folate metabolism as the mechanism for increased risk of MCM in children born to women taking antiepileptic drugs (AEDs) has been confirmed in multiple studies

C. Folic acid supplementation of at least 0.4 mg/day in the preconceptional period is recommended for all women with epilepsy (WWE) who are on AEDs

D. WWE who are on valproic acid should receive 4-mg folic acid supplementation daily as this has been shown to decrease the risk of neural tube defects

8. Which of the following statements best describes antiepileptic drug (AED) noncompliance in epilepsy patients?

A. In adults, noncompliance can be as high as 70%

B. In children, socioeconomic status is the major predictor of noncompliance

C. Mean compliance rate declines significantly after switching from a once-a-day to twice-a-day regimen

D. Compliance rate has no relation to clinic visits

9. A 22-year-old male with suspected juvenile myoclonic epilepsy is maintained on valproate monotherapy. Because of a recent increase in generalized tonic–clonic seizures, his neurologist decides to add carbamazepine and titrate it up to the target dose of 600 mg/day over 1 week. When the patient is seen in follow-up 6 weeks after initiation of carbamazepine, all of the following can be expected EXCEPT:

A. Decreased frequency of generalized tonic–clonic seizures

B. Increased frequency of myoclonic seizures

C. Supratherapeutic serum level of carbamazepine

D. Low serum sodium

10. Which of the following statements is true regarding carbamazepine?

  A. It has no active metabolites
  B. It has less efficacy than valproate in controlling partial seizures
  C. It is better tolerated than lamotrigine in the elderly
  D. It is more likely to cause rash in patients of Asian descent

11. A 30-year-old woman, seizure free for 18 months on lamotrigine monotherapy, wants to plan pregnancy in the next 6 months. In counseling her regarding what to expect during pregnancy, all of the following statements are true EXCEPT:

  A. She has >80% chance of remaining seizure free during pregnancy
  B. Her chances of having status epilepticus (SE) during pregnancy is <2%
  C. She needs a minimum folic acid supplementation of 4 mg/day
  D. Her lamotrigine level should be monitored carefully during pregnancy

12. A 50-year-old male, previously healthy, was admitted with new-onset focal seizures of 3 weeks duration. His seizures were characterized by motionless staring, unresponsiveness, and left facial twitching. He continued to have 5 to 6 seizures per day despite being on high doses of phenytoin, levetiracetam, and lacosamide administered intravenously. Over the past 2 weeks, he was noted to have increasing memory loss, agitation, auditory hallucinations, and confusion. Continuous video-EEG monitoring showed right temporo-occipital periodic lateralized epileptiform discharges (PLEDs) and seizures of right temporal onset. Cerebrospinal fluid (CSF) analysis was normal. Polymerase chain reaction (PCR) test for herpes simplex virus (HSV) was negative. A coronal T2 image of his MRI is shown. Which of the following interventions would be appropriate in this patient?

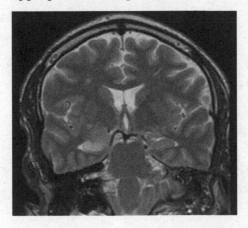

  A. Phenobarbital
  B. Rituximab
  C. Propofol-induced burst suppression
  D. Right temporal lobe biopsy

13. Which of the following is true regarding perampanel?

    A. It acts by opening the potassium channels
    B. It is metabolized by the cytochrome P450 system
    C. It has a half-life of 20 hours
    D. It has no effect on oral contraceptives

14. Which of the following visual disturbances is associated with vigabatrin treatment?

    A. Irreversible homonymous hemianopia
    B. Irreversible, bilateral, concentric peripheral visual field constriction
    C. Irreversible, bilateral, bull's eye maculopathy
    D. Reversible, bilateral, concentric peripheral visual field constriction

15. Which of the following statements is true regarding the 2012 American Academy of Neurology's practice parameters for the treatment of infantile spasms?

    A. Low-dose adrenocorticotropic hormone (ACTH) is probably as effective as high-dose ACTH
    B. Vigabatrin (VGB) is more effective than ACTH for short-term treatment
    C. VGB should be preferred over hormonal therapy in infants with cryptogenic infantile spasms
    D. Lag time to treatment has no impact on long-term developmental outcome

16. Which of the following is NOT a risk factor for development of valproate-induced hyperammonemic encephalopathy?

    A. Concomitant phenobarbital therapy
    B. Protein-deficient diet
    C. Urea cycle defects
    D. Carnitine deficiency

17. A patient with epilepsy is receiving carbamazepine monotherapy. What can be expected in terms of drug levels and metabolism when primidone is added?

    A. Phenobarbital clearance may decrease
    B. Phenobarbital level may increase
    C. Primidone level may increase
    D. None of the above

18. Which of the following can occur as a complication of the ketogenic diet?

    A. Hypercoagulability
    B. Obesity
    C. Hypertrophic cardiomyopathy
    D. Optic neuropathy

19. A ketogenic diet at a ratio of 4:1 represents which of the following?

    A. Proportion of carbohydrates is 4 in relationship to 1 of fat

    B. Proportion of fats is 4 in relationship to 1 of carbohydrates

    C. Proportion of fats is 4 in relationship to 1 of protein and carbohydrates combined

    D. Proportion of protein and carbohydrates combined is 4 in relationship to 1 of fats

20. What is the incidence of electro-clinical dissociation or subclinical seizures in neonates during continuous EEG monitoring after administration of antiepileptic drugs (AEDs)?

    A. 10% to 20%

    B. 30% to 40%

    C. 50% to 60%

    D. 70% to 80%

21. A 2-year-old boy with intractable epilepsy is started on the ketogenic diet, resulting in a dramatic improvement in seizure control by more than 70%. However, for the past 2 days, he has had an increase in seizures. Which of the following scenarios could be the most likely reason for this?

    A. He has an ear infection

    B. He ate seven macadamia nuts instead of three

    C. His caretaker applied a suntan lotion

    D. Any of the above

22. Which of the following is true regarding the use of antiepileptic drugs (AEDs) and contraception in women with epilepsy (WWE)?

    A. Estrogen-containing oral contraceptives can worsen seizure control

    B. Valproate can reduce the efficacy of oral contraceptives

    C. Oral contraceptives can significantly reduce lamotrigine level

    D. Efficacy of transdermal patches is not affected by AEDs

23. The strategies that can be routinely recommended to enhance compliance to antiepileptic drug (AED) therapy in new-onset epilepsy include all of the following EXCEPT:

    A. Provide a microelectronic monitoring system for patients who live alone

    B. Select once-a-day or twice-a-day regimen, if possible

    C. Instruct the patient to take the daytime missed dose at bedtime

    D. Instruct the patient to take the medication around meal times

24. Which of the following adverse effects are associated with the use of felbamate?

    A. Thrombocytopenia and liver failure

    B. Aplastic anemia and liver failure

    C. Aplastic anemia and renal failure

    D. Hemolytic anemia and liver failure

25. Treatment of status epilepticus (SE) can be divided into categories, which include emergent initial treatment and urgent control treatment. Guidelines for the urgent control treatment of SE include all of the following statements EXCEPT:

A. It is needed for patients whose seizures have stopped after benzodiazepine emergent initial treatment in order to achieve rapid therapeutic antiepileptic drug (AED) levels
B. It is needed for patients who fail emergent initial treatment in order to stop SE
C. It is not needed if emergent initial treatment results in termination of SE
D. It is not needed if the immediate cause of SE is known and definitively corrected

26. A 12-year-old boy with chronic renal disease presents with status epilepticus (SE) that is refractory to treatment with benzodiazepines, fosphenytoin, phenobarbital, and valproic acid. He is started on an intravenous (IV) pentobarbital drip and burst suppression is achieved on EEG. About 24 hours later, the seizures recur, and he is found to have hypotension, arrhythmia, and increased anion gap. Which of the following statements is most accurate regarding the diagnosis and course of action?

A. He has sepsis and needs broad-spectrum antimicrobial coverage
B. He has propylene glycol toxicity and needs discontinuation of pentobarbital
C. He has worsening SE and needs an increase in the pentobarbital drip rate
D. He has worsening SE and needs a change to another treatment agent such as propofol

27. The adverse effects of medications used to treat refractory status epilepticus (RSE) include all of the following EXCEPT:

A. Pentobarbital can cause cardiac instability and hypotension
B. Midazolam can cause hyperammonemia
C. Propofol can cause metabolic acidosis and rhabdomyolysis
D. Ketamine can cause cardiac arrhythmias

28. Which of the following statements best describes the evidence for effectiveness of resective epilepsy surgery in terms of seizure outcome?

A. About two thirds of patients become free of disabling seizures after anteromedial temporal resection
B. About three fourths of patients become free of disabling seizures after anteromedial temporal resection
C. About one third of patients become free of disabling seizures after localized neocortical resection
D. About two thirds of patients become free of disabling seizures after localized neocortical resection

29. Neuropsychological outcome after anteromedial temporal lobectomy can be summarized by all of the following statements EXCEPT:

    A. Above-average preoperative memory can be associated with postoperative decline after dominant temporal lobectomy
    B. Verbal memory improves after nondominant temporal lobectomy
    C. Visuospatial memory improves after dominant temporal lobectomy
    D. Naming declines after dominant temporal lobectomy

30. Determination of postoperative seizure outcome using the International League Against Epilepsy (ILAE) classification system takes into account all of the following EXCEPT:

    A. It requires specification of a 12-month preoperative baseline period
    B. It distinguishes complete seizure freedom
    C. It distinguishes postoperative seizure worsening
    D. It defines outcome classes based on both absolute and relative number of seizures

31. Which of the following statements is true regarding treatment for refractory status epilepticus (RSE)?

    A. Pentobarbital is more effective than midazolam or propofol in the short-term seizure control
    B. Incidence of breakthrough seizures is similar regardless of titration of the agent to seizure suppression or EEG background suppression
    C. Propofol is associated with a higher rate of hypotension than pentobarbital
    D. Mortality rate is significantly higher with pentobarbital

32. Which of the following is true regarding the use of lorazepam and diazepam in treating seizures?

    A. Lorazepam is more lipophilic than diazepam
    B. Lorazepam has longer antiseizure effect than diazepam
    C. Lorazepam redistributes to fatty tissues faster than diazepam
    D. Lorazepam has quicker onset of action in the brain than diazepam

33. A 70-year-old woman with newly diagnosed epilepsy secondary to right middle cerebral artery infarction was started on oxcarbazepine. The initial dose was 300 mg/day, and it was titrated up to 2,400 mg/day over 1 week because of breakthrough seizures. Routine lab tests at her 4-week appointment showed serum sodium level of 126 mEq/L. She was also receiving treatment with aspirin and losartan for hypertension. Possible contributing factors to her hyponatremia include all of the following EXCEPT:

    A. Patient's age
    B. Concomitant treatment with losartan
    C. Titration schedule of oxcarbazepine
    D. Dose of oxcarbazepine

34. Administration of oxcarbazepine can be associated with:

A. Autoinduction
B. No significant change in efficacy of oral contraceptives
C. Increase in plasma phenytoin level
D. No significant change in plasma valproic acid level

35. Which of the following statements best describes the properties of eslicarbazepine?

A. It stabilizes the inactivated state of the sodium channels
B. It has no active metabolites
C. It does not affect the efficacy of oral contraceptives
D. It reduces the efficacy of warfarin

36. The ketogenic diet is the treatment of choice for which of the following inborn errors of metabolism?

A. Carnitine palmitoyl transferase deficiency
B. Very long chain acyl CoA dehydrogenase deficiency
C. Pyruvate dehydrogenase (PDH) deficiency
D. Acute intermittent porphyria

37. According to the practice parameter put forth by the American Academy of Neurology (AAN), which of the following antiepileptic drugs transfers into breast milk in clinically significant amounts?

A. Phenytoin
B. Phenobarbital
C. Carbamazepine
D. Levetiracetam

38. According to the practice parameter put forth by the American Academy of Neurology (AAN), which of the following statements is true regarding pregnancy in women with epilepsy (WWE) taking antiepileptic drugs?

A. There is higher risk of cesarean delivery
B. There is higher risk of late pregnancy bleeding
C. There is higher risk of premature labor and delivery in WWE who smoke
D. Seizure freedom prior to pregnancy is not associated with seizure freedom during pregnancy

39. Which of the following statements is true regarding the interaction between hormones and epilepsy?

A. Progesterone and its metabolites are proconvulsant
B. Estrogens are both proconvulsant and anticonvulsant
C. Androgens are mainly proconvulsant
D. Progesterone supplement may benefit women whose seizures show perimenstrual exacerbation

40. Topiramate (TPM) therapy is associated with an increased risk for kidney stones. Which of the following is true regarding this?

    A. TPM is associated with an increase in urinary citrate, leading to increased risk of stone formation

    B. TPM is associated with a decrease in urinary citrate, leading to increased risk of stone formation

    C. TPM is associated with an alkaline urine, leading to increased risk of stone formation

    D. TPM inhibits carbonic anhydrase, making alkali therapy ineffective to prevent stone formation

41. Which of the following therapies is in the clinical stage of development for epilepsy?

    A. Ganaxolone for treatment of intractable generalized epilepsy syndromes

    B. Triheptanoin for treatment of ring chromosome 20 disorder

    C. Inhaled alprazolam for treatment of acute repetitive seizures

    D. Cannabidiol for treatment of intractable childhood focal epilepsy syndromes

42. Which of the following alternative or complementary therapies has been shown in a randomized trial to be beneficial in controlling seizures?

    A. Yoga

    B. Biofeedback

    C. Atkins diet

    D. Acupuncture

43. A 35-year-old man presents to the emergency department after a witnessed generalized tonic–clonic seizure. Initially, he was confused, but returned to baseline subsequently. Neurological exam was nonfocal. According to the practice parameter put forth by the American Academy of Neurology (AAN) regarding evaluation of an apparent unprovoked first seizure in adults, which of the following tests is recommended as part of the routine evaluation?

    A. Toxicology screen

    B. Lumbar puncture

    C. EEG

    D. Laboratory tests such as blood counts and electrolyte panel

44. A 27-year-old male presented to the emergency department after having two seizures. He has no history of epilepsy, but recently started an unknown medication. Which of the following medication classes is NOT known to increase the risk of seizures?

    A. Opiate analgesics

    B. Beta-lactam antibiotics

    C. Quinolones

    D. Carbonic anhydrase inhibitors

45. Two Veterans Affairs (VA) cooperative trials compared traditional antiepileptic drugs (AEDs) as initial monotherapy for partial seizures. Which of the following statements best supports the findings of these studies with respect to the efficacy of AEDs?

A. Carbamazepine is more efficacious than phenobarbital for generalized tonic–clonic seizures

B. Primidone is more efficacious than phenobarbital

C. Valproate is more efficacious than carbamazepine for secondarily generalized seizures

D. There is no statistical difference in efficacy between carbamazepine and phenytoin

46. Combining antiepileptic drugs can lead to therapeutic challenges. In that context, all of the following statements are true EXCEPT:

A. Phenobarbital and valproate combination leads to sedation and weight gain

B. Lacosamide and oxcarbazepine combination leads to dizziness and diplopia

C. Valproate and lamotrigine combination requires valproate dose adjustment

D. Topiramate and carbamazepine combination increases topiramate clearance

47. A 50-year-old female with intractable primary generalized seizures on valproate monotherapy presented to the emergency department with encephalopathy. EEG ruled-out nonconvulsive seizures. When reviewing the history, it was noted that a new antiepileptic drug (AED) was added to her regimen recently. Which of the following AEDs could be the most likely cause of her encephalopathy?

A. Lamotrigine

B. Phenytoin

C. Topiramate

D. Carbamazepine

48. Which of the following best describes the effect of felbamate (FBM) on the levels of concomitant antiepileptic drugs?

A. Increases phenytoin, increases carbamazepine, increases valproate

B. Increases phenytoin, decreases carbamazepine, decreases valproate

C. Decreases phenytoin, decreases carbamazepine, increases valproate

D. Increases phenytoin, decreases carbamazepine, increases valproate

49. A patient without known history of epilepsy was admitted with acute renal failure. The next morning, he was noted to have fluctuating mental status, for which he was started on continuous video-EEG monitoring. Within 10 minutes of the recording, an equivocal periodic EEG pattern was noted. Reasonable treatment options at this time include all of the following EXCEPT:

A. Trial of a rapidly acting benzodiazepine

B. Trial of small incremental doses of a nonsedating antiepileptic drug (AED)

C. Intubation followed by administration of an anesthetic medication

D. Continued observation and reassessment of the EEG in 2 hours

50. A 17-year-old girl was carried into the emergency department by a friend, who stated that she became unresponsive after a generalized convulsion lasting more than 10 minutes. Which of the following is NOT considered part of the initial evaluation?

A. Noncontrast head CT
B. Checking blood sugar
C. EKG
D. EEG

51. A 28-year-old male presents with intractable epilepsy since age 8. Video-EEG monitoring showed semiology and electrical onset consistent with right temporal lobe seizures. Neuropsychological testing showed mild nonlateralizing deficits. The Wada test showed left hemispheric language and memory dominance. The figure shows his MRI images (T2 on the left and gradient echo on the right). Which of the following procedures is LEAST likely to provide the best postoperative seizure outcome in this patient?

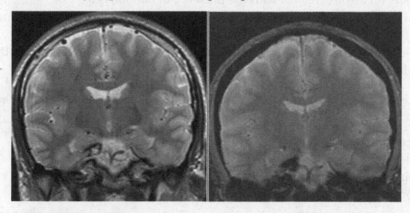

A. Pure lesionectomy
B. Lesionectomy and removal of surrounding brain tissue
C. Lesionectomy, removal of surrounding brain tissue, and selective amygdalo-hippocampectomy
D. Standard anteromedial temporal resection

52. A 19-year-old male presents with intractable epilepsy. His past history is notable for mild head trauma at age 2 when he fell out of his crib and hit his head on a tiled floor. MRI was normal. Positron emission tomography (PET) scan was nondiagnostic. Semiology consisted of an aura of fear followed by agitation, initial head turning to the right or left, lip smacking, right-hand automatisms, figure-of-4 posturing with left-arm extension and right-arm flexion, and generalized tonic–clonic activity. Scalp ictal EEG consisted of semirhythmic delta activity lateralized to the right hemisphere in some seizures and nonlateralized in others. In localizing the seizure onset by invasive recording, sampling of the electrical activity from which of the following areas is LEAST likely to be helpful?

A. Right fronto-temporal region
B. Left fronto-temporal region
C. Right medial frontal region
D. Right medial temporal region

53. A 22-year-old male presents with seizures characterized by versive head deviation to the left, left-arm extension, right-arm flexion, and vocalization followed by tonic–clonic activity. His MRI did not show a lesion. Which of the following factors needs to be considered in evaluating this patient for surgery?

    A. Scalp interictal epileptiform discharges are likely to be concordant with ictal onset
    B. Hypometabolism on positron emission tomography (PET) scan is likely to be smaller than the ictal onset zone
    C. Outcome of surgical resection with respect to freedom from disabling seizures is around 70%
    D. Presence of beta activity at ictal onset predicts favorable outcome

54. All of the following statements regarding focal cortical dysplasia (FCD) are true EXCEPT:

    A. FCD presents with epilepsy in nearly 80% of patients
    B. T2 hyperintensity on MRI correlates with the presence of balloon cells
    C. Repetitive ictal spiking pattern on electrocorticography correlates with the anatomical lesion
    D. Postsurgical seizure outcome is independent of the extent of resection of the anatomical lesion

55. Visual disturbance associated with ezogabine can be characterized by all of the following statements EXCEPT:

    A. It is due to pigmentary retinopathy
    B. It is irreversible
    C. It can be seen in up to one third of patients
    D. It can occur concurrently with skin discoloration

56. A 20-year-old female presents with history of epilepsy since age 6. Her seizures are described as staring with loss of consciousness and loss of awareness, lasting a few seconds with occasional generalized convulsions. However, over the past 2 years, the staring spells have been well controlled, but the generalized convulsions have become more frequent, occurring two to three times per month. She is currently on a combination of valporic acid and levetiracetam. Her neurologist wants to substitute valporic acid with a different medication. Her routine EEG is shown (filter: 1–70 Hz). All of the following medications would be appropriate EXCEPT:

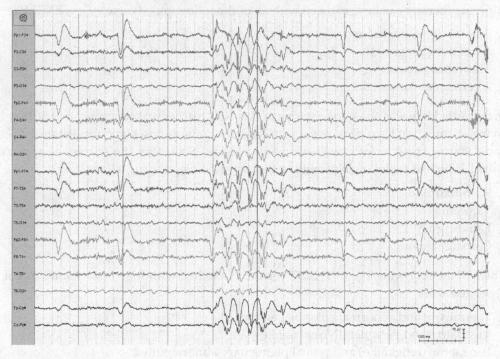

A. Topiramate
B. Lamotrigine
C. Perampanel
D. Ethosuximide

57. Adrenocorticotropic hormone (ACTH) therapy can result in all of the following side effects EXCEPT:

A. Cardiomyopathy
B. Nephrocalcinosis
C. Agitation
D. Hypotension

58. Which of the following is true regarding the metabolic profile of rufinamide?

A. It is metabolized by cytochrome P450 enzymes
B. It undergoes substantial metabolism via carboxylesterases
C. Valproic acid may decrease its plasma concentration
D. It has significant pharmacodynamic interactions with lamotrigine

59. Clobazam differs from clonazepam in all of the following ways EXCEPT:

A. Clobazam is a 1,5 benzodiazepine, whereas clonazepam is a 1,4 benzodiazepine
B. Penetration of clobazam into the central nervous system (CNS) is significantly higher than clonazepam
C. Clobazam has greater binding affinities to the alpha 2 versus alpha 1 subunit of GABA receptors, whereas clonazepam has equal binding affinity to alpha 1 and 2 receptors
D. If substituted, clobazam dosage is roughly 15-fold higher than that of clonazepam

60. Valproate therapy can be associated with all of the following adverse effects EXCEPT:

A. Secondary nocturnal enuresis
B. Excessive hair growth
C. Thrombocytopenia
D. Altered platelet function

61. An 8-year-old boy was noted to be staring in class. His teacher was concerned that he may be having seizures, but his parents never witnessed any convulsions. Hyperventilation induced a brief staring episode with swallowing automatisms. Soon after the seizure, he appeared normal. Which of the following would be the best antiepileptic drug to start?

A. Ethosuximide
B. Valproate
C. Lamotrigine
D. Carbamazepine

62. Which of the following agents is NOT correctly matched with the visual disturbance it is associated with?

A. Topiramate and abnormal color perception
B. Vigabatrin and peripheral visual field loss
C. Ezogabine (retigabine) and retinal pigmentary abnormalities
D. Phenytoin and ophthalmoplegia

63. A 32-year-old woman with partial epilepsy would like to be on oral contraception to prevent pregnancy. Which of the following antiepileptic drugs (AEDs) is likely to affect the contraceptive efficacy?

A. Valproate
B. Topiramate
C. Lamotrigine
D. Zonisamide

64. Multiple subpial transections (MST) is a disconnection procedure often used to treat intractable epilepsy. The MST procedure can be described by all of the following statements EXCEPT:

A. MST prevents the initiation and propagation of epileptic activity
B. Transection is carried out to a depth of 1 mm at 5-mm intervals
C. MST is indicated for Landau–Kleffner syndrome
D. Seizure freedom is unlikely with pure MST

65. A 22-year-old male has a history of multiple febrile seizures until age 4 years followed by intractable epilepsy starting at age 12. Video-EEG monitoring showed semiology and electrical onset consistent with left temporal lobe seizures. Neuropsychological testing showed impaired verbal memory. A fluid attenuated inversion recovery (FLAIR) image of his MRI is shown. If he were to undergo standard left anterior temporal lobectomy, which of the following structures would NOT be included as part of the procedure?

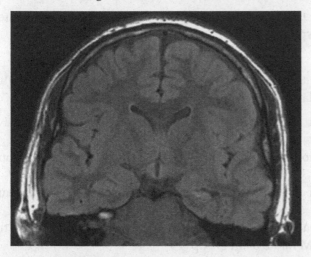

A. Amygdala
B. Head, body, and tail of the hippocampus up to the posterior margin of midbrain
C. Parahippocampal gyrus
D. 4 cm of the lateral temporal neocortex including the superior, middle, and inferior temporal gyri

66. Inadvertent injury to which of the following vessels is the most likely cause of stroke during anteromedial temporal resection?

A. Middle cerebral artery
B. Vein of Labbe
C. Anterior choroidal artery
D. Thalamoperforating artery

67. The Veterans Affairs (VA) Cooperative Trial compared four therapies for initial treatment for status epilepticus (SE): diazepam followed by phenytoin, lorazepam, phenobarbital, and phenytoin. Based on the results of the trial, all of the following statements are correct EXCEPT:

A. About 55% patients with overt generalized convulsive SE and 15% with subtle generalized convulsive SE respond to the initial therapy
B. Lorazepam is more likely to be effective than phenytoin as the initial therapy for overt generalized convulsive SE
C. Diazepam plus phenytoin is more likely to be effective than lorazepam as initial therapy for subtle generalized convulsive SE
D. The 30-day outcome is likely to be similar with respect to the four treatments

68. Which of the following statements is true regarding treatment of prehospital status epilepticus (SE)?

    A. Efficacy of lorazepam is superior to diazepam in terminating the SE by the time of arrival at the hospital
    B. Posttreatment cardiopulmonary complications are likely to be higher with lorazepam compared with placebo
    C. Rate of ICU admission is likely to be similar regardless of whether SE was terminated by the time of arrival to the hospital or not
    D. All of the above

69. Which of the following statements is true regarding prehospital treatment of status epilepticus (SE) using intramuscular (IM) and intravenous (IV) benzodiazepines?

    A. IM midazolam was superior to IV lorazepam in terminating generalized convulsive SE prior to arrival at the hospital
    B. Need for endotracheal intubation was significantly higher in the IV lorazepam group than the IM midazolam group
    C. Seizure recurrence was higher in the IM midazolam group than the IV lorazepam group
    D. Median time from active treatment to cessation of seizures was longer in the IV lorazepam group than the IM midazolam group

70. A 45-year-old male presented with generalized convulsive status epilepticus (SE) that ended after the second dose of a benzodiazepine. He is noted to be responding appropriately although mildly confused. While going through his chart, it was noted that he has a history of brain tumor, for which he is on steroids and chemotherapy. He also has coronary artery disease with preexisting cardiac conduction delay. What is the most appropriate therapy at this point?

    A. Observe and treat only if he has another seizure
    B. Load with fosphenytoin
    C. Load with lacosamide
    D. Load with valproate

71. Bilateral stimulation of the anterior nuclei of the thalamus shows statistically significant seizure reduction in which of the following?

    A. Unilateral temporal lobe seizures
    B. Unilateral or bilateral temporal lobe seizures
    C. Frontal lobe seizures
    D. Multifocal- or diffuse-onset seizures

72. Complications of epilepsy surgery are feared by patients and referring physicians, which limits the selection of this treatment option for intractable epilepsy. Which of the following statements is true regarding the complications of epilepsy surgery?

    A. Invasive monitoring is associated with major complications in >10% of patients
    B. The most common medical complication after resective surgery is infection
    C. The most common neurologic complication after resective surgery is hemiparesis
    D. Perioperative mortality associated with epilepsy surgery is about 1%

73. Which of the following is a predictor of successful reoperation after failed epilepsy surgery?

    A. Presence of seizures with a different semiology
    B. Concordance between postsurgical MRI and ictal EEG
    C. Head trauma as a risk factor for epilepsy
    D. Brain infection as a risk factor for epilepsy

74. A 36-year-old male is being evaluated for possible epilepsy surgery. His seizures started at age 18, about 2 years after head trauma in which he suffered from right frontal hematoma, requiring evacuation. His seizures are characterized by a weird sensation in the head, well-formed words at onset, lip smacking, deep breathing, howling, agitation, and rapid postictal recovery. Ictal EEG shows rhythmic delta activity in the right fronto-temporal region. Two representative fluid attenuated inversion recovery (FLAIR) images of his MRI are shown. The most appropriate intervention would be:

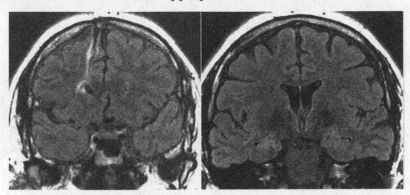

    A. Standard right anterior temporal lobectomy
    B. Stereotactic, MRI-guided laser ablation of right medial frontal structures
    C. Implantation of right temporal depth and right frontal subdural electrodes
    D. No surgical intervention because of widespread ictal EEG onset

75. Which of the following predicts favorable seizure outcome after temporal lobectomy for intractable temporal lobe epilepsy (TLE) due to mesial temporal sclerosis (MTS)?

    A. Age at seizure onset
    B. Gender
    C. History of febrile seizures
    D. Duration of epilepsy

76. Which of the following is true regarding long-term postoperative seizure outcome for medically refractory nonlesional extratemporal lobe epilepsy in adults?

    A. About 10% of those who undergo resection after intracranial monitoring have excellent outcome
    B. About 60% of those who undergo resection after intracranial monitoring have excellent outcome
    C. Scalp interictal epileptiform discharges predict excellent outcome
    D. Intracranial interictal epileptiform discharges predict excellent outcome

77. An 8-month-old boy with a large right fronto-parietal focal cortical dysplasia (FCD) has medically intractable epilepsy with infantile spasms and complex partial seizures. His EEG is shown (sensitivity: 10-mcV/mm, interval between vertical lines: 1 second; filter: 1–70 Hz). Which of the following is true regarding his candidacy for epilepsy surgery?

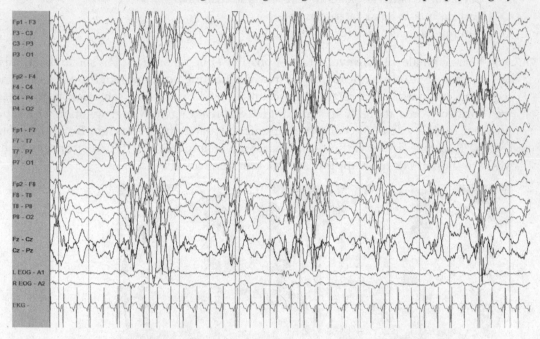

A. He is not a good surgical candidate because he has infantile spasms
B. He is a good surgical candidate because he has complex partial seizures
C. He is not a good surgical candidate because he has generalized EEG abnormalities
D. He is a good surgical candidate because he has an early epileptogenic focal lesion

78. A 9-year-old boy with bilateral frontal cortical dysplasia and developmental delay has medically intractable epilepsy. Vagus nerve stimulation was not beneficial. He undergoes anterior corpus callosotomy. The anticipated complications include all of the following EXCEPT:

A. Tactile and visual transfer deficits
B. Mutism
C. Left leg paresis
D. Urge urinary incontinence

79. Which of the following is the most common adverse effect of vagus nerve stimulation (VNS) 3 months after implant?

A. Cough
B. Palpitation
C. Dyspnea
D. Hoarseness

80. In the pivotal trial for vagus nerve stimulation (VNS), the average percent reduction in seizures at 3 months compared with baseline was:

    A. 10% to 15%
    B. 20% to 25%
    C. 50% to 55%
    D. 60% to 65%

81. Typical vagus nerve stimulation (VNS) settings include all of the following EXCEPT:

    A. Output current: 3 mA
    B. Pulse width: 500 mcs
    C. Signal frequency: 20 Hz
    D. On time: 7 seconds; Off time: 18 seconds

82. All of the following statements regarding ethosuximide are true EXCEPT:

    A. It is effective against both typical and atypical absence seizures
    B. It reduces L-type calcium currents in thalamic neurons
    C. It can cause forced normalization reaction and psychosis
    D. It can cause lupus-like syndrome

83. Ethosuximide associated lupus-like syndrome is characterized by which of the following?

    A. Arthralgia and fever
    B. Elevated ANA and antidouble strand DNA antibodies
    C. Both A and B
    D. Neither A or B

84. Which of the following is true regarding hepatic enzyme induction as seen with phenobarbital?

    A. Enzyme induction is a slow regulatory process that is dose and time dependent
    B. Induction only affects metabolism of drugs but not the endogenous compounds
    C. If a drug metabolized by the induced enzyme has an active metabolite, then induction leads to a decrease in metabolite concentration and decreased efficacy
    D. Induction is specific to cytochrome P450 (CYP) enzymes

85. Which of the following is true regarding pharmacokinetics in the elderly?

    A. Increased hepatic metabolism
    B. Increased enzyme inducibility
    C. Decreased renal elimination
    D. Increased protein binding

86. Which of the following antiepileptic drugs has Level A evidence establishing it as efficacious or effective as initial monotherapy in elderly adults with partial-onset seizures?

    A. Gabapentin
    B. Carbamazepine
    C. Topiramate
    D. Valproate

87. What of the following is NOT a common side effect of lacosamide?

    A. Incoordination
    B. Diplopia
    C. Ataxia
    D. Cognitive slowing

88. Which of the following statements is true regarding the risk of seizure recurrence after the first unprovoked seizure?

    A. Risk of recurrence is 10% within 2 years
    B. Risk of recurrence is 25% within 2 years when the EEG and neurological exam are normal
    C. Risk of recurrence is higher if the initial seizure event is status epilepticus regardless of etiology
    D. Risk of recurrence is higher in adults who present with multiple seizures within 24 hours as opposed to a single seizure

89. Which of the following statements is true regarding the comparison of older and newer antiepileptic drugs in the Standard and New Antiepileptic Drugs (SANAD) trial?

    A. Lamotrigine is significantly better than carbamazepine with respect to time to treatment failure for partial seizures
    B. Gabapentin is significantly better than carbamazepine with respect to 12-month remission for partial seizures
    C. Lamotrigine is significantly better than valproate for idiopathic generalized epilepsy (IGE)
    D. Topiramate is significantly better than valproate for IGE

90. A 30-year-old woman with medically intractable epilepsy presents to the emergency department with bleeding from the mouth with sloughing of skin. She is on multiple antiepileptic drugs (AEDs) including carbamazepine, levetiracetam, valproate, and lamotrigine. She reports that she has been taking them erratically because of lack of consistent prescription medication insurance. Which of the following statements is important in guiding further management?

    A. All of her AEDs need to be stopped immediately
    B. There is well-established cross-reactivity between lamotrigine and carbamazepine
    C. There are no clear genetic markers to predict AED-induced hypersensitivity
    D. These symptoms could reflect AED changes made within the past few months

91. A 32-year-old male with intractable epilepsy due to left mesial temporal sclerosis (MTS) undergoes an MRI-guided stereotactic thermal laser ablation procedure. His postablation damage model is shown. Which of the following statements is true regarding this procedure in the treatment of temporal lobe epilepsy?

A. Irreversible tissue ablation occurs at temperatures of 60°C to 90°C
B. The amygdalo-hippocampal complex (AHC) is completely ablated
C. The parahippocampal gyrus is partially ablated
D. The typical laser exposure treatment time is about 1 minute

92. A 42-year-old male undergoes responsive neurostimulation (RNS) implantation with a subdural strip for treatment of intractable, nonlesional, left frontal lobe epilepsy. A sample of the stored electrocorticography (ECoG) tracing is shown (marker "B1" indicates the detected seizure; marker "Tr" indicates delivery of stimulation). What is the most appropriate conclusion?

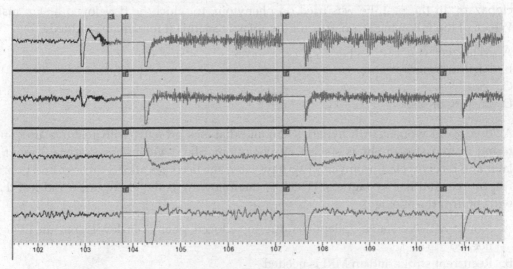

A. The system misses detection of seizure onset
B. Seizure is successfully terminated after the first stimulation
C. This patient needs a change in detector settings
D. This patient needs a change in stimulation parameters

93. Evidence-based guidelines regarding the role of vagus nerve stimulation (VNS) for the treatment of epilepsy include all of the following EXCEPT:

A. VNS is efficacious in treating generalized seizures in children
B. VNS is efficacious in treating seizures associated with Lennox–Gastaut syndrome (LGS)
C. VNS shows improved efficacy over time
D. VNS is associated with significant improvement in mood in children and adults with epilepsy

94. Neonatal seizures can be characterized by all of the following statements EXCEPT:

A. The most common cause is intracranial hemorrhage
B. Underlying etiology is a primary predictor of outcome
C. Focal clonic and tonic seizures have a relatively good outcome compared with generalized tonic posturing
D. Phenytoin is often used for acute treatment

95. Neonatal seizures can be extremely refractory to treatment with the commonly used first-line agent phenobarbital. This is believed to be due to:

A. Excitatory nature of GABA signaling in immature neurons
B. Inhibitory nature of GABA signaling in immature neurons
C. Both A and B
D. Neither A or B

96. A 9-year-old African American boy with Lennox–Gastaut syndrome and intractable epilepsy continues to have frequent convulsive seizures and atonic seizures despite trials of multiple antiseizure medications. He is currently on rufinamide, topiramate, and clobazam. In the past, he was tried on phenytoin, to which he developed a skin rash. Which of the following is a risk factor for aplastic anemia if felbamate is added?

A. Male gender
B. African American race
C. Age
D. History of rash

97. A 70-year-old woman with hypertension and diabetes presents with seizures after suffering from a stroke. She is started on phenytoin. She develops pneumonia 3 months later and receives clarithromycin. Two days later, she becomes ataxic, drowsy, and poorly responsive, and has nystagmus. Which of the following is the likely cause and test that will confirm the etiology?

A. Nonconvulsive status epilepticus due to reduced phenytoin levels and an EEG is needed
B. Recurrent stroke and an MRI is needed
C. Phenytoin toxicity due to clarithromycin addition and free and total phenytoin levels are needed
D. Clarithromycin toxicity and clarithromycin level is needed

98. Side effects of phenytoin and fosphenytoin administration include all of the following EXCEPT:

A. Osteoporosis
B. Irreversible gingival hyperplasia
C. Cerebellar atrophy
D. Limb ischemia

99. Which of the following is true regarding levetiracetam?

A. It is metabolized by the UDP-glucuronyl transferase isozyme (UGT) system
B. It has Food and Drug Administration (FDA) indications for both adjunctive therapy and monotherapy
C. It is available in a 3D-printable form
D. It has 50% to 60% bioavailability after oral administration

100. The pharmacologic profile of pregabalin can be described by all of the following statements EXCEPT:

A. It is effective in the maximum electroshock (MES) model
B. It binds to voltage-gated calcium (P/Q) channels
C. Its bioavailability drops with increasing dose within the clinical dosing range
D. It is excreted unchanged in the urine

101. A 17-year-old male honor student became confused after starting tiagabine for insomnia. Which of the following patterns is most likely to be seen on his EEG?

A. Generalized spike-wave discharges
B. Periodic lateralized epileptiform discharges (PLEDs)
C. Temporal intermittent rhythmic delta activity (TIRDA)
D. Frontal intermittent rhythmic delta activity (FIRDA)

102. Regarding the mechanism of action of the antiepileptic drugs, all of the following statements are correct EXCEPT:

A. Ezogabine inhibits voltage-gated calcium channels
B. Brivaracetam binds to synaptic vesicle protein 2A (SV2A)
C. Lacosamide acts on the sodium channels
D. Vigabatrin inhibits GABA-transaminase

103. A 55-year-old woman with long standing epilepsy fell and fractured her forearm. She underwent a bone density scan which showed osteoporosis. Which of the following antiepileptic drugs (AEDs) is LEAST likely to cause bone loss?

A. Phenytoin
B. Lamotrigine
C. Primidone
D. Valproate

104. Which of the following benefits can be seen after hemispherectomy for Rasmussen syndrome?

A. Seizure freedom or occasional nondisabling seizures in a majority of patients
B. Improvement of the hemiparesis
C. Cognitive stabilization
D. Both A and C

105. Responsive neurostimulation (RNS) differs from deep brain stimulation (DBS) in all of the following ways EXCEPT:

A. In RNS, the stimulation target is the epileptogenic zone
B. In RNS, stimulations are delivered when the seizure is detected
C. In DBS, knowledge of the precise location of the epileptogenic zone is crucial
D. In DBS, the stimulations are delivered at predefined intervals

106. A 35-year-old female has had epilepsy since she was a teenager. A presurgical workup, done a decade ago, was consistent with MRI-negative dominant temporal lobe epilepsy. She deferred surgical resection. Seizures have remained medically intractable, and she has developed a new type of seizures with a different semiology along with verbal memory loss. Positron emission tomography (PET) scan demonstrates bilateral temporal hypometabolism. Which of the following options is most appropriate at this stage?

A. Dominant temporal lobectomy
B. MRI-guided stereotactic laser ablation of the dominant hippocampus
C. Vagus nerve stimulation (VNS)
D. Bitemporal responsive neurostimulation (RNS)

107. A full-term boy is born with a low Apgar score. He starts to have bilateral, independent clonic seizures that are refractory to phenobarbital and phenytoin. On examination, he is hypotonic with poor sucking. He has large open anterior and posterior fontanelles, broad nasal bridge, micrognathia, and high forehead. Liver is enlarged. EEG shows multifocal spikes and mild voltage attenuation of the background interictally. CT scan shows colpocephaly. Which of the following is the most likely diagnosis?

A. Prader–Willi syndrome
B. Myotonic dystrophy
C. Ohtahara syndrome
D. Zellweger syndrome

108. An 18-year-old, intellectually disabled, girl with epilepsy is on phenobarbital and topiramate. She is nonverbal and nonambulatory. She receives physical therapy for spasticity. After a therapy session, she starts to cry incessantly and cannot be calmed. Which of the following is indicated in the evaluation of this patient?

A. Renal ultrasound
B. X-ray of extremities and 25-OH vitamin D level
C. EEG
D. Upper gastrointestinal endoscopy

109. A 25-year-old woman, on levetiracetam monotherapy for management of primary generalized epilepsy, is started on lamotrigine. Two weeks after initiation of medication, she calls to report a rash. Prior to this, she had developed a rash to zonisamide, which was discontinued. Which of the following characteristics of her clinical profile is a predictor of hypersensitivity to lamotrigine?

   A. Age
   B. History of developing rash while on zonisamide
   C. Concomitant treatment with levetiracetam
   D. Primary generalized epilepsy

110. An 18-year-old girl with primary generalized epilepsy continues to have breakthrough seizures on lamotrigine (LTG) monotherapy. In the past, she has failed monotherapy trials with topiramate, zonisamide, and levetiracetam. A decision is made to start valproic acid (VPA) after discussing the risks and side effects of this medication in a young woman of child-bearing age. Two days after starting valproic acid, she is dizzy, ataxic, and nauseous. What is the most likely cause?

   A. Valproic acid is an enzyme inducer and this led to toxic levels of lamotrigine
   B. Lamotrigine is an enzyme inhibitor and this led to toxic levels of valproic acid
   C. Valproic acid is an enzyme inhibitor and this led to toxic level of lamotrigine
   D. Lamotrigine is an enzyme inhibitor and this led to toxic levels of valproic acid

111. Mechanism of action of levetiracetam can be described by all of the following statements EXCEPT:

   A. It is effective in kindled animals
   B. It is ineffective in maximal electroshock (MES) model
   C. It is ineffective in pentylenetetrazol (PTZ) model
   D. It inhibits presynaptic sodium channels

112. Which of the following is true regarding felbamate (FBM)?

   A. It binds to the NR2B subunit of N-methyl-D-aspartate (NMDA) receptors
   B. It decreases the level of phenytoin
   C. Its level is increased by concomitant phenytoin
   D. Its idiosyncratic reactions are due to its toxic metabolite fluorofelbamate

113. Felbamate has a specific Food and Drug Administration (FDA) indication for treatment of which of the following syndromes?

   A. Lennox–Gastaut syndrome
   B. Dravet syndrome
   C. Juvenile myoclonic epilepsy
   D. Landau–Kleffner syndrome

114. Which of the following statements is true regarding gabapentin?

   A. It acts on the voltage-gated sodium channels
   B. Its bioavailability is independent of its dose
   C. It is contraindicated in patients with porphyria
   D. It may worsen myoclonus

115. All of the following statements regarding gabapentin are true EXCEPT:

   A. It follows dose-dependent absorption
   B. It is highly protein bound
   C. It crosses the blood–brain barrier
   D. It can cause weight gain

116. Early antiepileptic drug (AED) treatment after the first unprovoked seizure:

   A. Prevents epileptogenesis
   B. May be reasonable in some patients with low seizure recurrence risk
   C. Favorably impacts the long-term prognosis of epilepsy
   D. Reduces the risk of subsequent seizure recurrence by 80%

117. A 16-year-old girl with an unknown epilepsy syndrome has been seizure free for 2 years and would like to stop her antiepileptic medication (AED). Which of the following statements is most accurate in terms of counseling her regarding the risk of seizure recurrence after medication withdrawal based on syndrome?

   A. Cryptogenic epilepsy is more likely to remit than remote symptomatic epilepsy
   B. Juvenile myoclonic epilepsy has a low recurrence risk
   C. All focal epilepsies have a high relapse rate
   D. Seizure recurrence risk is independent of the epilepsy syndrome in children

118. A 17-year-old female with a 10-year history of epilepsy wants to discontinue her antiepileptic drug (AED). She graduated from high school and received an academic scholarship for college. She has been seizure free for the past 4 years despite having a poor initial AED response. She is currently on lamotrigine monotherapy, with a recent serum trough level of 1.2 mcg/mL (normal: 2.5–15 mcg/mL). She has had a number of subtherapeutic levels at prior visits in the past 3 years, which she attributes to having a busy lifestyle and forgetting to take the medication. Which of the following factors is most predictive of seizure recurrence in her?

   A. Age at epilepsy onset
   B. Neurological state
   C. Low drug levels
   D. Poor initial AED response

119. Which of the following best approximates the proportion of newly diagnosed, untreated epilepsy patients who can be expected to become seizure free for 1 year on initial therapy with an antiepileptic drug (AED)?

    A. 25%
    B. 35%
    C. 45%
    D. 65%

120. A 20-year-old male, on 300 mg of phenytoin monotherapy, presents to the emergency department after an unprovoked seizure. His random serum phenytoin level is 15 mcg/mL. He is otherwise healthy. Which of the following properties of phenytoin is most important when adjusting his dose?

    A. Auto-induction
    B. Zero-order kinetics
    C. Protein binding
    D. Bioavailability

121. A 6-year-old girl is about to start the ketogenic diet. All of the following statements regarding the patient's existing antiepileptic drug (AED) regimen are true EXCEPT:

    A. AEDs must be reduced prior to diet initiation
    B. AED solutions may need to be changed to tablets or capsules prior to diet initiation
    C. AEDs with carbonic anhydrase inhibiting properties require careful monitoring after diet initiation
    D. AED toxic effects are particularly likely during the fasting phase

122. A 33-year-old female with a 7-year history of epilepsy recently got married and would like to start a family in the next couple of years. She is currently on lamotrigine and levetiracetam, and has been seizure free for 6 months, her longest seizure-free interval. Which of the following would be the most appropriate recommendation regarding her antiepileptic drug (AED) therapy and monitoring?

    A. As she is seizure free, continue current AED doses and reassess once she becomes pregnant
    B. Attempt complete withdrawal of AEDs now to ensure that she remains seizure free prior to getting pregnant
    C. Attempt to simplify therapy to monotherapy at the lowest possible effective dose prior to pregnancy
    D. As she is seizure free, defer checking the AED levels until after she becomes pregnant

123. A 19-year-old female with MRI-negative epilepsy with focal and generalized tonic–clonic seizures is being evaluated for epilepsy surgery. She suffered from a single febrile seizure at age 4 years before developing seizure recurrence at age 15. She was initially tried on ethosuximide for 3 years, which she failed. Currently, she is on carbamazepine and levetiracetam, and has 1 to 2 focal seizures per month. Her recent video-EEG monitoring documented right temporal seizure onset. She can be considered to have medically refractory epilepsy because:

    A. She has history of single febrile seizure at age 4
    B. She has failed three antiepileptic medications
    C. She has failed two antiepileptic medications
    D. She has temporal lobe epilepsy

124. A 23-year-old female is being evaluated for epilepsy surgery. Her MRI shows a lesion in the right middle and inferior temporal gyri, felt to be a low-grade glioma. Her scalp EEG shows sharp waves distributed over the right mid-frontal and anterior temporal leads. Scalp ictal onset was localized to the right fronto-temporal region. Which of the following statements is true of her presurgical evaluation?

    A. Irritative zone is smaller than the epileptic lesion
    B. Ictal onset zone is smaller than the epileptic lesion
    C. Epileptogenic zone consists of the right middle and inferior temporal gyri and the right hippocampus
    D. Neuropsychological testing is likely to be a good measure of the functional deficit zone

125. Which of the following is a predictor of seizure recurrence after frontal lobectomy for refractory epilepsy?

    A. MRI-visible frontal lobe lesion
    B. Occurrence of acute postoperative seizures
    C. Younger age at onset of epilepsy
    D. Duration of epilepsy prior to surgery

126. Which of the following clinical seizure characteristics is of localizing value during surgical planning for intractable frontal lobe epilepsy?

    A. Seizures with hyperkinetic automatisms localize to the medial frontal lobe
    B. Early forced head/eye version lateralizes to the contralateral frontal lobe
    C. Tonic seizures most often localize to the medial frontal lobe
    D. Oroalimentary automatisms always indicate extra-frontal seizure onset

127. Which of the following statements best describes the epileptogenic zone?

    A. It corresponds to the area from which the recorded seizures arise
    B. It corresponds to the cortical area, removal of which will result in seizure freedom
    C. Its extent is the same across patients as long as they have the same pathological condition
    D. Its location cannot be determined without a structural lesion

128. In which of the following patients would resective epilepsy surgery be contraindicated?

A. A 30-year-old male with two focal seizures with secondary generalization per year and mesial temporal sclerosis (MTS) on MRI

B. A 44-year-old female with frequent left temporal lobe seizures, left anterior neocortical temporal cavernoma, and left hemispheric dominance for language and memory

C. A 24-year-old male with frequent left-sided seizures with Jacksonian march following head trauma, and right frontal lobe gliosis on MRI

D. A 49-year-old male with bilateral MTS, frequent left temporal lobe focal seizures, and mild global memory impairment

129. Intracranial EEG helps predict the outcome of epilepsy surgery in patients with nonlesional extratemporal lobe epilepsy. Seizure-free outcome is likely to be seen with all of the following intracranial EEG findings EXCEPT:

A. Ictal onset with a restricted focal pattern

B. Ictal onset pattern with fast rhythmic activity

C. Long latency to onset of seizure spread

D. Infrequent interictal epileptiform discharges

130. A 9-month-old boy, with left-hand preference, presents with daily infantile spasms consisting of clusters of flexion of neck and extremities, involving the right side more than the left since 4 months age. Spasms have been refractory to treatment with steroids, vigabatrin, and the ketogenic diet. On examination, he has right gaze preference and right hemiparesis. A T2 image of his MRI is shown. Which of the following options is most likely to improve his long-term outcome?

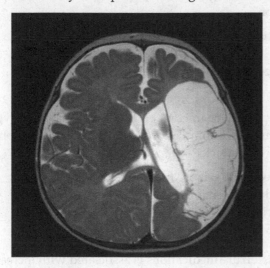

A. Functional hemispherotomy

B. Lobar resection

C. Vagus nerve stimulation (VNS) implant

D. Continued medical therapy

131. Corpus callosotomy is indicated in which of the following patients?

A. A 2-year-old boy with multiple seizure types including tonic seizures and unilateral cortical dysplasia

B. A 5-year-old boy with severe intellectual disability and medically intractable complex partial and generalized tonic–clonic seizures and normal MRI

C. A 17-year-old girl with medically intractable Lennox–Gastaut syndrome and daily atypical absence seizures

D. A 16-year-old boy with medically intractable Lennox–Gastaut syndrome and daily drop attacks

132. A 57-year-old female with history of intractable, focal epilepsy recently underwent vagus nerve stimulation (VNS) implantation. All of the following safety precautions are true EXCEPT:

A. Pulse generator should be kept more than 8 inches from electromagnetic sources

B. MRI is safe with a send-and-receive coil

C. Holding the magnet over the pulse generator stops the stimulation

D. Holding a cell phone close to the pulse generator can cause inadvertent stimulation

133. A 63-year-old male developed epilepsy 17 years ago after sustaining a traumatic brain injury. He has failed seven medications. The clinical semiology consists of an aura of anxiety and fear progressing to bimanual and oral automatisms and infrequent right hemifacial twitching. EEG shows left temporal ictal discharge in the setting of bitemporal, independent interictal epileptiform discharges, and slowing. Brain MRI shows bilateral mesial temporal sclerosis (MTS), with greater atrophy on the left. Which of the following would be the best next option?

A. MRI-guided stereotactic laser ablation of the left hippocampus

B. Ketogenic diet

C. Selective left amygdalo-hippocampectomy

D. Vagus nerve stimulation (VNS)

134. A 12-year-old female has childhood epilepsy characterized by multiple seizure types, including drop attacks. How does vagus nerve stimulation (VNS) compare with corpus callosotomy (CC) for the treatment of drop attacks?

A. VNS is more effective than CC in reducing seizure frequency

B. VNS is less effective than CC in reducing seizure frequency

C. Adverse events are less common with VNS than CC

D. Efficacy is immediate for both VNS and CC

135. Addition of which of the following antiseizure medications is associated with increased risk of acute encephalopathy in patients on valproate monotherapy?

A. Levetiracetam

B. Felbamate

C. Ethosuximide

D. Topiramate

4

TREATMENT OF SEIZURES AND EPILEPSY

ANSWERS

1. **C.** The figure shows that the seizure arises from multiple contacts in the temporal neocortex (LT and ST) and then spreads to the hippocampus (LD). Therefore, it is not a focal onset in the hippocampus. Although part of the ST strip could be located in the parahippocampal gyrus, the seizure onset is not focal in the ST strip, and therefore, it is unlikely to be confined just to the parahippocampal gyrus.

   Mihara T, Baba K. Combined use of subdural and depth electrodes. In: Luders HO, Comair YG, eds. *Epilepsy Surgery*. 2nd ed. Philadelphia, PA: Lippincott Williams & Wilkins; 2001:613–621.

2. **D.** The seizure onset in the figure in Question 1 localizes to the left temporal neocortex. Thus, features of temporal lobe epilepsy constitute the semiology, including cold sensation all over the body (an autonomic phenomenon) and oroalimentary automatisms. Neocortical temporal seizures can spread to the operculum resulting in contralateral facial twitching. Well-formed speech at seizure onset is unlikely in left temporal lobe seizures unless the left hemisphere is nonlanguage dominant; among the options given, this would be the least likely feature.

   Foldvary N. Ictal electroencephalography in neocortical epilepsy. In: Luders HO, Comair YG, eds. *Epilepsy Surgery*. 2nd ed. Philadelphia, PA: Lippincott Williams & Wilkins; 2001:431–439.

3. **D.** This patient has left neocortical temporal seizure onset. Lack of hippocampal structural abnormality (normal imaging) and intact left-sided memory (Wada result) suggest a high risk of postoperative memory deficit if hippocampal or temporal resection is performed. Thus, neither standard anteromedial temporal resection nor selective amygdalo-hippocampectomy would be appropriate. Neocortical temporal resection corresponding to the lateral temporal electrodes showing ictal onset would also be risky given the proximity of those contacts to the language area. Thus, multiple subpial transections would be the most appropriate procedure as it can be performed over the eloquent speech cortex without necessarily causing permanent speech impairment. Another potential option would responsive neurostimulation.

   Wyler A. Multiple subpial transections. In: Luders HO, Comair YG, eds. *Epilepsy Surgery*. 2nd ed. Philadelphia, PA: Lippincott Williams & Wilkins; 2001:807–811.

4. D. The MRI shows T2 hyperintense lesions in the right insula and right parieto-occipital region (white arrows), and at the foramen of Monro (arrowhead). These are suspicious for tubers and a subependymal nodule as seen in tuberous sclerosis (TS). For further confirmation of the diagnosis, a Wood's lamp examination is appropriate to look for ash leaf spots, which are hypopigmented macules that are best seen with a Wood's lamp. Genetic testing for TSC1 and TSC2 mutations would also be appropriate. MEG is helpful for further localization of the epileptogenic areas, and is indicated if surgery is contemplated. Biopsy is not appropriate at this stage given the imaging findings.

Lachhwani DK, Pestana E, Gupta A, et al. Identification of candidates for epilepsy surgery in patients with tuberous sclerosis. *Neurology*. 2005;64:1651–1654.

5. A. Ictal SPECT shows hyperperfusion in the right parieto-occipital region, suggesting the presence of an epileptogenic tuber there. However, the possibility of the right insular tuber being epileptogenic cannot be excluded. That becomes a distinct possibility if this patient has seizures with different semiologies. Tuberous sclerosis (TS) itself or the presence of multiple tubers should not be considered a contraindication for epilepsy surgery. Seizures tend to be refractory to medical therapy in 50% to 80% of patients with TS. Frequent and uncontrolled seizures have a negative effect on development and cognition. It has been shown that resection of epileptogenic regions can lead to significant seizure reduction or elimination. Tuberous sclerosis complex (TSC) is characterized by several features that commonly complicate epilepsy surgery including multifocal or generalized epileptiform abnormalities, frequent extratemporal location, and appearance of secondary epileptogenic foci following resection of the dominant lesion. Multimodality imaging using MRI, positron emission tomography (PET), SPECT, and magnetoencephalography (MEG) are often necessary to confirm and better define an area for resection. At this stage, it would be most appropriate to proceed with intracranial EEG monitoring with subdural strips over bilateral lateral fronto-temporal regions, and medial frontal regions, and a subdural grid over the right parieto-occipital region. This will help determine the epileptogenic tuber and the eloquent cortex. If necessary, multistage surgery can be considered if it turns out that there are multiple epileptogenic tubers.

Lachhwani DK, Pestana E, Gupta A, et al. Identification of candidates for epilepsy surgery in patients with tuberous sclerosis. *Neurology*. 2005;64:1651–1654.

Romanelli P, Najjar S, Weiner HL, et al. Epilepsy surgery in tuberous sclerosis: multistage procedures with bilateral or multilobar foci. *J Child Neurol*. 2002;17:689–692.

6. B. The incidence of MCM in WWE is 7.1%, whereas it is 2.3% in healthy women. Incidence is highest for AED polytherapy (17%). Valproate monotherapy is associated with the highest incidence of MCM (11%), which is highest among all other AEDs. Overall, the incidence of MCM in children born of WWE is about threefold that of healthy women. The risk is increased for all AED monotherapy and further increased for AED polytherapy compared with women without epilepsy. The risk is significantly higher for children exposed to valproate monotherapy and to polytherapy with two or more AEDs when the polytherapy combination consists of phenobarbital, phenytoin, or valproate. The most common MCM in children born to mothers without epilepsy are malformations of the cardiovascular system, in particular, ventricular septal defects; musculoskeletal defects and urinary malformations are less common, but still prominent. In children born to WWE, cardiovascular and musculoskeletal systems are the most common types of MCM, but some rare defects, such as defects of the ear, neck, and face and cleft lip, are significantly greater in children of WWE compared with those without epilepsy. Of note, the incidence of spina bifida is 15-fold higher for those children born to WWE.

Meador K, Reynolds MW, Crean S, et al. Pregnancy outcomes in women with epilepsy: a systematic review and meta-analysis of published pregnancy registries and cohorts. *Epilepsy Res.* 2008;81:1–13.

7. **C.** For WWE, a folic acid dose of 0.4 to 5 mg/day has been suggested, but there is no convincing evidence for the effectiveness of folic acid in this population. The recommendation for women who have a history of neural tube defects in an earlier pregnancy is 4 mg/day. Some studies have suggested that low maternal folate levels are a risk factor for fetal malformations, but other studies do not support this. Higher dose folate supplementation (1–4 mg/day) for women taking valproate and enzyme-inducing AEDs has been suggested, but there is no evidence to show that it decreases the risk of neural tube defects. The mechanism by which anticonvulsants cause congenital malformations is not known. Folic acid deficiency is one suspected cause, as some AEDs are known to affect folate metabolism.

Harden C, Pennel PB, Koppel BS, et al. Practice parameter update: management issues for women with epilepsy—focus on pregnancy (an evidence-based review): vitamin K, folic acid, blood levels, and breastfeeding. Report of the Quality Standards Subcommittee and Therapeutics and Technology Assessment Subcommittee of the American Academy of Neurology and American Epilepsy Society. *Neurology.* 2009;73:142–149.

Kluger B, Meador K. Teratogenicity of antiepileptic medications. *Semin Neurol.* 2008;28:328–335.

Noe K, Pack A. Women's issues and epilepsy. *Continuum* (Minneap Minn). 2010;16:159–178.

8. **B.** Retrospective studies have shown the rate of noncompliance to AEDs in adult patients is 26% to 41%. However, a prospective study in children showed the noncompliance rate to be higher at 58%. In this study, only lower socioeconomic status emerged as the sole predictor of noncompliance; none of the seizure-related factors (seizure type, seizure freedom, number of AEDs, or frequency of adverse events), or the demographic factors (age, gender, or caregiver marital status) predicted the compliance pattern. In a survey of 55 patients, the overall compliance rate was 75%; mean compliance rates declined as the dosing frequency increased: once a day, 86%; twice a day, 80%; three times a day, 76; and four times a day, 53%, with a significant decrease of compliance with the latter. It has been shown that the compliance rate declines significantly from 82% during the 5-day peri-clinic visit time to 67% between visits (*P* < .05).

Cramer JA. Compliance. Engel J, Jr, Pedley TA, eds. *Epilepsy: A Comprehensive Textbook.* 2nd ed. Philadelphia, PA: Lippincott Williams & Wilkins; 2008:1291–1293.

Modi AC, Rausch JR, Glauser TA. Patterns of nonadherence to antiepileptic drug therapy in children with newly diagnosed epilepsy. *JAMA.* 2011;305:1669–1676.

Modur PN. Failure to take antiepileptic drugs as prescribed: a socioeconomic issue after all. *Arch Neurol.* 2011;68:1320–1322.

9. **C.** The second Veterans Affairs (VA) Cooperative Trial showed that carbamazepine and valproate were equally efficacious for generalized tonic–clonic seizures, but carbamazepine was more efficacious for partial seizures. Other reports have shown that carbamazepine can worsen absence and myoclonic seizures. Thus, in this patient, the

addition of carbamazepine could result in an increase in myoclonic seizures, while the generalized tonic–clonic seizures may improve. Carbamazepine induces the activity of CYP3A4 because of autoinduction, which occurs 2 to 6 weeks after starting therapy. As a result, the serum level of carbamazepine is likely to be subtherapeutic, not supratherapeutic. Low serum sodium (hyponatremia) is a known side effect of carbamazepine, and can be expected.

Guerreiro CAM, Guerreiro MM. Carbamazepine and oxcarbazepine. In: Wyllie E, ed. *Wyllie's Treatment of Epilepsy: Principles and Practice*. 5th ed. Philadelphia, PA: Lippincott Williams & Wilkins; 2011:614–621.

10. **D.** Carbamazepine is oxidized by CYP3A4 and CYP2C8 to carbamazepine-epoxide, which is an active metabolite. The second Veterans Affairs (VA) Cooperative Trial showed that carbamazepine and valproate were equally efficacious for generalized tonic–clonic seizures, but carbamazepine was more efficacious for partial seizures. Another study showed that in elderly patients with new onset seizures, carbamazepine, gabapentin, and lamotrigine were equally efficacious, but the retention rate was higher with gabapentin and lamotrigine, suggesting that carbamazepine may not be well tolerated in that population. Hypersensitivity to carbamazepine is related to the HLA-B*1502 allele, which occurs more commonly in people of Asian descent; as a result, rash can be more commonly seen in that ethnic group.

Guerreiro CAM, Guerreiro MM. Carbamazepine and oxcarbazepine. In: Wyllie E, ed. *Wyllie's Treatment of Epilepsy: Principles and Practice*. 5th ed. Philadelphia, PA: Lippincott Williams & Wilkins; 2011:614–621.

11. **C.** It has been shown the women with epilepsy (WWE) who remain seizure free for at least 9 to 12 months prior to pregnancy have 84% to 92% chance of remaining seizure free during pregnancy. There is insufficient evidence to support or refute an increased risk of SE in pregnant WWE; it is estimated that the annual frequency of SE in patients with varied epilepsy types is approximately 1.6%. Thus, SE does not occur more frequently during pregnancy. Folic acid supplementation is generally recommended to reduce the risk of major congenital malformations during pregnancy despite insufficient data to show that it is effective in WWE. Therefore, the current recommendation is to provide at least 0.4 mg of folic acid daily supplementation to all women of childbearing potential, with or without epilepsy, prior to conception and during pregnancy. Data are insufficient to address the dosing of folic acid and whether higher doses offer greater protective benefit to WWE taking AEDs. Reduction in AED levels occur because of physiologic changes of pregnancy including activation of hepatic P450 enzymes, alterations of serum protein binding, increased renal clearance, and increased volume of drug distribution. Thus, monitoring of lamotrigine, carbamazepine, and phenytoin levels during pregnancy should be considered (Level B) and monitoring of levetiracetam and oxcarbazepine levels may be considered (Level C).

Harden C, Hopp J, Ting TY, et al. Practice parameter update: management issues for women with epilepsy—focus on pregnancy (an evidence-based review): obstetrical complications and change in seizure frequency: report of the Quality Standards Subcommittee and Therapeutics and Technology Assessment Subcommittee of the American Academy of Neurology and American Epilepsy Society. *Neurology*. 2009;73:126–132.

Harden C, Pennel PB, Koppel BS, et al. Practice parameter update: management issues for women with epilepsy—focus on pregnancy (an evidence-based review): vitamin K, folic acid, blood levels, and breastfeeding. Report of the Quality Standards Subcommittee and Therapeutics and Technology

Assessment Subcommittee of the American Academy of Neurology and American Epilepsy Society. *Neurology*. 2009;73:142–149.

12. **B.** The MRI shows right medial temporal T2 hyperintensity. This finding, along with history of new-onset intractable seizures in a previously healthy person, normal CSF, and negative HSV PCR, strongly points to limbic encephalitis. The latter is generally considered to be a paraneoplastic condition with antibodies directed against the intracellular antigens (Hu, Ma2, CRMP5, and amphiphysin) or against the cell membrane or synaptic receptors (e.g., VGKC, NMDAR, LGI1, Caspr, $GABA_B$, GAD). The clinical picture of temporal lobe seizures and neuropsychiatric manifestations further supports the diagnosis. The patient is already on three conventional antiepileptic drugs (AEDs). Therefore, the addition of another AED such as phenobarbital, is not likely to be of much benefit. Temporal lobe biopsy would likely reveal nonspecific inflammatory changes and is not likely to be of great diagnostic value. Testing the paraneoplastic panel for the above antibodies and workup for an unknown primary tumor would be beneficial. Propofol-induced burst suppression would be appropriate if there is clear evidence of status epilepticus, which is not the case in this patient. Given the underlying autoimmune basis for limbic encephalitis, the most appropriate intervention would be immunosuppressive therapy such as rituximab. Other reasonable options include methylprednisolone, intravenous immunoglobulin, and plasmapheresis.

Dubey D, Konikkara J, Modur PN, et al. Effectiveness of multimodality treatment for autoimmune limbic epilepsy. *Epileptic Disord*. 2014;16:494–499.

Toledano M, Pittock SJ. Autoimmune epilepsy. *Semin Neurol*. 2015;35:245–258.

13. **B.** Perampanel is a noncompetitive antagonist of the ionotropic α-amino-3-hydroxy-5-methyl-4-isoxazolepropionic acid (AMPA) glutamate receptor present on the postsynaptic neurons. Glutamate is the primary excitatory neurotransmitter in the central nervous system. Perampanel has no effect on potassium channels. It is extensively metabolized via primary oxidation and glucuronidation, primarily mediated by CYP3A4/5. The half-life of perampanel is about 105 hours, so it takes 2 to 3 weeks to reach steady state. At low doses (4–8 mg/day), perampanel has no significant effect on oral contraceptives, but at high doses (12 mg), it decreases the C_{max} of ethinylestradiol and levonorgestrel by 18% and 42%, respectively.

Fycompa (perampanel) prescribing information. https://www.fycompa.com/sites/all/themes/fycompa/pdf/fycompa_prescribing_information.pdf. Accessed January 11, 2016.

14. **B.** Vigabatrin is an irreversible inhibitor of GABA transaminase. Retinopathy, characterized by irreversible, bilateral, concentric peripheral visual field constriction, is associated with vigabatrin treatment. Routine ophthalmologic evaluation is recommended. Retinopathy characterized by irreversible, bilateral, bull's eye maculopathy is associated with chloroquine toxicity.

Fecarotta C, Sergott R. Vigabatrin-associated visual field loss. *Int Ophthalmol Clin*. 2012;52:87–94.

15. **A.** There is insufficient evidence to determine whether other forms of corticosteroids are as effective as ACTH for short-term treatment of infantile spasms. However, low-dose ACTH is probably as effective as high-dose ACTH, so low-dose ACTH should be considered for treatment of infantile spasms. ACTH is more effective than VGB for

short-term treatment of children with infantile spasms (excluding those with tuberous sclerosis complex), so ACTH should be considered preferentially over VGB. Hormonal therapy (ACTH or prednisolone) may be considered for use in preference to VGB in infants with cryptogenic infantile spasms, to possibly improve developmental outcome. Short lag time to treatment leads to better long-term developmental outcome. Successful short-term treatment of cryptogenic infantile spasms with ACTH or prednisolone leads to better long-term developmental outcome than treatment with VGB.

Go CY, Mackay MT, Weiss SK, et al. Evidence-based guideline update: medical treatment of infantile spasms. Report of the Guideline Development Subcommittee of the American Academy of Neurology and the Practice Committee of the Child Neurology Society. *Neurology*. 2012;78:1974–1980.

16. **B.** Valproic acid is a branched-chain carboxylic acid that undergoes hepatic metabolism through glucuronidation and mitochondrial beta-oxidation. Carnitine is an essential cofactor in mitochondrial beta-oxidation and carnitine depletion from valproic acid treatment results in a shift to omega oxidation; this increases the production of toxic metabolites, which inhibit the mitochondrial enzyme involved in ammonia elimination, resulting in ammonia accumulation and encephalopathy. Urea cycle defects predispose to development of valproate-induced hyperammonemic encephalopathy. In addition, carnitine deficiency, protein-rich diets, and hypercatabolic states may also increase ammonia production. Polytherapy with drugs, such as phenobarbital and topiramate, seems to contribute to hyperammonemia. Carnitine is used for treatment of valproate-induced hyperammonemic encephalopathy due to overdoses or usual dosages of valproic acid.

Mock CM, Schwetschenau KH. Levocarnitine for valproic-acid-induced hyperammonemic encephalopathy. *Am J Health Syst Pharm*. 2012;69:35–39.

Segura-Bruna N, Rodriguez-Campello A, Puente V, et al. Valproate-induced hyperammonemic encephalopathy. *Acta Neurol Scand*. 2006;114:1–7.

17. **B.** Primidone therapy results in two active metabolites: phenobarbital and phenylethylmalonamide. When primidone is added to carbamazepine, the latter induces the phenobarbital-producing pathway of primidone metabolism, resulting in an increase in phenobarbital level. Phenobarbital clearance remains unchanged.

Michelucci R, Pasini E, Tassinari CA. Phenobarbital, primidone and other barbiturates. In: Shorvon SD, Perucca E, Engel J, Jr, eds. *The Treatment of Epilepsy*. 3rd ed. Oxford, UK: Wiley-Blackwell; 2009:585–604.

18. **D.** Optic neuropathy due to thiamin deficiency has been reported in patients on the ketogenic diet. This resolves following thiamin administration. Bleeding abnormalities, prolonged bleeding times, and abnormalities of platelet aggregation but not hypercoagulability, can occur on the ketogenic diet. Linear growth may be retarded while on the ketogenic diet. Obesity is not a complication of the ketogenic diet as the total daily calories are calculated based on age, activity level, and requirements; those calories are then divided into the required ratio of fats to protein and carbohydrates. Cardiac abnormalities including dilated cardiomyopathy and prolonged QT interval have been reported while on the ketogenic diet. Other complications include renal calculi, increased infections, pancreatitis, hypoproteinemia, and potentiation of valproate toxicity.

Ballaban-Gill KR. Complications of the ketogenic diet. In: Stafstrom CE, Rho JM, eds. *Epilepsy and the Ketogenic Diet*. Totowa, NJ: Humana Press; 2004:123–128.

19. C. In a 4:1 ratio ketogenic diet, there are four times as many grams of fat for every 1 g of protein and carbohydrate combined. The ratio regulates the degree of ketosis, with higher ratios inducing greater ketosis. Different individuals, matched for age and weight, may develop different levels of ketosis on the same ratio, due to individual variations in energy metabolism and energy expenditure.

Zupec-Kania B, Werner RR, Zupanc ML. Clinical use of the ketogenic diet: the dietician's role. In: Stafstrom CE, Rho JM, eds. *Epilepsy and the Ketogenic Diet*. Totowa, NJ: Humana Press; 2004:63–82.

20. C. 50% to 60% of neonates will have subclinical seizures detected on EEG monitoring after AED administration. Neonatal seizures are often brief, subtle, and difficult to recognize in terms of clinical manifestations. In addition, a significant percentage of electrographic seizures may not have clinical manifestations, especially after AED administration. The persistence of electrographic seizures is termed uncoupling or decoupling.

Clancy RR. Summary proceedings from the neurology group on neonatal seizures. *Pediatrics*. 2006;117:S23–S27.

Scher MS, Alvin J, Gaus L, et al. Uncoupling of EEG-clinical neonatal seizures after antiepileptic drug use. *Pediatr Neurol*. 2003;28:277–280.

21. D. Infections, new medications, and foods that contain even small amounts of carbohydrates can induce seizures in children carefully titrated for seizure control on the ketogenic diet. Suntan lotions, hair gels, ointments containing sorbitol can reverse the ketosis and induce seizures. Small changes in dietary intake can also induce seizures.

Kosoff EH, Freeman JM. The ketogenic diet: the physician's perspective. In: Stafstrom CE, Rho JM, eds. *Epilepsy and the Ketogenic Diet*. Totowa, NJ: Humana Press; 2004:53–62.

22. C. Despite the well-known effects of estrogen on lowering seizure threshold, observational studies do not support that estrogen-containing oral contraceptives worsen seizure control in WWE. Enzyme-inducing AEDs can reduce estrogen and progesterone to subtherapeutic levels, leading to decreased efficacy of oral contraception. AEDs known to reduce the efficacy of oral contraceptives include carbamazepine, eslicarbazepine, oxcarbazepine, perampanel, phenobarbital, phenytoin, primidone, rufinamide, and topiramate. AEDs without significant effects on oral contraceptive efficacy include ethosuximide, gabapentin, lacosamide, lamotrigine, levetiracetam, tiagabine, valproate, and zonisamide. Although the effect of oral contraceptives on AEDs is less concerning, it is important to note that the oral contraceptives can significantly reduce the lamotrigine level, resulting in loss of efficacy and breakthrough seizures. The transdermal patch and vaginal ring formulations also have higher failure rates with enzyme-inducing AEDs. Intramuscular (IM) medroxyprogesterone provides higher dosages of progestin, but it may still require dosing at 8- to 10-week intervals rather than 12-week intervals. Efficacy of intrauterine devices is not typically affected by the AEDs.

Pennell P. Hormonal aspects of epilepsy. *Neurol Clin*. 2009;27:941–965.

23. A. A microelectronic monitoring system has been shown to improve AED compliance in epilepsy patients. However, the benefit of providing such a system routinely for patients is unclear. Such systems are typically indicated for patients whose seizures are uncontrolled or occur randomly despite adequate treatment. The other listed strategies can be recommended routinely: prescribing the fewest number of dose times;

instructing when to take missed doses; and providing cues on how to take the medication (e.g., taking medications at specific times, around meal times, or around specific activities, using pill boxes, using log sheets).

Cramer JA. Compliance. In: Engel J, Jr, Pedley TA, eds. *Epilepsy: A Comprehensive Textbook.* 2nd ed. Philadelphia, PA: Lippincott Williams & Wilkins; 2008:1291–1293.

24. **B.** Felbamate is associated with increased risk of aplastic anemia and liver failure. Risk of aplastic anemia associated with felbamate is estimated to be 127 cases per million exposures. In comparison, the risk of aplastic anemia with carbamazepine is 5 to 20 cases per million exposures, and the risk in the general population is 2 to 6 per million per year. Risk factors for felbamate-associated aplastic anemia include history of cytopenia, history of allergy or significant toxicity to an antiepileptic drug (AED), prior history of autoimmune disorder (i.e., systemic lupus erythematosus, rheumatoid arthritis, Hashimoto's thyroiditis, panhypogammaglobulinemia, idiopathic thrombocytopenia purpura), and a positive antinuclear antibody titer. In patients who developed aplastic anemia while on felbamate, 42% had a history of cytopenia previous to felbamate use, 52% had a history of allergy or significant toxicity to an AED, and 33% had evidence of an underlying autoimmune disease. Due to the limited number of reported cases, the true incidence of liver failure related to felbamate use cannot be determined. The estimated incidence is between 1 per 26,000 and 1 per 34,000 exposures. In comparison, in patients taking valproate, the risk of death due to liver failure is between 1 in 10,000 and 1 in 49,000; in children <2 years of age who are taking valproate, the risk of fatal liver toxicity is 1 in 500.

Pellock JM, Fraught E, Leppick IE, et al. Felbamate: consensus of current clinical experience. *Epilepsy Res.* 2006;71:89–901.

25. **C.** The preferred agents for emergent initial treatment of SE are intravenous (IV) lorazepam, intramuscular (IM) midazolam (which can also be administered via the buccal or nasal routes), and rectal diazepam. IM midazoalm has been found to be at least as effective as IV lorazepam for out-of-hospital treatment of SE. The preferred agents for urgent control treatment of SE are IV phenytoin/fosphenytoin, phenobarbital, valproate, or continuous midazolam infusion. There are two potential goals of urgent control treatment. For patients who respond to emergent initial treatment and have complete resolution of SE, the goal is rapid attainment of therapeutic AED levels and continued dosing for maintenance therapy. For patients who fail emergent initial therapy, the goal of urgent control therapy is to stop SE. However, urgent control treatment is not needed if the immediate cause of SE is known and definitively corrected (e.g., severe hypoglycemia).

Brophy GM, Bell R, Claassen J, et al. Guidelines for the evaluation and management of status epilepticus. *Neurocrit Care.* 2012;17:3–23.

26. **B.** Pentobarbital contains 40% v/v of propylene glycol, which is the likely cause of the patient's metabolic derangements. Propylene glycol toxicity is a potentially life-threatening iatrogenic complication that is common and preventable. It should be considered when a patient has an unexplained anion gap, unexplained metabolic acidosis, hyperosmolality, and clinical deterioration. IV lorazepam- and diazepam-related propylene glycol toxicity has also been described.

Bledsoe KA, Kramer AH. Propylene glycol toxicity complicating use of barbiturate coma. *Neurocrit Care.* 2008;9:122–124.

27. **B.** Treatment of RSE is challenging. Pentobarbital, midazolam, propofol, and ketamine are often used. Pentobarbital can cause cardiac instability and hypotension. Midazolam is a short-acting benzodiazepine and can cause respiratory depression, sedation, and hypotension. Propofol can cause propofol-related infusion syndrome (PRIS), characterized by metabolic acidosis, rhabdomyolysis, hyperkalemia, and lipemia. Children may be at higher risk for this potentially fatal syndrome. Patients may also have an allergic response to soybean oil, egg phospholipid, or glycerol in the propofol emulsion. Continuous infusion of propofol involves a large lipid and caloric load. Although ketamine has been found to be well-tolerated, cardiac arrhythmias such as supraventricular tachycardia and atrial fibrillation have been reported.

Brophy GM, Bell R, Claassen J, et al. Guidelines for the evaluation and management of status epilepticus. *Neurocrit Care*. 2012;17:3–23.

Gaspard N, Foreman B, Judd LM, et al. Intravenous ketamine for the treatment of refractory status epilepticus: a retrospective multicenter study. *Epilepsia*. 2013;54:1498–1503.

28. **A.** Based on the Practice Parameter published in 2003, the evidence for effectiveness of resective epilepsy surgery is as follows: about two thirds of patients become free of disabling seizures after anteromedial temporal resection, and about half of patients become free of disabling seizures after localized neocortical resection. The outcome of temporal lobectomy assessed by uncontrolled studies was similar to the one found in a randomized, controlled trial of surgery versus antiepileptic drug treatment.

Engel J Jr., Wiebe S, French J, et al. Practice parameter: temporal lobe and localized neocortical resections for epilepsy: report of the Quality Standards Subcommittee of the American Academy of Neurology, in association with the American Epilepsy Society and the American Association of Neurological Surgeons. *Neurology*. 2003;60:538–547.

Wiebe S, Blume WT, Girvin JP, et al. A randomized, controlled trial of surgery for temporal lobe epilepsy. *N Engl J Med*. 2001;345:311–318.

29. **D.** Anteromedial temporal lobectomy results in material-specific language and memory deficits. Although no significant changes in mean scores are noted in large groups of patients postoperatively, individual patients show either improvement or impairment. Average or high preoperative memory performance can be associated with a 10% or more postoperative decline in some components of Wechsler Memory Scale (WMS) scores after dominant temporal lobectomy; in contrast, patients with below-average preoperative memory performance are likely to improve in the WMS scores ($P < .05$). Verbal memory has been shown to improve after nondominant temporal lobectomy and decline after dominant temporal lobectomy ($P < .05$). Visuospatial memory has been shown to improve after dominant temporal lobectomy and decline after nondominant temporal lobectomy ($P < .05$). In terms of language outcome, naming does not change after dominant or nondominant temporal lobectomy, although individual patients may experience improvement or impairment. Only the Token Test, a measure of receptive comprehension, shows laterality effects: patients with dominant temporal lobectomy show a greater pre- to postoperative improvement in this measure than patients with nondominant temporal lobectomy ($P < .001$).

Engel J, Jr, Wiebe S, French J, et al. Practice parameter: temporal lobe and localized neocortical resections for epilepsy: report of the Quality Standards Subcommittee of the American Academy of Neurology, in association with the American Epilepsy Society and the American Association of Neurological Surgeons. *Neurology*. 2003;60:538–547.

30. **D.** The ILAE seizure outcome classification system has six classes: class 1, completely seizure free and no auras; class 2, only auras and no other seizures; class 3, 1 to 3 seizure days per year with or without auras; class 4, 4 seizure days per year to 50% reduction of baseline seizure days with or without auras; class 5, <50% reduction of baseline seizure days to 100% increase of baseline seizure days with or without auras; and class 6, >100% increase of baseline seizure days with or without auras. In this scheme, the number of "seizure days" is counted instead of the absolute number of seizures; a "seizure day" is defined as a 24-hour period. For the baseline, the number of "seizure days" during the 12-month period before surgery is considered. For classes 1 to 3, the absolute number of seizure days is counted, whereas for classes 4 to 6, relative changes with respect to the preoperative baseline are counted.

Wieser HG, Blume WT, Fish D, et al. ILAE Commission Report. Proposal for a new classification of outcome with respect to epileptic seizures following epilepsy surgery. *Epilepsia*. 2001;42:282–286.

31. **A.** There are no randomized controlled studies assessing the treatment for RSE. However, a systemic review (not meta-analysis) was done on the published articles on midazolam, propofol, and pentobarbital for RSE. It was found that the mortality was not significantly associated with the choice of agent or titration goal. Pentobarbital was usually titrated to EEG background suppression by using intermittent EEG monitoring, whereas midazolam and propofol were more often titrated to seizure suppression with continuous EEG monitoring. Compared with midazolam or propofol, pentobarbital was associated with a lower frequency of short-term treatment failure (8% vs. 23%; $P < .01$), breakthrough seizures (12% vs. 42%; $P < .001$), and changes to a different continuous intravenous (IV) antiepileptic drug (AED) (3% vs. 21%; $P < .001$), and a higher frequency of hypotension (systolic blood pressure <100 mmHg; 77% vs. 34%; $P < .001$). Compared with seizure suppression, titration of treatment to EEG background suppression was associated with a lower frequency of breakthrough seizures (4% vs. 53%; $P < .001$) and a higher frequency of hypotension (76% vs. 29%; $P < .001$). These findings led to the conclusion that treatment with any continuous IV AED infusion to attain EEG background suppression may be more effective than other strategies for treating RSE.

Claassen J, Hirsch LJ, Emerson RG, et al. Treatment of refractory status epilepticus with pentobarbital, propofol, or midazolam: a systematic review. *Epilepsia*. 2002;43:146–153.

32. **B.** Diazepam is highly lipophilic and enters the brain on first pass, but it also redistributes quickly to other fatty tissues. Therefore, brain concentrations of diazepam decline rapidly, requiring repeated doses (as frequent as every 15–30 minutes) to prevent seizure recurrence in a patient with status epilepticus. On the other hand, lorazepam has slower onset of action and slower redistribution from the brain. This is probably the reason for the longer antiseizure effect of lorazepam despite its shorter serum half-life compared with diazepam (14 vs. 30 hours).

Alldredge BK, Treiman DM, Bleck TP, et al. Treatment of status epilepticus. In: Engel J, Jr, Pedley TA, eds. *Epilepsy: A Comprehensive Textbook*. 2nd ed. Philadelphia, PA: Lippincott Williams & Wilkins; 2008:1357–1363.

33. **B.** Hyponatremia from oxcarbazepine occurs in 2.5% of patients. The degree of hyponatremia is related to age (7.3% incidence for patients >65 years), dose of oxcarbazepine, and rapid titration. A recent study showed that concomitant treatment

with diuretics is a risk factor for symptomatic hyponatremia. There is no clear association between hyponatremia and the use of losartan. Oxcarbazepine-induced hyponatremia is felt to be due to direct effect of the drug on the renal tubules and increased sensitivity of the tubules to antidiuretic hormone (ADH).

Guerreiro CAM, Guerreiro MM. Carbamazepine and oxcarbazepine. In: Wyllie E, ed. *Wyllie's Treatment of Epilepsy: Principles and Practice*. 5th ed. Philadelphia, PA: Lippincott Williams & Wilkins; 2011:614–621.

Kim Y-S, Kim DW, Jung K-H, et al. Frequency of and risk factors for oxcarbazepine-induce severe and symptomatic hyponatremia. *Seizure*. 2014;23:208–212.

34. **C.** Unlike, carbamazepine, no autoinduction has been observed with oxcarbazepine. Oxcarbazepine is a weak inducer of CYP3A4/5; so the concentration of ethinyl estradiol and levonorgestrel can be decreased, resulting in decreased efficacy of oral contraceptives. Oxcarbazepine is a weak inhibitor of CYP2C19, which metabolizes phenytoin; so the phenytoin level may increase by up to 40% with administration of large doses of oxcarbazepine (>1,200 mg/day). No significant change in plasma valproic acid level has been noted with the administration of oxcarbazepine.

Guerreiro CAM, Guerreiro MM. Carbamazepine and oxcarbazepine. In: Wyllie E, ed. *Wyllie's Treatment of Epilepsy: Principles and Practice*. 5th ed. Philadelphia, PA: Lippincott Williams & Wilkins; 2011:614–621.

35. **A.** Eslicarbazepine acts by blocking the sodium channels and stabilizing the inactivated state of the sodium channels. It undergoes first-pass hepatic hydrolysis to S-licarbazepine, which is the major active metabolite. S-licarbazepine is the active enantiomer of the monohydroxy derivative (MHD), which is the active metabolite of oxcarbazepine (note that R-licarbazepine is the inactive enantiomer of MHD). Eslicarbazepine is a weak inducer of CYP3A4, and can cause decreased plasma concentrations of ethinyl estradiol and levonorgestrel. Thus, eslicarbazepine can decrease the efficacy of oral contraceptives, but its effect is less than that of oxcarbazepine. Eslicarbazepine does not affect warfarin level.

Gazzola DM, Delanty N, French JA. Newer antiepileptic drugs. In: Wyllie E, ed. *Wyllie's Treatment of Epilepsy: Principles and Practice*. 5th ed. Philadelphia, PA: Lippincott Williams & Wilkins; 2011:771–778.

36. **C.** PDH is the rate limiting enzyme connecting glycolysis with the tricarboxylic acid cycle, and plays a key role in energy metabolism, and the ketogenic diet is beneficial in treating PDH deficiency. The other three disorders are contraindications to the ketogenic diet. Carnitine palmitoyl transferase deficiency and very long-chain acyl-CoA dehydrogenase deficiency are disorders of beta oxidation and fat metabolism that require high carbohydrate contents and the ketogenic diet may result in increased morbidity and mortality. Porphyrias are diseases caused by blocks in heme synthesis. Carbohydrates reduce porphyrin synthesis, and are used at high doses during an attack. The ketogenic diet can worsen this condition.

Gunhild A, Bergquist C. Indications and contraindications of the ketogenic diet. In: Stafstrom CE, Rho JM, eds. *Epilepsy and the Ketogenic Diet*. Totowa, NJ: Humana Press; 2004:111–122.

37. **D.** According to AANs practice parameter, primidone and levetiracetam probably transfer into breast milk in clinically significant amounts. Valproate, phenobarbital, phenytoin, and carbamazepine probably are not transferred into breast milk in clinically important amounts.

Harden C, Pennel PB, Koppel BS, et al. Practice parameter update: management issues for women with epilepsy—focus on pregnancy (an evidence-based review): vitamin K, folic acid, blood levels, and breastfeeding. Report of the Quality Standards Subcommittee and Therapeutics and Technology Assessment Subcommittee of the American Academy of Neurology and American Epilepsy Society. *Neurology*. 2009;73:142–149.

38. **C.** According to AAN's practice parameter for WWE taking antiepileptic drugs, there is probably no substantially increased risk (>2 times expected) of cesarean delivery or late pregnancy bleeding, and probably no moderately increased risk (>1.5 times expected) of premature contractions or premature labor and delivery. However, there is possibly a substantially increased risk of premature contractions and premature labor and delivery during pregnancy for WWE who smoke. Seizure freedom for at least 9 months prior to pregnancy is probably associated with a high likelihood (84%–92%) of seizure freedom during pregnancy.

Harden C, Hopp J, Ting TY, et al. Practice parameter update: management issues for women with epilepsy—focus on pregnancy (an evidence-based review): obstetrical complications and change in seizure frequency: report of the Quality Standards Subcommittee and Therapeutics and Technology Assessment Subcommittee of the American Academy of Neurology and American Epilepsy Society. *Neurology*. 2009;73:126–132.

39. **D.** Catamenial epilepsy refers to the cyclic exacerbation of seizures in relation to the menstrual cycle. Three patterns of catamenial epilepsy are described: perimenstrual, periovulatory, and luteal. Monthly fluctuations in hormone levels of estrogen and progesterone are the basis for catamenial epilepsy. Progesterone and its metabolites are anticonvulsant, whereas estrogens are mainly proconvulsant. Androgens are mainly anticonvulsant, but their metabolism to estradiol and other substances makes their effects more varied. There is a bidirectional relationship between hormones and epilepsy, such that the hormones influence epilepsy, and epilepsy affects hormones. Antiepileptic drugs (AEDs) can interact both with epilepsy and with hormones. Sex hormones influence brain excitability. Epileptic activity, especially mediated via the amygdala, alters reproductive function. In women with partial epilepsy, progesterone was not beneficial over placebo when tested in the catamenial and noncatamenial groups. However, the level of perimenstrual seizure exacerbation was a significant predictor of the responder rate with progesterone therapy so that progesterone may provide clinically important benefit for a subset of women with perimenstrually exacerbated seizures.

Herzog AG, Fowler KM, Smithson SD, et al. Progesterone vs placebo therapy for women with epilepsy: a randomized clinical trial. *Neurology*. 2012;78:1959–1966.

Taubøll E, Sveberg L, Svalheim S. Interactions between hormones and epilepsy. *Seizure*. 2015;28:3–11.

40. **B.** In the pivotal trial, TPM was associated with 1% to 2% incidence of renal stones. Later study has shown higher prevalence of nephrolithiasis with long-term TPM use (10.7% symptomatic and 20% asymptomatic). TPM inhibits carbonic anhydrase, which is felt to be the cause for increased risk of stone formation. Inhibition of proximal renal tubule carbonic anhydrase results in systemic acidosis because of reduced bicarbonate reabsorption; this leads to an increase in the urine pH, which increases the risk for calcium phosphate stone formation. Furthermore, the proximal tubule intracellular acidosis enhances renal citrate reabsorption and metabolism, resulting in hypocitraturia, which in turn increases the risk of both calcium oxalate and calcium phosphate stone formation. Recently, alkali

therapy has been shown to raise urinary citrate excretion in patients who form renal stones while being treated with TPM, suggesting that such a treatment might be beneficial in reducing the risk of kidney stones in patients taking TPM.

Jhagroo RA, Wertheim ML, Penniston KL. Alkali replacement raises urinary citrate excretion in patients with topiramate-induced hypocitraturia. *Br J Clin Pharmacol.* 2015;81:131–136..

Maalouf NM, Langston JP, Van Ness PC, et al. Nephrolithiasis in topiramate users. *Urol Res.* 2011;39:303–307

41. **C.** Inhaled alprazolam is being investigated as a potential novel treatment for acute repetitive seizures using the Staccato system to deliver it to the lung in a single breath, with no coordination required. With this system, excipient-free pure drug is transformed (through heating) into fine aerosolized particles to get into the deep lung. Vaporization takes <1 second and results in high bioavailability with intravenous-like pharmacokinetics. Peak plasma concentrations are obtained faster than intranasal or rectal routes of administration. Ganaxolone is a neurosteroid that is a synthetic analog of allopregnanolone. It is a positive allosteric modulator of the GABA-A receptor, and is active at synaptic and extrasynaptic receptors. Ganaxolone is under investigation for treatment of intractable partial onset seizures. Triheptanoin is a triglyceride of medium-chain fatty acids with an odd number chain length of seven carbons. It is broken into heptanoate and later metabolized to four and five carbon ketone bodies, which provide multiple energy substrates to the brain. Triheptanoin is being evaluated for treatment of Glut1 deficiency disorder. A liquid form of highly purified, plant-derived cannabidiol (CBD) is under investigation in children with Dravet syndrome and Lennox–Gastaut syndrome.

French JA, Schachter SC, Sirven J, et al. The Epilepsy Foundation's 4th biennial epilepsy pipeline update conference. *Epilepsy Behav.* 2015;46:34–50.

42. **C.** The Atkins diet has been shown in one randomized trial to be beneficial in controlling seizures. None of the other therapies was found to be beneficial, suggesting a need for further investigation.

Cheuk DK, Wong V. Acupuncture for epilepsy. *Cochrane Database Syst Rev.* 2008;4:CD005062.

Levy RG, Cooper PN, Giri P. Ketogenic diet and other dietary treatments for epilepsy. *Cochrane Database Syst Rev.* 2012;3:CD001903.

Panebianco M, Sridharan K, Ramaratnam S. Yoga for epilepsy. *Cochrane Database Syst Rev.* 2015;5:CD001524.

Ramaratnam S, Baker GA, Goldstein LH. Psychological treatments for epilepsy. *Cochrane Database Syst Rev.* 2008;3:CD002029.

43. **C.** For adults presenting with a first unprovoked seizure, a routine EEG reveals epileptiform abnormalities in approximately 23% of patients, which are predictive of seizure recurrence. A brain imaging study (CT or MRI) is significantly abnormal in 10% of patients, which indicates a possible seizure etiology. Laboratory tests such as blood counts, blood glucose, and electrolyte panels are abnormal in approximately 15% of patients, but the abnormalities are minor and do not indicate the cause for the seizure. Clinical signs of infection such as fever predict significant cerebrospinal fluid (CSF) abnormalities on lumbar puncture. Toxicology screening studies are only occasionally positive. Based on these results, EEG and brain imaging (CT or MRI) should be considered as part of the routine evaluation of adults presenting with an apparent unprovoked first seizure (Level B). Laboratory tests, lumbar puncture, and toxicology screening may

be helpful as determined by the specific clinical circumstances, but the data are insufficient to support or refute recommending any of these tests for the routine evaluation of adults presenting with an apparent first unprovoked seizure (Level U).

Krumholz A, Wiebe S, Gronseth G, et al. Practice parameter: evaluating an apparent unprovoked first seizure in adults (an evidence-based review): report of the Quality Standards Subcommittee of the American Academy of Neurology and the American Epilepsy Society. *Neurology*. 2007;69:1996–2007.

44. D. Acute symptomatic seizures could be caused by a medication, and discontinuing the medication may be more appropriate than starting an antiepileptic drug. Examples of medications with low threshold for causing seizures include opiate and nonopiate analgesics, quinolones, high-dose beta lactam antibiotics, antidepressants, and antipsychotics. Carbonic anhydrase inhibitors are not known to cause seizures. On the contrary, a few antiepileptic drugs (topiramate, zonisamide, acetazolamide) actually have carbonic anhydrase inhibitor properties.

Britton JW. Antiepileptic drug therapy: when to start, when to stop. *Continuum* (Minneap Minn). 2010;16:105–120.

45. D. There is no class I evidence to support that one AED is clearly more efficacious than another for initial monotherapy of partial-onset seizures, but there were two landmark VA cooperative trials that compared traditional AEDs as initial monotherapy for partial seizures. The first study in 1985 compared carbamazepine, phenytoin, phenobarbital, and primidone. "Efficacy" was defined as a combination of seizure control and tolerability. Overall treatment success was highest with carbamazepine and phenytoin, intermediate with phenobarbital, and lowest with primidone ($P < .002$). Carbamazepine provided complete control of partial seizures more often than primidone or phenobarbital ($P < .03$). This led to carbamazepine and phenytoin being recommended as the first-line monotherapy agents for adults with partial and/or generalized tonic–clonic seizures. The second study in 1992 compared valproate and carbamazepine. For the control of secondarily generalized tonic–clonic seizures, carbamazepine and valproate were comparably effective. For complex partial seizures, four of five outcome measures favored carbamazepine over valproate. Carbamazepine was also superior according to a composite score. This led to the conclusion that valproate is as effective as carbamazepine for the treatment of generalized tonic–clonic seizures, but carbamazepine provides better control of complex partial seizures and has fewer long-term adverse effects.

Mattson RH, Cramer JA, Collins JF. A comparison of valproate with carbamazepine for the treatment of complex partial seizures and secondarily generalized tonic-clonic seizures in adults. *N Engl J Med*. 1992;327:765–771.

Mattson RH, Cramer JA, Collins JF, et al. Comparison of carbamazepine, phenobarbital, phenytoin, and primidone in partial and secondarily generalized tonic-clonic seizures. *N Engl J Med*. 1985;313:145–151.

46. C. When monotherapy fails, combination therapy is tried in an attempt to improve effectiveness by improving efficacy and/or tolerability. But combining drugs leads to pharmacokinetic and pharmacodynamic interactions. Phenobarbital and valproate combination leads to sedation and weight gain. Many combinations, especially of sodium channel blockers (e.g., carbamazepine, phenytoin, oxcarbazepine, lacosamide, and lamotrigine) can lead to dizziness and diplopia. Occasionally, dose adjustments need to be made. For example, enzyme-inducing drugs (e.g., carbamazepine, phenytoin, phenobarbital, and primidone) can increase the clearance of topiramate, lamotrigine, and zonisamide. In addition, valproate inhibits lamotrigine metabolism; therefore, when the two are combined, the lamotrigine dose (not the valproate dose) needs to be adjusted. Despite the therapeutic complexities, certain combinations, such as valproate and lamotrigine, are felt to have better efficacy than others. There are no widely accepted comparative efficacy trials of adjunctive therapies. However, there is evidence that polytherapy based on mechanisms of action (rational polytherapy) may enhance effectiveness. A retrospective review found that combining a sodium channel blocker with a drug enhancing GABAergic inhibition appears to be advantageous; combining two GABA-mimetic drugs or combining an α-amino-3-hydroxy-5-methyl-4-isoxazolepropionic acid (AMPA) antagonist with an N-methyl-D-aspartate (NMDA) antagonist may enhance efficacy, but tolerability may be reduced; and combining two sodium channel blockers seems less promising.

Deckers CL, Czuczwar SJ, Hekster YA, et al. Selection of antiepileptic drug polytherapy based on mechanisms of action: the evidence reviewed. *Epilepsia*. 2000;41:1364–1374.

Fountain NB. Choosing among antiepileptic drugs. *Continuum* (Minneap Minn). 2010;16:121–135.

French JA, Gazzola DM. Antiepileptic drug treatment: new drugs and new strategies. *Continuum* (Minneap Minn). 2013;19:643–655.

47. **C.** There have been multiple reports demonstrating that encephalopathy can result when valproate is used in conjunction with other AEDs, such as topiramate and phenobarbital. Other risk factors for valproate-induced encephalopathy include the presence of underlying inborn errors of metabolism, febrile states, and insufficient nutritional intake causing reduced carnitine levels leading to hyperammonemia.

Noh Y, Kim DW, Chu K, et al. Topiramate increases the risk of valproic acid-induced encephalopathy. *Epilepsia*. 2013;54:e1–e4.

48. **D.** Inhibition of CYP2C19 by FBM decreases phenytoin clearance, resulting in 30% to 50% increase in phenytoin level. Induction of CYP3A4 by FBM decreases carbamazepine level by 20% to 30%, but the carbamazepine epoxide level increases by 50% to 60%. FBM increases valproate levels by inhibiting its metabolism by beta-oxidation.

Faught E. Felbamate. In: Wyllie E, ed. *Wyllie's Treatment of Epilepsy: Principles and Practice*. 5th ed. Philadelphia, PA: Lippincott Williams & Wilkins; 2011:741–746.

49. **C.** The diagnosis of nonconvulsive seizures and status epilepticus can be challenging when there are equivocal patterns that fall on the interictal-ictal continuum. When this occurs, a number of possible options can be considered, including a trial of a rapidly acting benzodiazepine to see if there is an improvement in the EEG and/or clinical examination. Trial of small incremental doses of a nonsedating AED may be considered as it would not interfere with assessment of clinical improvement. Although the clinical significance of the EEG is unknown at this stage, continued observation and reassessment of the EEG at a later time are not unreasonable either. However, intubation followed by administration of an anesthetic medication without a clear diagnosis of refractory status epilepticus is not warranted.

Hirsch LJ, Gaspard N. Status epilepticus. *Continuum* (Minneap Minn). 2013;19:767–794.

50. **D.** The etiology of the patient's unresponsiveness is unclear, and although she may be in nonconvulsive status epilepticus, the initial management needs to include basic life

support measures. Monitoring of vital signs, assessing for rapidly reversible causes of status epilepticus, such as hypoglycemia or electrolyte imbalance, assessing the cardiac status, and assessing for an intracranial structural abnormality are part of this evaluation. Once these measures are completed, it is reasonable to do an EEG. Given the fact the patient's mental status is poor, it is reasonable to do continuous video-EEG monitoring.

Hirsch LJ, Gaspard N. Status epilepticus. *Continuum* (Minneap Minn). 2013;19:767–794.

51. **A.** The MRI shows a right medial temporal lesion with a low T2 signal but with a high T2 signal in the center; this low signal enlarges in the gradient echo images. This appearance is characteristic of cavernoma with surrounding hemosiderin deposition. Cavernomas are commonly treated by pure lesionectomies with reportedly good seizure-free rates of 70% to 90% in patients with sporadic seizures and epilepsy duration of <1 year. On the other hand, it has been argued that the seizures do not arise from the cavernoma itself (as it has no neurons), but from the surrounding gliosis and hemosiderin fringe. Accordingly, lesionectomy along with removal of surrounding brain tissue rather than pure lesionectomy is recommended to achieve better seizure outcome. Options C and D are also likely to provide better seizure control in this case because the lesion involves the hippocampus although the full extent of it is not discernible from the images.

Crandall PH, Mathern GW. Surgery for lesional temporal lobe epilepsy. In: Luders HO, Comair YG, eds. *Epilepsy Surgery*. 2nd ed. Philadelphia, PA: Lippincott Williams & Wilkins; 2001:653–665.

Rosenow F, Alonso-Vanegas MA, Baumgartner C, et al. Cavernoma-related epilepsy: review and recommendations for management—report of the Surgical Task Force of the ILAE Commission on Therapeutic Strategies. *Epilepsia*. 2013;54:2025–2035.

52. **C.** This patient has nonlesional (MRI-negative) epilepsy. Negative PET scan makes it even more challenging. Semiology suggests temporal lobe seizure onset, likely right temporal, because of right-hand automatisms. Subsequent manifestations suggest propagation to the right frontal region, giving rise to the figure-of-4 posturing with left-arm extension and right-arm flexion. Both semiology and ictal onset suggest possible neocortical temporal onset. Accordingly, for further localization, right fronto-temporal convexity needs to be sampled along with right medial temporal and right orbito-frontal regions. Given the nonlateralized seizure onset, sampling from the left fronto-temporal region is reasonable. The semiology does not suggest seizure onset in the medial frontal region, and therefore, sampling from the right medial frontal region is least likely to be helpful.

Khan SA, Yaqub BA, Al Deeb SM, et al. Surgery for neocortical temporal lobe epilepsy. In: Luders HO, Comair YG, eds. *Epilepsy Surgery*. 2nd ed. Philadelphia, PA: Lippincott Williams & Wilkins; 2001:667–673.

53. **D.** The semiology suggests right frontal seizure onset given versive head deviation to the left. Presence of asymmetric posturing of upper extremities suggests possible right supplementary motor area seizure onset. Thus, he seems to have nonlesional frontal lobe epilepsy, likely medial frontal. In medial frontal lobe epilepsy, the interictal epileptiform discharges can be midline-predominant or bilateral (secondary bilateral synchrony), whereas the ictal discharges can be nonlateralizing or even absent. PET scan typically shows hypometabolism larger than the ictal onset zone. Outcome of surgical resection in extratemporal epilepsy with respect to freedom from disabling seizures is around 50%. Presence of beta activity at ictal onset has been reported as a predictor of favorable outcome.

Engel J, Jr, Wiebe S, French J, et al. Practice parameter: temporal lobe and localized neocortical resections for epilepsy: report of the Quality Standards Subcommittee of the American Academy of Neurology, in association with the American Epilepsy Society and the American Association of Neurological Surgeons. *Neurology*. 2003;60:538–547.

So EL. Nonlesional cases. In: Wyllie E, ed. *Wyllie's Treatment of Epilepsy: Principles and Practice*. 5th ed. Philadelphia, PA: Lippincott Williams & Wilkins; 2011:964–972.

Sperling MR, Clancy RR. Ictal electroencephalogram. In: Engel J, Jr, Pedley TA, eds. *Epilepsy: A Comprehensive Textbook*. 2nd ed. Philadelphia, PA: Lippincott Williams & Wilkins; 2008:825–854.

54. **D.** The incidence of FCD in surgically treated epilepsy is 2% to 36%. The most common presentation of FCD is epilepsy, which is seen in 77% to 90% of patients. T2 hyperintensity on MRI correlates with more severe forms of FCD, including the presence of balloon cells. Repetitive ictal spiking pattern on electrocorticography in seen in nearly two thirds of patients with FCD; when present, such a pattern correlates with the anatomical lesion in >80% of patients. Postsurgical seizure outcome correlates with the completeness of resection of the anatomical lesion and the continuous electrical activity.

Bingaman WE, Cataltepe O. Epilepsy surgery for focal malformations of cortical development. In: Luders HO, Comair YG, eds. *Epilepsy Surgery*. 2nd ed. Philadelphia, PA: Lippincott Williams & Wilkins; 2001:781–791.

55. **B.** Ezogabine is associated with retinal pigmentary abnormalities resulting in damage to the photoreceptors and vision loss. About one third of patients who received ezogabine over a 4-year period developed retinal pigmentation. However, it is not clear if these abnormalities are progressive or reversible. Concurrent skin discoloration and retinal pigmentary abnormalities were seen in 25% of patients. Patients taking ezogabine should have baseline and periodic (every 6 months) monitoring by an ophthalmologist for visual acuity and dilated fundus photography. Additional testing may include fluorescein angiograms, optical coherence tomography, perimetry, and electroretinogram. If retinal pigmentary abnormalities or vision changes are detected, ezogabine should be discontinued.

Potiga (ezogabine) prescribing information. https://www.gsksource.com/pharma/content/dam/GlaxoSmithKline/US/en/Prescribing_Information/Potiga/pdf/POTIGA-PI-MG.PDF. Accessed January 11, 2016.

56. **D.** The figure shows 4-Hz generalized spike-wave discharge, an interictal finding consistent with primary generalized seizures. Both topiramate and lamotrigine are effective for primary generalized seizures and are Food and Drug Administration (FDA) approved for treating them. Perampanel, a noncompetitive α-amino-3-hydroxy-5-methyl-4-isoxazolepropionic acid (AMPA) glutamate receptor antagonist, was shown to be effective for primary generalized seizures, and was recently approved by the FDA for adjunctive treatment of such seizures. Ethosuximide is effective for absence seizures, but not generalized tonic–clonic seizures, and therefore, it would not be appropriate in this patient. Both valporic acid and levetiracetam that the patient is taking are also appropriate for the treatment of generalized convulsions.

Fycompa (perampanel) prescribing information. https://www.fycompa.com/sites/all/themes/fycompa/pdf/fycompa_prescribing_information.pdf. Accessed January 11, 2016.

57. **D.** ACTH therapy can cause hypertension, proteinuria, and bleeding. Cardiomyopathy and infectious diseases are the major causes of death. Salt retention, renal failure, and

nephrocalcinosis are the major electrolyte imbalance complications. Neuropsychiatric complications include agitation, insomnia, and apathy, which may occur in the second or third week of treatment. Brain atrophy on MRI is visible within 1 week of treatment, and reaches maximum within 4 weeks; it resolves within 1 to 4 weeks following completion of treatment.

Dulac O, Tuxhorn I. Infantile spasms and West syndrome. In: Roger J, Bureau M, Dravet C, et al., eds. *Epileptic Syndromes in Infancy, Childhood and Adolescence*. 4th ed. Montrouge, France: John Libbey Eurotext; 2005:53–72.

58. **B.** Rufinamide is indicated for the adjunctive treatment of seizures associated with Lennox–Gastaut syndrome in children 4 years and older and adults. It is metabolized by carboxylesterases, and is not cytochrome P450-dependent. It is well absorbed orally with a t_{max} of 4 to 6 hours. Steady state is reached within 2 days. Plasma elimination half-life is approximately 6 to 10 hours. There are no clinically significant pharmacodynamic interactions involving rufinamide. Valproic acid may increase the plasma concentration of rufinamide, so it is recommended that rufinamide be started at a lower dose and titrated slowly when adding rufinamide to valproic acid.

Banzel (rufinamide) prescribing information. http://www.banzel.com/pdfs/BanzelPI.pdf. Accessed January 16, 2016.

59. **B.** Clobazam is a 1,5 benzodiazepine, whereas clonazepam is a 1,4 benzodiazepine. Based on a combination of lipophilicity and protein binding, the CNS penetration of clonazepam and clobazam is believed to be comparable. Clobazam has greater binding affinities to the alpha 2 versus alpha 1 subunit of GABA receptors, whereas clonazepam has equal binding affinity to alpha 1 and 2 receptors. Alpha 1 GABA receptors mediate sedation, whereas anticonvulsant activity can be achieved by activation of alpha 2 subunits of GABA receptors. Clobazam is metabolized to N-desmethylclobazam by hepatic metabolism. If clobazam is being substituted for clonazepam, the final dosage of clobazam for each milligram of clonazepam is roughly estimated to be 15-fold. Development of tolerance with clobazam is variable, depending on the models in which it is tested.

Sankar R, Chung S, Perry MS, et al. Clinical considerations in transitioning patients with epilepsy from clonazepam to clobazam: a case series. *J Med Case Rep*. 2014;8:429.

60. **B.** Adverse effects of valproate treatment include dose-related tremor, hyperammonemic encephalopathy, hepatotoxicity, polycystic ovaries, thrombocytopenia, altered platelet function, and acute hemorrhagic pancreatitis. Excessive weight gain is another common side effect; this is not entirely due to increased appetite, but is felt to be due to decreased β-oxidation of fatty acids. Secondary nocturnal enuresis is a side effect of valproate treatment in children. Excessive hair loss (not hair growth) can occur; it is usually temporary, but the hair that grows back can be different in texture and color. Facial and limb edema are also noted. Lower IQ has been noted by age 3 years in children exposed to valproate in utero. Neural tube defects occur in 1% to 2% fetuses exposed to valproate in the first trimester of pregnancy and folate supplementation can be protective. The occurrence of rash with valproate therapy is very rare.

Birnbaum A, Marino S, Bourgeois BFD. Valproate. In: Wyllie E, ed. *Wyllie's Treatment of Epilepsy: Principles and Practice*. 5th ed. Philadelphia, PA: Lippincott Williams & Wilkins; 2011:622–629.

61. A. Based on the description, the patient most likely has new-onset absence seizures without generalized tonic–clonic seizures (GTCS). In a prospective comparative efficacy study of childhood absence seizures, ethosuximide and valproate were found to be more effective than lamotrigine, and ethosuximide had less effect on attention. Of note, the patient was not witnessed to have GTCS. If GTCS are present, ethosuximide would be ineffective, and valproate would be the next best choice. Motionless staring with eye blinking could also be seen in a partial seizure, in which case, carbamazepine would be appropriate. However, the patient's age, brief duration of the seizure, induction with hyperventilation, and the lack of postictal phase support childhood absence epilepsy with automatisms. Multiple AEDs have been shown to worsen absence seizures and should be avoided; these include carbamazepine, phenytoin, gabapentin, tiagabine, oxcarbazepine, and vigabatrin.

Fountain NB. Choosing among antiepileptic drugs. *Continuum* (Minneap Minn). 2010;16:121–135.

Glauser TA, Cnaan A, Shinnar S, et al. Ethosuximide, valproic acid, and lamotrigine in childhood absence epilepsy. *N Engl J Med*. 2010;362:790–799.

62. A. Visual disturbances can occur as a side effect of antiepileptic drugs (AEDs). Nonspecific visual abnormalities can occur with toxicity or with prolonged AED use, including diplopia, blurred vision, and nystagmus. Some visual problems are more specific and may be related to the drug itself. Topiramate has been associated with acute closed-angle glaucoma, acute myopia, suprachoroidal effusions, and conjunctivitis, but not abnormal color perception (which has been reported with carbamazepine, phenytoin, and tiagabine). Vigabatrin has been associated with bilateral concentric visual field loss, electrophysiological changes, reduced contrast sensitivity, abnormal color perception, and morphological alterations of the fundus and retina. Ezogabine has been associated with retinal pigmentary abnormalities. Ophthalmoplegia has been reported with phenytoin, phenobarbital, primidone, and carbamazepine.

Asadi-Pooya AA, Sperling MR. AEDs and ophthalmological problems. In: *Antiepileptic Drugs: A Clinician's Manual*. New York, NY: Oxford University Press; 2009:213–216.

Hilton EJ, Hosking SL, Betts T. The effect of antiepileptic drugs on visual performance. *Seizure*. 2004;13:113–128.

Potiga (ezogabine) product information. https://www.gsksource.com/pharma/content/dam/GlaxoSmith Kline/US/en/Prescribing_Information/Potiga/pdf/POTIGA-PI-MG.PDF. Accessed January 15, 2016.

63. B. Understanding the effect of AEDs on the efficacy of contraception is important in the treatment of women with epilepsy. AEDs that induce liver enzymes, such as carbamazepine, felbamate, phenytoin, phenobarbital, primidone, oxcarbazepine, rufinamide, and topiramate, tend to affect the efficacy of oral contraceptives. AEDs that are not known to change contraceptive efficacy include gabapentin, lacosamide, levetiracetam, lamotrigine, tiagabine, valproate, and zonisamide.

Pennell P. Hormonal aspects of epilepsy. *Neurol Clin*. 2009;27:941–965.

64. B. MST was developed based on the demonstration that epileptic discharges travel tangentially in the cortex, such that a surgical intervention that divides the short tangential (horizontal) fibers within the cortex will prevent the initiation and propagation of epileptic activity. It has been shown that the vertically oriented column is the key to cortical organization; as these fibers are preserved during MST, the normal cortical function is expected to be intact. For MST to be successful, the vertical cuts have to involve the entire depth of the cortical ribbon, which is about 4 mm (not 1 mm). These cuts are placed at 5-mm intervals. MST is indicated for focal seizures arising from eloquent motor, sensory, and speech areas. Other indications include epilepsia partialis continua (as seen in Rasmussen syndrome), and Landau–Kleffner syndrome characterized by continuous spike waves in slow-wave sleep and severe speech difficulty. MST is more effective for partial seizures than generalized seizures. Complete seizure freedom is seen only when MST is combined with resection. Seizure free rates of 31% to 56% are reported. In one report of pure MST, class I outcome was seen in 45% but only 10% of patients were seizure free. Better outcome was associated with absence of an MRI-defined lesion. Worse outcome was seen when the area of MST was greater.

Polkey CE, Smith MC. Multiple subpial transections and other interventions. In: Engel J, Jr, Pedley TA, eds. *Epilepsy: A Comprehensive Textbook*. 2nd ed. Philadelphia, PA: Lippincott Williams & Wilkins; 2008:1921–1928.

65. **D.** MRI shows atrophy and increased FLAIR signal of the left hippocampus. This finding in conjunction with the information given suggests that the patient has left mesial temporal sclerosis (MTS). Surgical approaches in such patients include standard left anterior temporal lobectomy and selective amygdalo-hippocampectomy. Standard left anterior temporal lobectomy involves resection of the amygdala, hippocampus (including the head, body, and tail up to the posterior margin of midbrain), parahippocampal gyrus, and up to 3.5 to 4 cm of the lateral temporal neocortex sparing the superior temporal gyrus. Limiting the neocortical temporal resection to <4 cm minimizes verbal memory deficits while sparing the superior temporal gyrus minimizes naming difficulties after dominant temporal resections. Selective amygdalo-hippocampectomy, on the other hand, involves resection of the amygdala and hippocampus along with limited resection of the parahippocampal gyrus while sparing the temporal neocortex.

Kim R, Spencer D. Surgery for mesial temporal sclerosis. In: Luders HO, Comair YG, eds. *Epilepsy Surgery*. 2nd ed. Philadelphia, PA: Lippincott Williams & Wilkins; 2001:643–652.

66. **C.** Injury to the anterior choroidal artery (AChA) is felt to be responsible for the majority of cases of stroke following anteromedial temporal resection, and can lead to hemiparesis. The AChA runs along the uncus within the semiannular sulcus before reaching the choroidal fissure, making it vulnerable to injury during coagulation of the arachnoid or the hippocampal arteries done during the procedure. Manipulation of the branches of the middle cerebral artery can lead to "manipulation hemiplegia" because of vasospasm and infarction but this is less common. The vein of Labbe is very easily identified during the surgery and is not likely to be injured inadvertently. Thalamoperforating arteries arise from the P1 segment of the posterior cerebral artery and are less likely to be injured during this procedure.

Kim R, Spencer D. Surgery for mesial temporal sclerosis. In: Luders HO, Comair YG, eds. *Epilepsy Surgery*. 2nd ed. Philadelphia, PA: Lippincott Williams & Wilkins; 2001:643–652.

67. **C.** The VA Cooperative Trial is the largest and most informative clinical trial to date comparing initial in-hospital therapies for SE. It was a randomized, double-blind study. Treatment was considered successful when all motor and EEG seizure activity stopped within 20 minutes after the beginning of the drug infusion and there was no recurrence of

seizure activity during the next 40 minutes. Overall, 56% patients with overt generalized convulsive SE (GCSE) and 15% with subtle GCSE responded to the initial therapy. Among patients with a verified diagnosis of overt GCSE, lorazepam was successful in 65%, phenobarbital in 58%, diazepam plus phenytoin in 56%, and phenytoin in 44% of patients who received them ($P = .02$ for the overall comparison among the four groups). Lorazepam was significantly superior to phenytoin in a pairwise comparison ($P = .002$). Among patients with a verified diagnosis of subtle GCSE, no significant differences among the treatments were seen (8%–24% success rates). In an intention-to-treat analysis, the differences among treatment groups were not significant among the patients with either overt SE or subtle SE. In the trial, there was little further response to the second or third treatment, and the majority of these appeared to respond only to intravenous (IV) general anesthesia. There were no differences among the treatments with respect to recurrence during the 12-hour study period, the incidence of adverse reactions, or the outcome at 30 days. This led to conclusion that lorazepam is more effective than phenytoin for the initial IV treatment for overt GCSE. Although lorazepam is no more efficacious than phenobarbital or diazepam plus phenytoin, it is easier to use.

Treiman DM, Meyers PD, Walton NY, et al. A comparison of four treatments for generalized convulsive status epilepticus. Veterans Affairs Status Epilepticus Cooperative Study Group. *N Engl J Med.* 1998;339:792–798.

68. **A.** There was a prospective prehospital SE treatment trial randomizing patients to receive up to two doses of intravenous (IV) diazepam, IV lorazepam, or placebo. The primary outcome was cessation of SE by the time of arrival to the emergency department. In this study, 51% of SE was terminated with active treatment by the time of arrival to the emergency department. Lorazepam (59%) was statistically better than diazepam (43%) or placebo (21%). The odds ratio (OR) for termination of SE in the lorazepam group was 4.8 compared with the placebo group; the OR was 1.9 in the lorazepam group compared with the diazepam group; the OR was 2.3 in the diazepam group compared with the placebo group. The rates of posttreatment cardiopulmonary complications were 23% in the placebo group, 11% in the lorazepam group, and 10% in the diazepam group, but they were not statistically significant. This suggests that cardiopulmonary compromise may be greater because of SE rather than administration of low doses of benzodiazepines. There were significantly fewer ICU admissions if SE was terminated in the field compared with persistent SE upon arrival (32% vs. 73%).

Alldredge BK, Gelb AM, Isaacs SM, et al. A comparison of lorazepam, diazepam, and placebo for the treatment of out-of-hospital status epilepticus. *N Engl J Med.* 2001;345:631–637.

69. **A.** The Rapid Anticonvulsant Medication Prior to Arrival Trial (RAMPART) was a randomized, double-blind, phase 3, noninferiority clinical trial, which evaluated prehospital treatment of SE using IM midazolam and IV lorazepam. This trial showed that IM midazolam was superior to IV lorazepam (73% vs. 63%) in controlling generalized convulsive SE when administered en route to the hospital by paramedics. The two treatment groups were similar with respect to need for endotracheal intubation (approximately 14% in either group) and recurrence of seizures (approximately 11% in either group). Among subjects whose seizures had terminated prior to arrival at the hospital, the median times to active treatment were 1.2 minutes in the IM midazolam group and 4.8 minutes in the IV lorazepam group, with corresponding median times from active

treatment to cessation of convulsions of 3.3 and 1.6 minutes, respectively. Adverse event rates were similar in the two groups. Thus, it took longer to establish IV access in patients, leading to delayed treatment, and may have accounted for this result. Of note, midazolam is being developed with newer formulations, including intranasal and buccal, which may be absorbed faster than intramuscular administration.

Silbergleit R, Durkalski V, Lowenstein D, et al. Intramuscular versus intravenous therapy for prehospital status epilepticus. *N Engl J Med*. 2012;366:591–600.

70. **D.** If a patient presents with SE, the recommendation is to immediately start an antiepileptic drug (AED) to help prevent early SE recurrence, which can happen after the effect of the benzodiazepine ends. Loading the patient with an intravenous (IV) AED may be warranted to rapidly achieve the desired level even if the patient is able to take oral medications. Current IV formulations include phenobarbital, fosphenytoin, phenytoin, valproate, leveltiracetam, and lacosamide. There is no clear evidence to show a difference in efficacy, so the choice of the AED is guided by etiology and comorbidities. Fosphenytoin and phenytoin are not the best options given their propensity to induce the cytochrome P450 system, which can reduce the efficacy of steroids and chemotherapy and also given the history of cardiac conduction abnormality. Other sodium channel drugs, such as carbamazepine and lacosamide, should also be avoided. Thus, the best option in this case appears to be valproate.

Hirsch LJ, Gaspard N. Status epilepticus. *Continuum* (Minneap Minn). 2013;19:767–794.

71. **B.** Deep brain stimulation (DBS) has been explored as a possible therapy for epilepsy for decades. Sites explored have included the cerebellum, centromedian (CM) thalamic nucleus, hippocampus, subthalamic nucleus, brainstem, corpus callosum, and the anterior nucleus of the thalamus (ANT). The ANT is part of the Papez circuit, which connects hippocampal output via the fornix and mammillary bodies to the ANT. Projections from the ANT travel to the cingulum and then around the wall of the lateral ventricle to the parahippocampal cortex, and return to the hippocampus to complete the circuit. All of these structures are commonly involved in seizures. Because of its small size and projections to limbic structures, the ANT is an attractive target for neurostimulation in epilepsy. Stimulation of the Anterior Nuclei of Thalamus for Epilepsy (SANTE) Trial showed that complex partial and "most severe" seizures were significantly reduced with bilateral stimulation. In the last month of the blinded phase, the stimulated group had a 29% greater reduction in seizures compared with the control group ($P = .002$). Unadjusted median seizure reduction at the end of the blinded phase was 14.5% in the control group and 40.4% in the stimulated group. By 2 years, there was a 56% median percent reduction in seizure frequency; 50% seizure reduction (responder rate) was seen in 54% of patients; and 12.7% of patients were seizure free for at least 6 months. Effectiveness of therapy depended upon the site of seizure origin. Patients with seizure onset in one or both temporal lobes showed the best response (median seizure reduction compared to baseline of 44.2% in the stimulated group versus 21.8% in the control group, $P = .025$). Stimulation in those with extratemporal lobe seizures (frontal, parietal, or occipital) did not show significant differences in seizure reduction. However, patients with multifocal or diffuse seizure onset showed a 35% reduction compared with a 14.1% reduction in the control group, which was not statistically different.

Fisher R, Salanova V, Witt T, et al. Electrical stimulation of the anterior nucleus of thalamus for treatment of refractory epilepsy. *Epilepsia*. 2010;51:899–908.

72. D. Invasive monitoring is associated with minor complications in 7.7% of patients and major complications in 0.6% of patients. Resective surgery is associated with minor and major medical complications in 5.1% and 1.5% of patients, respectively, with the most common medical complication being cerebrospinal fluid leak (8.5%), followed by aseptic meningitis (3.6%), bacterial infection (3%), and intracranial hematoma (2.5%). Minor neurologic complications are twice as frequent in children as adults (11.2% vs. 5.5%). The most common neurologic complication after resective surgery is a minor visual field deficit (one quadrant or less) seen in 12.9% of patients, the majority of which are asymptomatic; these are more likely to occur after temporal versus extratemporal resections (17.9% vs. 7.2%). Major visual field deficits (hemianopia) are seen in 2.1% of patients. Minor or temporary aphasia is seen in 3.7% of patients and major aphasia is seen in 0.8%, and is similar regardless of resection location. Minor or temporary hemiparesis occurs in 3.3% of all patients, but is more common after extratemporal than temporal resections (7.9% vs. 1.8%). Major or permanent hemiparesis is seen in 1.8% of patients overall, similar in frequency after temporal or extratemporal resections (1.8% vs. 2.3%). Perioperative mortality is uncommon after epilepsy surgery, occurring in only 0.4% of temporal lobe patients and 1.2% of extratemporal patients. In summary, the majority of complications after epilepsy surgery are minor or temporary. Major permanent neurologic complications are uncommon. Mortality as a result of epilepsy surgery in the modern era is rare.

Hader WJ, Tellez-Zenteno J, Metcalfe A, et al. Complications of epilepsy surgery: a systematic review of focal surgical resections and invasive EEG monitoring. *Epilepsia*. 2013;54:840–847.

73. B. Reoperation after thorough assessment of clinical, imaging, and EEG findings can be an efficacious and reasonably safe treatment option for sustained seizure control after failed resective epilepsy surgery. Over a third of patients can be expected to achieve seizure freedom ranging from 6 months to 4 years after the second operation. Postsurgical complications are seen in 13.5%, and consist of visual field defects and hemiparesis. The causes of failed first epilepsy surgery include incorrect localization of the seizure focus, incomplete resection of the seizure focus, presence of additional seizure foci, and progression of the underlying disease. Predictors of successful reoperation include: concordance of postsurgical imaging and electroclinical findings, and absence of brain trauma and cerebral infection prior to epilepsy onset.

Surges R, Elger CE. Reoperation after failed resective epilepsy surgery. *Seizure*. 2013;22:493–501.

74. C. His MRI shows evidence of right mesial temporal sclerosis (MTS) and a linear gliotic lesion in the right frontal lobe. His semiology suggests either a frontal or temporal onset, with the ictal EEG showing a rather widespread right hemispheric lateralization. Based on this, it is difficult to localize the seizure onset zone, and it is not possible to exclude two independent seizure onset zones. Accordingly, neither standard right anterior temporal lobectomy nor stereotactic, MRI-guided laser ablation of the right medial frontal structures can be recommended at this point. Implantation of right temporal depth and right frontal subdural electrodes for a more accurate localization seems to be the most appropriate option at this time. If the invasive evaluation localizes the seizure onset, he will still be a surgical candidate despite widespread scalp ictal EEG onset.

Hamer HM, Morris HH III. Indications for invasive video-electroencephalographic monitoring. In: Luders HO, Comair YG, eds. *Epilepsy Surgery*. 2nd ed. Philadelphia, PA: Lippincott Williams & Wilkins; 2001:559–566.

75. **B.** In TLE due to MTS, most studies have · not shown an association between postoperative seizure outcome and age at surgery, age at seizure onset, duration of epilepsy, history of febrile seizures, family history of epilepsy, history of secondary generalized seizures, or side of seizure. When an association was found, the effect size was small or the association was weak. However, male gender and ipsilateral interictal discharges have been found to be associated with favorable postoperative seizure outcome in MTS. Of note, in non-MTS lesional TLE (e.g., tumors, dysplasia, vascular lesions), longer duration of epilepsy is associated with poor postoperative seizure outcome; in nonlesional (MRI-negative) TLE, history of febrile seizures and focal temporal ictal EEG are associated with good postoperative seizure outcome.

Velasco TR, Mathern GW. Surgical treatment of refractory temporal lobe epilepsy. In: Wyllie E, ed. *Wyllie's Treatment of Epilepsy: Principles and Practice*. 5th ed. Philadelphia, PA: Lippincott Williams & Wilkins; 2011:922–936.

76. **C.** Long-term outcome for medically refractory nonlesional extratemporal lobe epilepsy was evaluated in a group of 85 patients. Based on the noninvasive diagnostic test results, a clear hypothesis for seizure origin was possible in 55%; of these, 66% proceeded to intracranial EEG monitoring. Of those who underwent intracranial EEG, a seizure focus was identified and surgically resected in 77%. Thus, out of 24 patients, 9 (38%) had an excellent outcome after resective epilepsy surgery. All patients with an excellent surgical outcome had at least 10 years of follow-up. The only predictor of excellent surgical outcome was the presence of localized interictal epileptiform discharges on scalp EEG. This suggests that scalp EEG is the most useful test for identifying patients with MRI-negative, extratemporal lobe epilepsy who are likely to have excellent outcomes after epilepsy surgery. It is important to note that although 9 of 24 patients undergoing resective surgery (38%) had excellent outcomes, only 9 of 31 patients undergoing intracranial EEG (29%) and only 9 of 85 patient with nonlesional extratemporal lobe epilepsy (11%) had long-term excellent outcomes.

Noe K, Sulc V, Wong-Kisiel L, et al. Long-term outcomes after nonlesional extratemporal lobe epilepsy surgery. *JAMA Neurol* 2013;70:1003–1008.

77. **D.** Interactions between early epileptogenic lesions and normal developmental processes may result in EEG patterns that are more diffuse than those seen in patients with lesions acquired after brain maturity. Therefore, generalized and contralateral EEG abnormalities in those cases represent maladaptive plasticity of the immature brain leading to hypersynchrony and generalized features. Thus, it is not uncommon for young children with congenital or early acquired focal lesions to present with hypsarrhythmia and infantile spasms, but can still have seizure free outcome after resective surgery.

Moosa A, Loddenkemper T, Wyllie E. Epilepsy surgery for congential or early lesions. In: Cataltepe O, Jallo G, eds. *Pediatric Epilepsy Surgery: Preoperative Assessment and Surgical Treatment*. New York, NY: Thieme Medical Publishers; 2010:14–23.

78. **A.** Mutism, left leg paresis, and urge urinary incontinence are features of acute disconnection syndrome and are caused by traction of the nondominant parasagittal

cortex. This is usually temporary. Tactile and visual transfer deficits are seen with posterior disconnection syndrome and may occur after splenial or posterior callosal disconnection. Split-brain syndrome may be seen after total or near-total callosotomy, in which patients have language impairment, disordered attention and memory sequencing, and hemisphere competition. Hydrocephalus, stroke, edema, and bleeding can occur, but are rare when performed by experienced neurosurgeons.

Wong T, Kwan S, Chang K. Corpus callosotomy. In: Cataltepe O, Jallo G, eds. *Pediatric Epilepsy Surgery: Preoperative Assessment and Surgical Treatment*. New York, NY: Thieme Medical Publishers; 2010:261–268.

79. **D.** Overall, VNS is fairly well tolerated. In general, the most common side effects noted at 3 months are hoarseness, cough, paresthesia, and dyspnea in that order. These symptoms tend to become less frequent over time. Other complications include cardiac arrhythmias (even asystole), bronchoconstriction, psychosis, vocal cord paralysis, and Horner's syndrome.

Schachter SC, Boon P. Vagus nerve stimulation. In: Engel J, Jr, Pedley TA, eds. *Epilepsy: A Comprehensive Textbook*. 2nd ed. Philadelphia, PA: Lippincott Williams & Wilkins; 2008: 1395–1399.

80. **B.** At 3 months postimplant, there was a 23% reduction in seizures compared to baseline in the pivotal trial for VNS. An increase in efficacy was noted over time, with 40% to 45% reduction in seizures over a period of 2 to 3 years.

Schachter SC, Boon P. Vagus nerve stimulation. In: Engel J, Jr, Pedley TA, eds. *Epilepsy: A Comprehensive Textbook*. 2nd ed. Philadelphia, PA: Lippincott Williams & Wilkins; 2008: 1395–1399.

81. **D.** Typical stimulator settings include: output current of 1 to 3 mA; signal frequency 20 to 30 Hz; pulse width 250 to 500 mcs; On time 14 to 30 seconds; Off time 3 to 5 minutes. There is a rapid cycling protocol with an On time of 7 seconds and Off time of 18 seconds. The efficacy of rapid cycling is still being evaluated, but it increases the duty cycle and hastens the need for battery replacement. The magnet output current is typically 0.25 to 0.5 mA higher than the stimulator output current and the magnet On time is typically 60 seconds.

Ardesch JJ, Buschman HP, Wagener-Schimmel LJ, et al. Vagus nerve stimulation for medically refractory epilepsy: a long-term follow-up study. *Seizure*. 2007;16:579–585.

Schachter SC, Boon P. Vagus nerve stimulation. In: Engel J Jr, Pedley TA, eds. *Epilepsy: A Comprehensive Textbook*. 2nd ed. Philadelphia, PA: Lippincott Williams & Wilkins; 2008: 1395–1399.

82. **B.** Ethosuximide is a first-line treatment for absence epilepsy. It is also beneficial for patients with both absence and generalized tonic–clonic seizures and for patients with atypical absence seizures. It acts by reducing the T-type calcium currents in thalamic neurons. There are reports of it being used for treatment of Lennox–Gastaut syndrome, juvenile myoclonic epilepsy, eyelid myoclonia with absences, and continuous spike wave of sleep. The common side effects are nausea and drowsiness, which are dose dependent. Rare, potentially life-threatening reactions include Stevens–Johnson syndrome, lupus-like syndrome, systemic lupus erythematosus, autoimmune thyroiditis, and decreased renal allograft survival. Psychosis and forced normalization reaction have been noted infrequently, concurrent with seizure and EEG improvement. It is metabolized by the CYP450 system, mainly CYP3A4.

Glauser T, Perucca E. Ethosuximide. In: Shorvon SD, Perucca E, Engel J, Jr, eds. *The Treatment of Epilepsy*. 3rd ed. Oxford, UK: Wiley-Blackwell; 2009:499–510.

Kanner AM, Glauser TA, Morita DA. Ethosuximide. In: Wyllie E, ed. *Wyllie's Treatment of Epilepsy: Principles and Practice*. 5th ed. Philadelphia, PA: Lippincott Williams & Wilkins; 2011:657–667.

83. **C.** Anticonvulsants have been linked to systemic lupus erythematosus (SLE) and lupus-like syndrome with arthralgia, fever, malar rash, and rarely, pleural effusion, and myocarditis. Carbamazepine, phenytoin, and ethosuximide have been causally linked, among some others. Discontinuation of medication leads to resolution of symptoms and normalization of labs, but recovery may be prolonged. Elevations of antinuclear antibodies and antidouble stranded DNA antibodies correlating with clinical symptoms of lupus have been reported on exposure to ethosuximide with relapse of symptoms when rechallenged.

Crespel A, Velizarova R, Agullo M, et al. Ethosuximide-induced de novo systemic lupus erythematosus with anti-double-strand DNA antibodies: a case report with definite evidence. *Epilepsia*. 2009;20:2003.

Glauser T, Perucca E. Ethosuximide. In: Shorvon SD, Perucca E, Engel J, Jr, eds. *The Treatment of Epilepsy*. 3rd ed. Oxford, UK: Wiley-Blackwell; 2009:499–510.

84. **A.** Enzyme induction is a slow regulatory process, which is dose and time dependent; this is unlike enzyme inhibition, which is an immediate process. Induction not only affects the metabolism of drugs but also the endogenous compounds such as cortisol, vitamin D3, and testosterone. Enzyme induction can affect the pharmacokinetics of a drug metabolized by the induced enzyme and lead to decreased serum concentration and efficacy. On the other hand, if a drug metabolized by the induced enzyme has an active metabolite, the induction leads to an increase in the metabolite concentration and toxicity. Induction not only affects CYP enzymes but also some UGT enzymes.

Michelucci R, Pasini E, Tassinari CA. Phenobarbital, primidone and other barbiturates. In: Shorvon SD, Perucca E, Engel J, Jr, eds. *The Treatment of Epilepsy*. 3rd ed. Oxford, UK: Wiley-Blackwell; 2009:585–604.

85. **C.** Pharmacokinetic changes in the elderly include reduction in protein binding, hepatic metabolism, enzyme inducibility, and renal elimination. In addition, pharmacodynamic changes can occur, including alterations in brain neurotransmitters, receptor function, autonomic pharmacology, and homoeostatic mechanisms.

Brodie MJ, Kwan P. Epilepsy in elderly people. *BMJ*. 2005;331:1317–1322.

86. **A.** According to the International League Against Epilepsy (ILAE) updated guidelines, only gabapentin and lamotrigine have Level A evidence establishing them as efficacious or effective as initial monotherapy in elderly adults with newly diagnosed or untreated partial-onset seizures. Carbamazepine has Level C (possibly) evidence. Topiramate and valproate have Level D (potentially) evidence. Level A evidence is based on one or more Class I studies or meta-analyses meeting class I criteria or two or more Class II studies.

Glauser T, Ben-Menachem E, Bourgeois B, et al. Updated ILAE evidence review of antiepileptic drug efficacy and effectiveness as initial monotherapy for epileptic seizures and syndromes. *Epilepsia*. 2013;54:551–563.

87. **D.** The most common side effects of lacosamide include dizziness, ataxia, vomiting, diplopia, nausea, vertigo, and blurred vision. Although memory impairment has been reported, no cognitive slowing is seen with lacosamide.

Zaccara G, Perucca P, Loiacono G, et al. The adverse event profile of lacosamide: a systematic review and meta-analysis of randomized controlled trials. *Epilepsia*. 2013;54:66–74.

88. **B.** After the first unprovoked seizure, the risk of recurrence within 2 years in untreated individuals is 40% to 50%. Treatment may reduce this risk by half. Abnormal EEG and an identifiable neurological condition are predictors of the risk. In individuals with normal EEG and normal neurological status, the risk of recurrence is approximately 20%, 25%, and 30% at 1, 2, and 4 years, respectively. In adults, status epilepticus can be associated with a substantially higher risk of recurrence within the subgroup of patients with remote symptomatic first seizures. There is no significant difference in seizure recurrence among adult patients who present with multiple seizures versus single seizure within 24 hours with respect to recurrence risk at 1 year, irrespective of the etiologic diagnosis and irrespective of whether they are treated. This suggests that a presentation with multiple seizures within 24 hours should be regarded as a single event, in keeping with the International League Against Epilepsy recommendations.

Berg AT. Risk of recurrence after a first unprovoked seizure. *Epilepsia*. 2008;49(suppl 1):13–18.

Kho LK, Lawn ND, Dunne JW, et.al. First seizure presentation: do multiple seizures within 24 hours predict recurrence? *Neurology*. 2006;67(6):1047–1049.

89. **A.** The SANAD trial was a two-part trial looking at the outcome of commonly used antiepileptic drugs as initial monotherapy as would be used in clinical practice. With respect to time to treatment failure, lamotrigine was found to be significantly better than carbamazepine, gabapentin, and topiramate, and had a nonsignificant advantage compared with oxcarbazepine. With respect to time to 12-month remission, carbamazepine was significantly better than gabapentin, and estimates suggested a nonsignificant advantage for carbamazepine against lamotrigine, topiramate, and oxcarbazepine. This led to the conclusion that lamotrigine is clinically better than carbamazepine for time to treatment failure outcomes and is therefore a cost-effective alternative for patients with partial seizures. With respect to time to treatment failure, valproate was significantly better than topiramate, but there was no significant difference between valproate and lamotrigine. For patients with IGE, valproate was significantly better than both lamotrigine and topiramate. With respect to time to 12-month remission, valproate was significantly better than lamotrigine overall and for the subgroup with IGE. But there was no significant difference between valproate and topiramate in either the overall analysis or for the subgroup with IGE. This led to the conclusion that valproate is better tolerated than topiramate and more efficacious than lamotrigine, and should remain the drug of first choice for patients with generalized and unclassified epilepsies. However, because of known potential adverse effects of valproate during pregnancy, the benefits of using valproate in women of childbearing age should be carefully considered.

Marson AG, Al-Kharusi AM, Alwaidh M, et al. The SANAD study of effectiveness of carbamazepine, gabapentin, lamotrigine, oxcarbazepine, or topiramate for treatment of partial epilepsy: an unblinded randomised controlled trial. *Lancet*. 2007;369:1000–1015.

Marson AG, Al-Kharusi AM, Alwaidh M, et al. The SANAD study of effectiveness of valproate, lamotrigine, or topiramate for generalised and unclassifiable epilepsy: an unblinded randomized controlled trial. *Lancet*. 2007;369:1016–1026.

90. **D.** This patient likely has a drug-related rash that could be life-threatening. Such potentially life-threatening hypersensitivity reactions include Stevens–Johnson syndrome (SJS), toxic epidermal necrolysis (TEN), erythema multiforme, exfoliatve dermatitis, and drug reaction with eosinophilia and systemic symptoms (DRESS), all of which require immediate discontinuation of the offending agent to prevent mortality. Of the listed AEDs, lamotrigine has been most associated with serious hypersensitivity reactions, followed by valproate. Note that valproate inhibits lamotrigine metabolism, increasing the risk of rash. There have been infrequent reports about gabapentin, levetiracetam, and topiramate leading to serious hypersensitivity reactions, but they are still generally considered safe. Stopping the possible offending agent(s) would be reasonable. However, stopping all AEDs could lead to adverse outcome (e.g., status epilepticus), and is therefore not warranted, unless absolutely necessary. In the latter situation, starting a nonoffending AED would be reasonable. A cross-reactivity of 40% to 60% has been noted between aromatic AEDs, such as phenytoin, phenobarbital, carbamazepine, and oxcarbazepine. However, there has been no clear cross-reactivity between lamotrigine and the aromatic AEDs. HLA-B*1502 allele has been the best defined genetic marker of increased risk of carbamazepine-induced hypersensitivity reaction. Although the hypersensitivity reactions can occur at any time during therapy, most of them occur within the first 4 months of therapy.

Amstutz U, Shear NH, Rieder MJ, et al. Recommendations for HLA-B*15:02 and HLA-A*31:01 genetic testing to reduce the risk of carbamazepine-induced hypersensitivity reactions. *Epilepsia*. 2014;55:496–506.

Gaeta F, Alonzi C, Valluzzi RL, et al. Hypersensitivity to lamotrigine and nonaromatic anticonvulsant drugs: a review. *Curr Pharm Des*. 2008;14:2874–2882.

Hirsch LJ, Arif H, Nahm EA, et al. Cross-sensitivity of skin rashes with antiepileptic drug use. *Neurology*. 2008;71:1527–1534.

91. **A.** MRI-guided steretotactic thermal laser ablation is a relatively new procedure to treat epilepsy. In this procedure, a 4-mm cranial incision and a 3.2-mm twist drill hole are made. Using a stereotactic approach, a laser applicator is placed in the seizure focus. Then, with real-time MRI guidance, a laser fiber is introduced into the applicator and heated to the desired temperature to achieve ablation. The fiber is gradually withdrawn, as needed, to achieve maximum tissue ablation. Tissue damage is verified in real time and confirmed by postablation contrast MRI. Effects of thermal ablation by laser is temperature dependent. At temperatures below 43°C, thermal damage does not occur regardless of exposure time. At 44°C to 59°C, time-dependent thermal damage occurs with thermal denaturation of critical enzymes and cell death. At 60°C to 100°C, there is instant denaturation of proteins and cellular components and tissue coagulation. At temperatures >100°C, vaporization of intra- and extra-cellular water occurs with rupture of cell membranes. Thus, a temperature in the range of 60°C to 100°C is optimum for causing irreversible tissue ablation. Because of the trajectory of insertion of the laser applicator postero-anteriorly in the axial plane, this procedure typically results in ablation of about 60% of the AHC, which includes about 58% of the amygdala and 63% of the hippocampus. Neither the parahippocampal gyrus nor the lateral temporal cortex is typically ablated. The laser treatment time is usually <20 minutes (9.6 ± 6.4 minutes in one study).

Willie JT, Laxpati NG, Drane DL, et al. Real-time magnetic resonance-guided stereotactic laser amygdalohippocampotomy for mesial temporal lobe epilepsy. *Neurosurgery*. 2014;74:569–584.

92. **D.** RNS involves placement of depth and/or subdural electrodes in close proximity to the seizure focus. The system detects seizure onset and then responds to it by delivering a series of stimulations to terminate the seizure. In this example, the RNS system detects the seizure in the top two channels, which is characterized by a sharp transient followed by low voltage, fast activity. Seizure detection occurs within 0.5 second of onset, as indicated by the "B1" marker. The first stimulation is delivered soon after seizure detection, as indicated by the "Tr" marker. However, the stimulations fail to terminate the seizure, which continues despite three stimulations. This suggests that although the seizure detection settings are optimal, the patient may need adjustment of the stimulation parameters for optimum control.

Morrell MJ. Responsive cortical stimulation for the treatment of medically intractable partial epilepsy. *Neurology*. 2011;77:1295–1304.

Sun FT, Morrell MJ. The RNS system: responsive cortical stimulation for the treatment of refractory partial epilepsy. *Expert Rev Med Devices*. 2014;11:563–572.

93. **D.** VNS is associated with a >50% seizure reduction in 55% of patients with LGS. VNS is associated with an increase in ≥50% seizure reduction rates of approximately 7% from 1 to 5 years postimplantation. VNS is associated with a significant improvement in standard mood scales in adults with epilepsy. Infection risk at the VNS implantation site is higher in children than adults (odds ratio 3:4). Based on these findings, VNS can be recommended for seizures in children (both partial and generalized), for LGS-associated seizures, and for improving mood in adults with epilepsy (Level C). VNS may be considered to have improved efficacy over time (Level C). There is no evidence to suggest improvement in mood in children with VNS. Children should be carefully monitored for site infection after VNS implantation.

Morris GL 3rd, Gloss D, Buchhalter J, et al. Evidence-based guideline update: vagus nerve stimulation for the treatment of epilepsy: report of the Guideline Development Subcommittee of the American Academy of Neurology. *Neurology*. 2013;81:1453–1459.

94. **A.** Hypoxic-ischemic encephalopathy is the most common cause of neonatal seizures, while intracranial hemorrhage is the second most common cause. Focal clonic and tonic seizures have a relatively good outcome as these are associated with relatively confined, nondiffuse brain injury compared with generalized tonic posturing and motor automatisms, which are associated with diffuse brain dysfunction. The underlying cause of the seizures is the most important predictor of outcome. Phenobarbital, phenytoin, and benzodiazepines are commonly used for acute treatment of neonatal seizures.

Mizrahi E, Watanabe K. Symptomatic neonatal seizures. In: Roger J, Bureau M, Dravet C, et al., eds. *Epileptic Syndromes in Infancy, Childhood and Adolescence*. 4th ed. Montrouge, France: John Libbey Eurotext; 2005:17–38.

95. **A.** In neonates, GABA-mediated excitation plays a role in neuronal development, and also renders the brain vulnerable to seizures. This excitatory nature of GABA signaling in immature neurons is believed to be the reason that GABA agonists are often ineffective in controlling neonatal seizures.

Kahle KK, Staley KJ. Neonatal seizures and neuronal transmembrane ion transport. In: Noebels JL, Avoli M, Rogawski MA, et al., eds. *Jasper's Basic Mechanisms of the Epilepsies*. 4th ed. New York, NY: Oxford University Press; 2012:1066–1076.

96. **D.** Risk factors associated with development of aplastic anemia due to felbamate include female gender, Caucasian race, adult age group, history of cytopenia, allergy or toxicity to other antiseizure medications, and diagnosis and or serological evidence of an auto-immune disorder. Dose does not appear to be a factor. Time to development of aplastic anemia is usually within 1 year of starting felbamate.

Pellock JM. Felbamate in epilepsy therapy: evaluating the risks. *Drug Saf.* 1999;21:225–239.

97. **C.** Phenytoin targets the voltage-gated sodium channels in the brain. It is extensively bound to serum plasma proteins (90%) and only the unbound fraction is pharmacologically active. It is metabolized by the hepatic cytochrome P450 enzymes (CYP2C9 and CYP2C19), and is susceptible to inhibitory drug interactions. Phenytoin has narrow therapeutic index, nonlinear kinetics, and multiple interactions with other medications. Inhibition of metabolism may produce significant increases in circulating phenytoin concentrations and enhance the risk of drug toxicity. Medications that displace phenytoin from albumin may also increase the free phenytoin levels and result in toxicity. Phenytoin exhibits zero-order kinetics at higher concentrations in the therapeutic range as the metabolic pathways become saturated such that small increases in dose result in nonlinear, large increases in total and free steady-state drug levels. Macrolide antibiotics such as clarithromycin inhibit cytochrome P450 hepatic metabolism, and addition of clarithromycin to a patient taking phenytoin can result in increased phenytoin concentration and drug toxicity.

Ament PW, Bertolino JG, Liszewski JL. Clinically significant drug interactions. *Am Fam Physician.* 2000;61:1745–1754.

Toledano R, Gil-Nagel A. Adverse effects of antiepileptic drugs. *Semin Neurol.* 2008;28:317–327.

98. **B.** Long-term phenytoin can cause folate deficiency and vitamin D deficiency due to cytochrome P450 induction and result in osteoporosis. Cerebellar atrophy has been reported after both long-term and acute use of high doses of phenytoin, although the underlying etiology (phenytoin versus seizures) remains unclear. Long-term phenytoin therapy has been associated with gingival hyperplasia, hirsutism, acne, and rash. The incidence of gingival hyperplasia is variable (approximately 13%–40%), but it is reversible and regresses after discontinuation of phenytoin. Acute intravenous administration of phenytoin and fosphenytoin can cause purple glove syndrome, characterized by pain, edema, and discoloration. The spectrum of tissue injury can range from mild local cutaneous reactions around the infusion site to frank limb ischemia.

Garbovsky LA, Drumheller BC, Perrone J. Purple glove syndrome after phenytoin or fosphenytoin administration: review of reported cases and recommendations for prevention. *J Med Toxicol.* 2015;11(4):445–459.

Morita DA, Glauser TA. Phenytoin and fosphenytoin. In: Wyllie E, ed. *Wyllie's Treatment of Epilepsy: Principles and Practice.* 5th ed. Philadelphia, PA: Lippincott Williams & Wilkins; 2011:630–647.

99. **C.** Levetiracetam has a number of different formulations, including pills, liquid, and intravenous solutions. Of note, in 2015, the FDA approved the first 3D-printable drug product, which happened to be of levetiracetam. Levetiracetam is 95% to 100% bioavailable. Within 24 hours of a dose of levetiracetam, 93% of the drug is excreted

unchanged in the urine with the rest being inactive metabolites. One of the main metabolites results from deamination that does not involve the cytochrome P450 or the UGT systems. It has FDA approval for use as adjunctive therapy for partial-onset seizures, myoclonic, and primary generalized tonic–clonic seizures. In the European Union, it is also approved for use as monotherapy in partial-onset seizures. Levetiracetam may destabilize mood, and over 10% of people experience agitation, hostility, apathy, anxiety, emotional lability, and depression. More serious symptoms such as hallucinations, suicidal ideations, or psychosis may occur in 1%. There is some evidence that pyridoxine (vitamin B6) may curtail some of these symptoms.

The First FDA Approved Drug Made by a 3D printer is levetiracetam. http://www.epilepsy.com/article/2015/8/first-fda-approved-drug-made-3d-printer-levetiracetam. Accessed January 14, 2016.

Privitera MD, Cavitt J. Levetiracetam. In: Engel J, Jr, Pedley TA, eds. *Epilepsy: A Comprehensive Textbook*. 2nd ed. Philadelphia, PA: Lippincott Williams & Wilkins; 2008:1583–1591.

100. **C.** Pregabalin is a structural analog of GABA and binds to alpha-2-delta subunit of the voltage-gated calcium (P/Q) channels. It is effective in the MES and pentylenetetrazole (PTZ) animal models, but not in the genetic absence epilepsy rats from Strasbourg (GAERS) model. Its bioavailability remains >90% across the clinical dosing range, unlike gabapentin, the bioavailability of which drops from 60% to 33% when the total daily dose is increased from 900 to 3,600 mg. Pregabalin is not metabolized in the liver, but >90% of it is excreted unchanged in the urine. It is approved for use in the United States as adjunctive therapy for partial seizures, neuropathic pain associated with diabetic neuropathy, and postherpetic neuralgia. In several other countries, there is an additional indication for generalized anxiety disorder.

Bergey GK. Pregabalin. In: Engel J, Jr, Pedley TA, eds. *Epilepsy: A Comprehensive Textbook*. 2nd ed. Philadelphia, PA: Lippincott Williams & Wilkins; 2008:1629–1637.

101. **A.** Tiagabine has been shown to induce spike-wave stupor, characterized by generalized spike-wave discharges. Patients with generalized epilepsy are predisposed to this. However, the same adverse effect has also been seen in patients without epilepsy who receive tiagabine for psychiatric or sleep disorders.

Kälviäinen R. Tiagabine. In: Engel J, Jr, Pedley TA, eds. *Epilepsy: A Comprehensive Textbook*. 2nd ed. Philadelphia, PA: Lippincott Williams & Wilkins; 2008:1655–1661.

102. **A.** Ezogabine (retigabine) is a potassium channel opener. Brivaracetam has an unknown mechanism of action, although it binds to SV2A with high affinity. Lacosamide selectively enhances the slow inactivation of the voltage-dependent sodium channels and binds to the collapsin response mediator protein 2 (CRMP2) as well. Vigabatrin is an irreversible inhibitor of GABA-transaminase.

White HS, Perucca E, Privitera MD. Investigational drugs. In: Engel J Jr, Pedley TA, eds. *Epilepsy: A Comprehensive Textbook*. 2nd ed. Philadelphia, PA: Lippincott Williams & Wilkins; 2008:1721–1740.

103. **B.** Maintaining bone health is an increasing concern in chronic epilepsy. Many studies have shown a reduction in bone mineral density and an increased fracture risk in patients treated with enzyme-inducing AEDs. This is felt to be related to upregulation of the enzymes that metabolize 25(OH)-vitamin D into inactive metabolites, resulting in reduced calcium absorption with consecutive secondary hyperparathyroidism.

Decreased bone density has also been seen in nonenzyme-inducing medications. Overall, phenobarbital, primidone, and phenytoin are most consistently associated with impaired bone health; carbamazepine and valproate are felt to have a negative effect, but the data are mixed; and lamotrigine has limited negative effect. Data on newer AEDs are limited, but changes in bone metabolism have been reported for oxcarbazepine, levetiracetam, and gabapentin. Bone health in children differs in that the focus is on bone growth, and not bone loss prevention. Few studies have looked into this, and it appears that bone growth may be impaired by AEDs. Specifically, polytherapy seems to be associated with a greater decrease in bone density than with monotherapy. Ketogenic diet may be associated with decreased bone density as well. Prophylactic administration of calcium and vitamin D is recommended for all patients. For patients with long-term AED exposure, bone mineral density measurement is recommended, especially for patients treated with enzyme-inducing AEDs. Bisphosphonate therapy is generally indicated for patients with a high fracture risk.

Meier C, Kraenzlin ME. Antiepileptics and bone health. *Ther Adv Musculoskelet Dis*. 2011;3:235–243.

Pack AM. Treatment of epilepsy to optimize bone health. *Curr Treat Options Neurol*. 2011;13:346–354.

Vestergaard P. Effects of antiepileptic drugs on bone health and growth potential in children with epilepsy. *Paediatr Drugs*. 2015;17:141–150.

104. **D.** Rasmussen syndrome is characterized by intractable focal motor seizures, progressive hemiparesis, declining cognitive function, visual field abnormality, and contralateral focal, predominantly perisylvian, cortical atrophy. Median age of onset is 6 years, with a range from infancy to adulthood. Epilepsia partialis continua (focal motor status epilepticus) occurs in 50% patients. The etiology is unknown, although there is growing evidence for an immunopathological basis. However, the role of central nervous system (CNS) autoantibodies (such as GluR3) in the pathogenesis of this condition remains unclear. Rasmussen's encephalitis is frequently refractory to medical treatment although intravenous immunoglobulins and steroids may provide short-term relief. Hemispherectomy remains the only cure for seizures caused by Rasmussen's encephalitis. According to one study, 88% of children who underwent hemispherectomy became seizure free or had only occasional, nondisabling seizures. Early hemispherectomy worsens the hemiparesis, but reduces the overall burden of illness because of a marked decrease in seizure frequency. Because hemiplegia is inevitable with surgery and likely without surgery, early surgery may allow the child to return to a more normal life by preventing the cognitive decline resulting from constant seizures.

Kossoff EH, Vining EP, Pillas DJ. Hemispherectomy for intractable unihemispheric epilepsy etiology vs. outcome. *Neurology*. 2003;18:228–232.

Varadkar S, Bien CG, Kruse CA, et al. Rasmussen's encephalitis: clinical features, pathobiology, and treatment advances. *Lancet Neurol*. 2014;13:195–205.

105. **C.** Both RNS and DBS differ from vagus nerve stimulation (VNS) in that the stimulation occurs in the brain rather than on a peripheral nerve that has projections to the brain. RNS allows for stimulation of the deeper structures (e.g., hippocampus) or the cortex, so the stimulation parameters need to be adjusted to prevent afterdischarges or any cognitive or sensorimotor responses. In RNS, it is important to implant the electrodes in close proximity to the seizure focus (i.e., the epileptogenic zone) to achieve maximum

efficacy. In DBS, knowledge of the exact location of the epileptogenic zone is not crucial as the stimulation target is a deeper brain structure, such as the anterior nucleus of the thalamus. RNS is a closed-loop system, where stimulations occur in response to a detected seizure. DBS is an open-loop system, where stimulations occur constantly at predefined intervals regardless of whether a seizure is detected.

Sun FT, Morrell MJ. The RNS system: responsive cortical stimulation for the treatment of refractory partial epilepsy. *Expert Rev Med Devices.* 2014;11:563–572.

106. **D.** This patient's presurgical workup is consistent with MRI-negative dominant temporal lobe epilepsy. Development of a new seizure type with a different semiology most likely suggests a second independent seizure focus. Presence of bitemporal hypometabolism supports bitemporal dysfunction. With these findings, neither resection nor ablation is likely to provide optimal seizure freedom because of the possibility of two seizure foci. Bitemporal RNS would be the best option for her. Although VNS can be considered, the chance of achieving favorable seizure outcome is less likely with VNS (an open-loop device) compared with RNS (a closed-loop device).

Jehi L. Responsive neurostimulation: the hope and the challenges. *Epilepsy Curr.* 2014;14:270–271.

Morrell MJ. Responsive cortical stimulation for the treatment of medically intractable partial epilepsy. *Neurology.* 2011;77:1295–1304.

107. **D.** Zellweger syndrome is one of the peroxisome biogenesis disorders caused by defects in the PEX genes, required for the normal formation and function of peroxisomes. Zellweger spectrum comprises three disorders that have considerable overlap of features. These include Zellweger syndrome, neonatal adrenoleukodystrophy, and infantile Refsum disease. Zellweger spectrum disorders result from dysfunctional lipid metabolism, including the over-accumulation of very long-chain fatty acids and phytanic acid. Symptoms include enlarged liver; characteristic facial features such as high forehead, underdeveloped eyebrow ridges, and wide-set eyes; and neurological abnormalities such as hypotonia, mental retardation, and seizures. The prognosis for infants with Zellweger syndrome is poor. Most infants do not survive past the first 6 months, and usually succumb to respiratory distress, gastrointestinal bleeding, or liver failure.

Peroxisome biogenesis disorder 1A (Zellweger). http://www.omim.org/entry/214100. Accessed January 12, 2016.

108. **B.** Intellectually and physically impaired adults and children with epilepsy are at increased risk for vitamin D deficiency, osteomalacia, osteoporosis, fractures with trivial trauma, and muscle weakness. Furthermore, enzyme-inducing antiepileptic drugs cause increased catabolism of vitamin D. 25-OH vitamin D levels should be monitored and vitamin D supplementation instituted in these high-risk patients. Topiramate can cause kidney stones, and a renal ultrasound would be helpful. Given that the patient became agitated after a physical therapy session, a fracture is more likely than a kidney stone. Because of the same reason, neither EEG nor upper gastrointestinal endoscopy would be helpful in the evaluation.

Copploa G, Fortunato D, Auricchio G, et al. Bone mineral density in children, adolescents, and young adults with epilepsy. *Epilepsia.* 2009;50:2140–2146.

Meier C, Kraenzlin ME. Antiepileptics and bone health. *Ther Adv Musculoskeletal Dis.* 2011;3:235–243.

109. **B.** There is a high degree of cross-reactivity (40%–80%) in patients with hypersensitivity or allergic reactions to antiepileptic drugs (AEDs). Patients with rash from another AED, have an approximate 14% risk of developing rash from lamotrigine, compared with approximately 5% for a person without a history of rash from another AED. Most rashes begin within the first 3 months of starting therapy. Aromatic AEDs, such as phenytoin, carbamazepine, oxcarbazepine, phenobarbital, zonisamide, and lamotrigine, are more frequently associated with hypersensitivity. Pharmacogenetic variations in drug biotransformation may also play a role. Children are more susceptible to lamotrigine rash than adults, but elderly patients are not. Concomitant treatment with valproic acid is a predictor of rash with lamotrigine, and may be due to inhibition of lamotrigine metabolism by valproic acid. Low initial dose and slow titration may help avoid this side effect. Avoidance of specific AEDs in populations at special risk, cautious dose titration, and careful monitoring of clinical response may reduce the consequences of such reactions.

Hirsch LJ, Weintraub DB, Buchsbaum R, et al. Predictors of lamotrigine-associated rash. *Epilepsia.* 2006;47:318–322.

110. **C.** The addition of VPA to LTG monotherapy regimen results in a decrease of LTG clearance. VPA inhibits the LTG clearance by approximately 30% at a dose of 125 mg/day and approximately 50% at doses of 250 mg and higher. There is a maximal inhibition of LTG clearance by VPA at doses of 500 mg/day. During conversion of LTG monotherapy to polytherapy regimen with LTG plus VPA, the inhibition of LTG clearance by VPA is immediate. The dose of LTG can be reduced by 50% on the day VPA is started at doses of 250 mg/day or higher. Although the addition of LTG to VPA may increase the risk of rash, the addition of VPA to an LTG regimen does not increase such risk, as the patient has already taken LTG for a long enough period to become desensitized to the effect of the drug. During conversion from a VPA plus LTG dual therapy to LTG monotherapy, the dose of LTG may be kept unchanged until the dose of VPA is lowered to 125 mg/day, at which point, the dose of LTG must be increased by 30% and, finally, doubled on the day VPA is discontinued.

Kanner AM. When thinking of lamotrigine and valproic acid, think "pharmacokinetically"! *Epilepsy Curr.* 2004;4:206–207.

111. **D.** Although the exact mechanism by which levetiracetam treats seizures is not known, it has been shown *in vitro* to inhibit presynaptic high-voltage-gated calcium channels, which is felt to reduce neurotransmitter release. It has no effect on sodium channels. It binds to synaptic vesicle protein 2A (SV2A). Levetiracetam differs from other antiepileptic drugs by lacking efficacy in the traditional animal models of MES and PTZ but showing potent broad-spectrum (partial and generalized) efficacy in kindled animals of chronic epilepsy.

Margineanu DG, Klitgaard H. Levetiracetam: mechanisms of action. In: Levy RH, Mattson RH, Meldrum BS, Perucca E, eds. *Antiepileptic Drugs.* 5th ed. Philadelphia, PA: Lippincott Williams & Wilkins; 2002:419–427.

112. **A.** FBM binds to the NR2B subunit of the N-methyl-D-aspartate (NMDA) receptors. This selective binding causes reduction of NMDA-mediated sodium and calcium excitatory conductances without the neurobehavioral complications typical of other NMDA-receptor blockers. FBM inhibits CYP2C19 and induces CYP3A4. Inhibition of

CYP2C19 decreases phenytoin clearance, resulting in 30% to 50% increase in phenytoin level. FBM is metabolized by CYP3A4 and CYP2E1. As a result, CYP3A4 inducers such as phenytoin, carbamazepine, and phenobarbital increase FBM clearance and lower its serum level. Serious adverse effects of FBM include hepatic failure and aplastic anemia (black box warning from the FDA). FBM is metabolized to atropaldehyde, which is cytotoxic and immunogenic. It is believed that the individuals who form more of this compound on a genetic basis are prone to the idiosyncratic reactions. On the other hand, fluorofelbamate is a potent antiepileptic compound that is not metabolized to atropaldehyde, and has been proposed as a safer alternative to FBM. FBM is approved by the FDA for adjunctive therapy and monotherapy for partial seizures as well as for treatment of seizures associated with Lennox–Gastaut syndrome.

Faught E. Felbamate. In: Wyllie E, ed. *Wyllie's Treatment of Epilepsy: Principles and Practice*. 5th ed. Philadelphia, PA: Lippincott Williams & Wilkins; 2011:741–746.

113. **A.** Felbamate is approved by the FDA for adjunctive therapy and monotherapy for partial seizures as well as for treatment of seizures associated with Lennox–Gastaut syndrome.

Faught E. Felbamate. In: Wyllie E, ed. *Wyllie's Treatment of Epilepsy: Principles and Practice*. 5th ed. Philadelphia, PA: Lippincott Williams & Wilkins; 2011:741–746.

114. **D.** Gabapentin acts on voltage-gated calcium channels, not sodium channels. The bioavailability of gabapentin decreases with increasing dose. One way to avoid this is to give more frequent but lower doses. Gabapentin is not metabolized by the liver and can be used for long-term seizure control in patients with porphyria. There are some reports of exacerbation of absence seizures and myoclonus by gabapentin.

Chadwick DW, Browne TR. Gabapentin. In: Engel J, Jr, Pedley TA, eds. *Epilepsy: A Comprehensive Textbook*. 2nd ed. Philadelphia, PA: Lippincott Williams & Wilkins; 2008:1569–1574.

115. **B.** Gabapentin follows nonlinear, dose-dependent absorption in the proximal small bowel by the L-amino acid transport system. It does not have significant protein binding. It is transported across the blood–brain barrier by the L-amino acid transport system. Its side effects include weight gain and pedal edema.

Chadwick DW, Browne TR. Gabapentin. In: Engel J, Jr, Pedley TA, eds. *Epilepsy: A Comprehensive Textbook*. 2nd ed. Philadelphia, PA: Lippincott Williams & Wilkins; 2008:1569–1574.

116. **B.** There is no clear evidence that early AED treatment prevents epileptogenesis. However, clinical trials have shown that early AED treatment after a first seizure reduces the risk of subsequent seizures compared with delayed treatment. The First Seizure Trial (FIRST) showed that the 24-month recurrence rate was 25% in the early treatment group versus 51% in the delayed group, amounting to a 60% reduction in the rate of relapse in the treated group. The Multicenter Trial for Early Epilepsy and Single Seizures (MESS) showed that the risk of relapse in the early-treated group was lower compared with the delayed-treated group, amounting to a 30% reduction in the rate of relapse in the treated group. The MESS trial showed that early treatment delayed the time to the first seizure, the second seizure, and the first tonic–clonic seizure. Early treatment also reduced the time it took to achieve 2-year seizure remission. Neither trial showed significant differences in the eventual attainment of 2-year remission,

supporting that delayed AED treatment may not alter the natural history and prognosis for seizure control. The MESS trial, on subsequent analysis, showed that early treatment may be preferable for those at a higher risk of seizure recurrence, including those with abnormal EEG, more than one seizure, and in those with an underlying neurological disease. Early treatment is also reasonable for those patients that might be considered low risk but would have to face significant consequences (e.g., driving, work, and general safety) if seizure recurred.

Berg AT. Risk of recurrence after a first unprovoked seizure. *Epilepsia*. 2008;49(suppl 1):13–18.

Britton JW. Antiepileptic drug therapy: when to start, when to stop. *Continuum* (Minneap Minn). 2010;16:105–120.

117. **A.** Idiopathic and cryptogenic seizures are more likely to remit than remote symptomatic seizures. Juvenile myoclonic epilepsy has a favorable prognosis for remission on medication but has a high relapse rate after medication withdrawal. Although focal epilepsies tend to have higher relapse rates, the childhood syndrome of benign rolandic epilepsy does not. Thus, syndromic diagnosis is important in assessing the seizure recurrence risk after stopping AEDs.

Tsur VG, O'Dell C, Shinnar S. Initiation and discontinuation of antiepileptic drugs. In: Wyllie E, ed. *Wyllie's Treatment of Epilepsy: Principles and Practice*. 5th ed. Philadelphia, PA: Lippincott Williams & Wilkins; 2011:527–539.

118. **D.** A number of risk factors have been associated with high seizure recurrence risk following AED discontinuance, including poor initial AED response, age of onset >10 to 12 years, symptomatic etiology, mental retardation, abnormal neurological examination, juvenile myoclonic epilepsy, symptomatic partial epilepsy, >1 AED at the time of discontinuance, EEG abnormalities, and family history of epilepsy. Certain factors have been associated with a low seizure recurrence risk after discontinuation, including prompt initial AED response, age of onset >2 years and <10 to 12 years, idiopathic etiology, normal mentation, normal neurological examination, childhood absence epilepsy, benign rolandic epilepsy, infrequent seizures, low drug levels at the time of decision to discontinue, and seizure-free interval much greater than 2 years.

Britton JW. Antiepileptic drug therapy: when to start, when to stop. *Continuum* (Minneap Minn). 2010;16:105–120.

119. **C.** The response to AEDs in patients with newly diagnosed epilepsy showed that among 470 previously untreated patients, 47% became seizure-free for 1 year during treatment with the first AED and 14% became seizure-free during treatment with a second or third AED. In 3%, epilepsy was controlled by treatment with two drugs. Among patients who had no response to the first AED, only 11% became seizure free subsequently.

Kwan P, Brodie MJ. Early identification of refractory epilepsy. *N Engl J Med*. 2000;342:314–319.

120. **B.** Phenytoin has zero-order kinetics, so a small increment in dose can lead to a large change in serum level. Therefore, in most patients, incremental total daily dose increases of 30 mg could be sufficient. Carbamazepine has auto-induction (a transient effect), so serum levels may fall with increased doses. Phenytoin is highly protein bound, and therefore, free serum level of phenytoin will be helpful when serum protein levels are low or when the patient is on other medications that are protein bound. Bioavailability is

more important for a medication such as gabapentin because it decreases with increased doses due to saturable absorption, so giving smaller doses more frequently may be needed; this is not relevant in this patient.

Tatum WO, IV. Antiepileptic drugs: adverse effects and drug interactions. *Continuum* (Minneap Minn). 2010;16;136–158.

121. **A.** AED dosages and formulations may need to be adjusted for a child starting the ketogenic diet due to a number of reasons including limiting the amount of carbohydrate intake; AED side effects that can compound effects from the diet; and tapering AED doses once seizure control is achieved. The diet has strict dietary restrictions, and adherence to the carbohydrate limits will help achieve ketosis goals. Medications are a source of carbohydrates. In general, the carbohydrate content is the highest in suspensions and solutions, lower in chewable and disintegrating tablets, and lowest in tablets and capsules that are meant to be swallowed. Specifically, carbamazepine suspension, ethosuximide syrup, phenobarbital elixir, and valproic acid syrup contain the highest amounts of carbohydrate, and should be avoided in diet patients. Choosing their tablet or capsule equivalents will reduce the daily carbohydrate intake while still providing the same dose. AED suspensions that are labeled "sugar free" often contain carbohydrates, such as sorbitol. Such "sugar free" labeling is used primarily for diabetics as they may contain carbohydrate-containing excipients that will not affect glycemia, but might affect ketosis in the diet. A patient's current AED regimen is typically compatible with the ketogenic diet although there are a few interactions that need to be carefully monitored. For example, if the patient is on an AED with carbonic anhydrase inhibiting properties (e.g., topiramate, zonisamide, acetazolamide), the bicarbonate levels need to be monitored because of the risk of metabolic acidosis. AED toxicities can also occur, especially during the fasting phase, if the ketogenic diet is introduced with an initial period of fasting. The diet may start to show an anticonvulsant effect within several days, but it usually takes at least 6 weeks to determine the efficacy. Therefore, if seizure control is optimized after a few months, AEDs may be tapered or discontinued at that point. Diet efficacy may be affected by the AED regimen. It has been reported that some AEDs lead to better success with the diet (e.g., zonisamide) and some lead to less success (e.g., phenobarbital).

Runyon AM, So T. The use of ketogenic diet in pediatric patients with epilepsy. *ISRN Pediatr.* 2012;2012:Article ID 263139.

122. **C.** Planning for pregnancy for women with epilepsy (WWE) is important to decrease the risks to the fetus and to the mother. Preconception management of WWE includes attempting to simplify the AED therapy to monotherapy; tapering dosages of AEDs to the lowest possible effective dose; attempting complete withdrawal of pharmacotherapy in women who have been seizure-free for more than 2 to 5 years; establishing the total and free AED levels necessary for achieving good clinical control; considering preconception genetic counseling; and supplementing the diet with folate at 4 mg/day. In this case, the patient has a couple of years to plan for the pregnancy; if the patient continues to remain seizure free, then decreasing to monotherapy and tapering to the lowest possible effective dose would be most appropriate. If the patient wants to get pregnant immediately, then continuing at the current AED doses would be reasonable given that the current regimen has led to her longest seizure-free interval thus far. The patient has had only 6 months of seizure control, so complete AED withdrawal is not prudent. Given that the

patient currently has good seizure control, this would be an optimal time to measure serum AED levels to use as a baseline during future pregnancy. The free levels are more important for the heavily protein bound AEDs.

Caughey AB. Seizure disorders in pregnancy. http://emedicine.medscape.com/article/272050-overview. Accessed January 15, 2016.

Pennell P. Pregnancy, epilepsy, and women's issues. *Continuum* (Minneap Minn). 2013;19:697–714.

123. **C.** In 2010, the International League Against Epilepsy (ILAE) provided a definition for drug resistant epilepsy. According to that definition, failing two antiepileptic medications satisfies the criterion for medically refractory epilepsy. History of febrile seizures or the location of seizure onset is not considered part of the definition.

Kwan P, Arzimanoglou A, Berg AT, et al. Definition of drug resistant epilepsy: consensus proposal by the ad hoc Task Force of the ILAE Commission on Therapeutic Strategies. *Epilepsia*. 2010;51(6):1069–1077.

124. **D.** The concept of the epileptogenic zone is abstract; it is the cortical area that is indispensable for the generation of seizures. The true extent of the epileptogenic zone can only be inferred when the removal or disconnection of that area results in subsequent seizure freedom. However, the extent of the epileptogenic zone can be estimated indirectly based on concordant data that define the other cortical zones. These include the ictal onset zone (from which the recorded seizures arise), the irritative zone (where the interictal epileptiform discharges are localized), the epileptogenic lesion (the lesion that is presumed to the cause of seizures), the symptomatogenic zone (the eloquent area that produces the clinical symptoms when activated by a seizure), and the functional deficit zone (the area that is responsible for deficits during the interictal period). It is important to note that the epileptogenic zone includes not only the primary seizure onset zone (from which the recorded seizures arise) but also the potential seizure onset zone (which is the adjacent or distant cortex that may cause seizures once the actual seizure onset zone is removed). Although the epileptogenic zone tends to be the same for an underlying pathological condition, subtle differences can exist from one patient to another; for example, tumors and vascular malformations often have abnormal perilesional areas that are responsible for generating seizures. Presence of an epileptogenic structural lesion makes it easier to identify the epileptogenic zone but this can exist without a lesion. In this patient, the localization of interictal activity and seizure onset seem to be larger than the visible lesion. Without invasive monitoring, it is not possible to infer if the hippocampus is part of the ictal onset zone, and therefore, may be part of the epileptogenic zone. Regardless, the neuropsychological testing will be helpful in determining the functional deficit zone.

Datta A, Loddenkemper T. The epileptogenic zone. In: Wyllie E, ed. *Wyllie's Treatment of Epilepsy: Principles and Practice*. 5th ed. Philadelphia, PA: Lippincott Williams & Wilkins; 2011:818–827.

125. **B.** After frontal lobectomy, the probability of complete seizure-freedom is 55.7 at 1 year, 45.1% at 3 years, and 30.1% at 5 years. The majority (80%) of seizure recurrences occur within the first 6 months after surgery. Late remissions and relapses are rare. Based on multivariate analysis, the independent predictors of seizure recurrence are MRI-negative

malformation of cortical development as disease etiology, any extrafrontal MRI abnormality, generalized/nonlocalized ictal EEG patterns, occurrence of acute postoperative seizures, and incomplete surgical resection. MRI-visible frontal lobe lesion and completeness of surgical resection of the lesion correlate with postoperative seizure-freedom. There is no correlation of postoperative seizure outcome with gender, side of surgery, age at onset of epilepsy, age at surgery, epilepsy duration, preoperative seizure frequency, history of generalized tonic–clonic seizures, multiple clinical seizure types, or family history of epilepsy.

Jeha LE, Najm I, Bingaman W, et al. Surgical outcome and prognostic factors of frontal lobe epilepsy surgery. *Brain*. 2007;130:574–584.

126. **C.** In frontal lobe seizures, early forced head/eye deviation is not a consistent lateralizing sign, whereas late head/eye deviation is consistently contralateral to the side of seizure origin. Early asymmetric tonic posturing is consistently contralateral to the side of seizure origin. Focal clonic seizures are associated with seizure origin in the frontal convexity; tonic seizures are most often associated with supplementary motor area (SMA) seizure onset, but they can also be associated with seizure onset in other parts of the frontal lobe; seizures resembling typical temporal lobe seizures with oroalimentary automatisms are associated with seizure onset in the orbitofrontal region; and seizures with hyperactive, frenetic automatisms do not localize to any specific region within the frontal lobes.

Jobst BC, Siegel AM, Thadani VM, et al. Intractable seizures of frontal lobe origin: clinical characteristics, localizing signs, and results of surgery. *Epilepsia*. 2000;41:1139–1152.

127. **B.** The concept of the epileptogenic zone is abstract, that is, it is the cortical area that is indispensable for the generation of seizures. The true extent of the epileptogenic zone can only be inferred when the removal or disconnection of that area results in subsequent seizure freedom. However, the extent of the epileptogenic zone can be estimated indirectly based on concordant data that define the other cortical zones. These include the ictal onset zone (from which the recorded seizures arise), the irritative zone (where the interictal epileptiform discharges are localized), the epileptogenic lesion (the lesion that is presumed to be the cause of seizures), the symptomatogenic zone (the eloquent area that produces the clinical symptoms when activated by a seizure), and the functional deficit zone (the area that is responsible for deficits during the interictal period). It is important to note that the epileptogenic zone includes not only the primary seizure onset zone (from which the recorded seizures arise) but also the potential seizure onset zone (which is the adjacent or distant cortex that may cause seizures once the actual seizure onset zone is removed). Although the epileptogenic zone tends to be the same for an underlying pathological condition, subtle differences can exist from one patient to another; for example, tumors and vascular malformations often have abnormal perilesional areas that are responsible for generating seizures. Presence of an epileptogenic structural lesion makes it easier to identify the epileptogenic zone but the latter can exist without a lesion.

Datta A, Loddenkemper T. The epileptogenic zone. In: Wyllie E, ed. *Wyllie's Treatment of Epilepsy: Principles and Practice*. 5th ed. Philadelphia, PA: Lippincott Williams & Wilkins; 2011:818–827.

128. **D.** Patient A has infrequent seizures, which affect his quality of life (driving, work, etc.) and he has a surgically remediable syndrome (right MTS); right temporal lobectomy would be appropriate in him. Patient B has frequent seizures and a surgically remediable syndrome (left neocortical temporal cavernoma); although she has left hemispheric dominance for language and memory, lesionectomy (without resection of left mesial temporal structures, which could potentially cause memory decline) can still be an option in her. Patient C has frequent seizures, with the semiology suggestive of primary motor cortex seizure onset; however, given the gliosis, it is possible that the seizures could originate outside the motor strip, the latter being the symptomatogenic zone. Based on this, patient C could still be a candidate for resective surgery. Patient D has bilateral MTS and global memory impairment; left temporal resection in this patient could cause worsening of memory impairment. Thus, based on the information given, resective surgery would be contraindicated in patient D.

Duchowny MS, Harvey AS, Sperling MR, et al. Indications and criteria for surgical intervention. In: Engel J, Jr, Pedley TA, eds. *Epilepsy: A Comprehensive Textbook*. 2nd ed. Philadelphia, PA: Lippincott Williams & Wilkins; 2008:1751–1759.

129. **D.** Widespread (>2 cm) rather than focal ictal onset pattern is associated with postoperative seizure recurrence. Fast rhythmic activity in the beta to gamma range at seizure onset is found more often in the seizure-free patients compared with residual seizure patients. Short latency to onset of seizure spread is associated with higher risk of seizure recurrence after surgery. Short latency to seizure spread may indicate an extended area of increased epileptogenicity beyond the actual seizure onset zone. Failure to resect this tissue may then result in greater probability of relapse. Alternatively, rapid spread could be a marker of defective network inhibitory mechanisms and indicate more widely distributed pathology in cortical and subcortical structures. Resection of tissue that shows ictal discharges in the first 3 seconds after onset is associated with the best chance of a seizure-free outcome. Neither the frequency nor the distribution of the intracranial interictal epileptiform discharges has been consistently found to correlate with seizure-free outcome.

Holtkamp M, Sharan A, Sperling MR. Intracranial EEG in predicting surgical outcome in frontal lobe epilepsy. *Epilepsia*. 2012;53:1739–1745.

Kim DW, Kim HK, Lee SK, et al. Extent of neocortical resection and surgical outcome of epilepsy: intracranial EEG analysis. *Epilepsia*. 2010;51:1010–1017.

Norden AD, Blumenfeld H. The role of subcortical structures in human epilepsy. *Epilepsy Behav*. 2002;3:219–231.

130. **A.** Infants and children with early acquired brain lesions that have intractable epilepsy within the first 2 years of life have significant risk for intellectual disability, especially if seizures are frequent. Recurrent seizures may affect the contralateral normal hemisphere as well. Early successful surgery may prevent damage to the contralateral side and has been shown to improve cognition, development, and quality of life. Hemispherotomy is an effective surgical procedure in hemispheric epilepsy syndromes in a child with hemiplegia that is the result of a congenital or early acquired lesion such as this case.

Cataltepe O. Hemisperectomy and hemispherotomy techniques in pediatric epilepsy surgery: an overview. In: Cataltepe O, Jallo G, eds. *Pediatric Epilepsy Surgery: Preoperative Assessment and Surgical Treatment*. New York, NY: Thieme Medical Publishers; 2010:205–215.

Moosa A, Loddenkemper T, Wyllie E. Epilepsy surgery for congential or early lesions. In: Cataltepe O, Jallo G, eds. *Pediatric Epilepsy Surgery: Preoperative Assessment and Surgical Treatment.* New York, NY: Thieme Medical Publishers; 2010:14–23.

131. D. The main indication for corpus callosotomy is medically refractory seizures without an identifiable or resectable epileptogenic focus. Drop attacks are the most responsive seizure type to callosotomy.

Wong T, Kwan S, Chang K. Corpus callosotomy. In: Cataltepe O, Jallo G, eds. *Pediatric Epilepsy Surgery: Preoperative Assessment and Surgical Treatment.* New York, NY: Thieme Medical Publishers; 2010:261–268.

132. D. Electromagnetic fields can trigger the VNS, including those from hair clippers, loudspeakers, and so on. Thus, it is recommended that the generator be kept 8 inches or more from an electromagnetic source. MRI with a transmit-only coil is contraindicated as it can lead to device overheating. However, MRI can be done in a patient with VNS using transmit-and-receive head coil. The VNS should be turned off prior to MRI to avoid misfiring or changes in programming. Holding the magnet over the pulse generator stops the stimulation. This is useful when the patient desires to turn it off temporarily (e.g., singing). Based on testing to date, cellular phones have no effect on pulse generator operation.

VNS Therapy® System Physician's Manual. http://us.livanova.cyberonics.com/en/vns-therapy-for-epilepsy/healthcare-professionals/vns-therapy/manuals-page. Accessed January 17, 2016.

133. D. The patient is not an ideal candidate for surgical resection or ablation given the findings of bilateral MTS. Although alternative diet therapies could be considered, initiating ketogenic diet therapy in an adult is not practical. Device therapy for seizure control with either VNS or responsive neurostimulation (RNS) is reasonable at this stage.

Morrell MJ. Responsive cortical stimulation for the treatment of medically intractable partial epilepsy. *Neurology.* 2011;77:1295–1304.

Schachter SC, Boon P. Vagus nerve stimulation. In: Engel J, Jr, Pedley TA, eds. *Epilepsy: A Comprehensive Textbook.* 2nd ed. Philadelphia, PA: Lippincott Williams & Wilkins; 2008: 1395–1399.

134. B. Drop attacks (atonic seizures) can be debilitating and refractory to medications. Surgical options to treat drop attacks include CC and VNS. Studies show that patients are more likely to achieve a >50% reduction in seizure frequency with CC versus VNS (85.6% vs. 57.6%, respectively relative risk: 1.5). Adverse events are more common with VNS, but are typically mild (e.g., 22% hoarseness and voice changes), compared with CC, where the most common complication is disconnection syndrome (13.2%). Both CC and VNS are well tolerated for the treatment of refractory atonic seizures. Evidence suggests that CC is probably more effective than VNS in reducing seizure frequency, but there is no direct comparison study. The seizure reduction effect for corpus callosotomy is more immediate, whereas the efficacy of VNS increases over time, even for controlling the drop attacks.

Rolston JD, Englot DJ, Wang DD, et al. Corpus callosotomy versus vagus nerve stimulation for atonic seizures and drop attacks: a systematic review. *Epilepsy Behav.* 2015;51:13–17.

135. **D.** Addition of topiramate increases the risk of valproate-induced encephalopathy by approximately 10-fold compared with valproate alone. It is believed that the combination of valproate and topiramate results in synergistic action on ornithine metabolism in the liver leading to hyperammonemia and encephalopathy.

Latour P, Biraben A, Polard E, et al. Drug induced encephalopathy in six epileptic patients: topiramate? valproate? or both? *Hum Psychopharmacol*. 2004;19:193-203.

Noh Y, Kim DW, Chu K, et al. Topiramate increases the risk of valproic acid-induced encephalopathy. *Epilepsia* 2013;54:e1-e4.

Index

Printed in the United States
By Bookmasters